HUMAN ANATOMY
for Allied and Healthcare Sciences

HUMAN ANATOMY
for Allied and Healthcare Sciences

Previously Known as Basics in Human Anatomy for BSc Paramedical Courses

THIRD EDITION

Priya Ranganath MBBS MS (Anatomy)
Professor and Head
Department of Anatomy
Bangalore Medical College and Research Institute
Bengaluru, Karnataka, India

Leelavathy N MSc (Anatomy) PhD
Professor
Department of Anatomy
East Point College of Medical Sciences and Research Center
Bengaluru, Karnataka, India

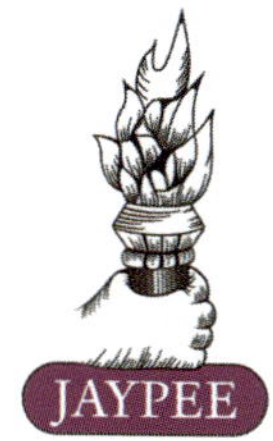

JAYPEE BROTHERS MEDICAL PUBLISHERS
The Health Sciences Publisher
New Delhi | London

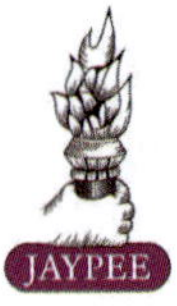

Jaypee Brothers Medical Publishers (P) Ltd

Headquarters
EMCA House
23/23-B, Ansari Road, Daryaganj
New Delhi 110 002, India
Landline: +91-11-23272143, +91-11-23272703
+91-11-23282021, +91-11-23245672
E-mail: jaypee@jaypeebrothers.com

Corporate Office
4838/24, Ansari Road, Daryaganj
New Delhi 110 002, India
Phone: +91-11-43574357
Fax: +91-11-43574314
E-mail: jaypee@jaypeebrothers.com

Overseas Office
J.P. Medical Ltd
83 Victoria Street, London
SW1H 0HW (UK)
Phone: +44 20 3170 8910
E-mail: info@jpmedpub.com

EU GPSR Authorised Representative
Logos Europe, 9 rue Nicolas Poussin
17000, La Rochelle, France
Phone: +33 (0) 6 67 93 73 78
E-mail: contact@logoseurope.eu

Website: www.jaypeebrothers.com
Website: www.jaypeedigital.com

Human Anatomy for Allied and Healthcare Sciences

First Edition: 2008
Second Edition: 2018
Third Edition: **2026**

ISBN: 978-93-6616-849-4

Printed in India

Preface to the Third Edition

Allied healthcare sciences colleges are on the rise not only in Karnataka, but also in other states in India. This book has had a very good response because of its simple explanations, tables and diagrams. We had done some additions for nursing students in the second edition. We have added histology photomicrographs and a chapter for BPT students in the third edition of this book.

Priya Ranganath
Leelavathy N

Preface to the First Edition

Anatomy is a vast subject. Learning the structure of each and every part of the human body separately is impossible. The books which are usually followed by the paramedical students at present, contain anatomy, physiology and biochemistry in combination which they find difficult to study. This book contains a simplified version of all systems and it is hoped that this will be understood by all paramedical students.

The text is simple and the line diagrams are easy to follow. Each chapter starts with a list of topics covered and ends with a list of most frequently asked questions. The gross, microscopic and applied anatomical features of each system are given together so that it becomes easy for the students to understand and correlate.

We have tried to present a comprehensive overview of anatomy required by the paramedical students. We have also added a section of general embryology to make the book a complete guide for students and hope that this book will be of great help to them.

The responsibilities of mistakes and omissions, if any, are ours alone. Suggestions from students and our colleagues are welcome.

Priya Ranganath
Suruchi Singhal
Leelavathy N
Vani Vijay Rao
Roopa R

Acknowledgments

We express our appreciation to our colleagues and friends for their valuable contribution and discussion during the period of preparation of the manuscript.

We express our grateful thanks to Dr Prem Pais, Dean, Father Thomas Kalam, Director, staff of Department of Anatomy, St John's Medical College, Bengaluru, and Dr Roopa R, Dr Suruchi Singhal, and Ms Vani Vijay Rao for their support, guidance and help in the first edition of this book.

We express our sincere thanks to Dr Uma SV, Sapthagiri Institute of Medical Sciences and Research Center, and Dr Deepa C, for their valuable suggestions which are incorporated in the second edition.

We express our heartfelt thanks to the whole team of M/s Jaypee Brothers Medical Publishers (P) Ltd, New Delhi, India, who helped and guided me, Shri Jitendar P Vij (Group Chairman), Mr Ankit Vij (Managing Director), Mr MS Mani (Group President), Dr Madhu Choudhary (Director-Educational Publishing), Ms Pooja Bhandari [Director-Production (Books and Journals)], Mr Ajay Kumar Sharma [Deputy General Manager (Books and Journals)], Ms Sunita Katla (Executive Assistant to Group Chairman and Publishing Manager), Ms Samina Khan (Executive Assistant to Director-Educational Publishing), Dr Upma Tomar (Managing Editor), Mr Vijay Kumar Bhatia (Manager-Production), Ms Seema Dogra (Cover Visualizer), Ms Neha Verma (Graphic Designer-Cover), Mr Bishan Singh (Production Manager-Press), Mr Mithilesh Kumar Singh (Quality Analyst), Ms Uma Adhikari (Typesetter), Mr Sumit Kumar (Team Lead-Graphic Designer) and their team members, for all their support to work in this project and make it a success. Without their cooperation, we could not have completed this project.

Contents

CHAPTER 1

Introduction

LEARNING OBJECTIVES

The student should be able to:

- Define anatomy and its divisions.
- Describe terms of location, positions and planes.
- Describe cell and its organelles with functions.

DEFINITION

- The term 'anatomy' is derived from a Greek word, '*anatome*', meaning cutting up.
- **Anatomical position:** Descriptive terms of position are used as though the body is standing upright with the upper limbs hanging by the sides and the palms of the hands, foot, eyes directed forwards.

Subdivisions in Anatomy

- **Macroscopic anatomy:** Study of anatomy on cadavers by dissection and observation of structures by naked eye. It can be studied by regional anatomy or systemic anatomy.
  - *Regional:* Head and neck, brain, thorax, abdomen and pelvis, upper limb, lower limb.
  - *Systemic:* An approach in which all structures forming a system are studied together at the same time, that is, integumentary, skeletal, articular, muscular, nervous, cardiovascular, lymphatic, endocrine, digestive, respiratory, urinary, reproductive.
- **Microscopic anatomy (histology):** Study of body structures with the help of a microscope.
- **Surface anatomy:** Study of a deeper structure on skin surface.
- **Comparative anatomy:** Study of changes in body that have taken place during evolution.
- **Physical anthropology:** Study of physical characteristics of humans and their ancestors, and of variability among and within different racial groups. This knowledge helps to solve medicolegal problems of identification of individuals.
- **Clinical anatomy:** Use of anatomical knowledge for anatomical basis, diagnosis and treatment of diseases.
- **Radiological anatomy:** Visualization of structures and their relations with neighboring structures inside the body by taking radiographs.

- **Developmental anatomy (embryology):** Study of intrauterine development of an individual, which begins with fertilization and ends with birth.
- **Genetics:** Study of principles of heredity.

TERMS OF POSITION

- **Sagittal plane**—a vertical imaginary plane passing anteroposteriorly through the midline of the body forming two symmetrical halves.
- **Parasagittal plane**—an imaginary plane passing anteroposteriorly through any part of the body parallel to median plane.
- **Coronal plane**—a vertical imaginary plane passing side to side at right angles to the sagittal plane.
- **Transverse or horizontal plane**—an imaginary plane passing parallel to the ground at right angles to vertical plane.
- **Superior** or **cephalic**—part that is nearer to the head.
- **Inferior** or **caudal**—part nearer the feet.
- **Anterior (ventral)**—part nearer the front of the body.
- **Posterior (dorsal)**—part nearer the back.
- **Median**—part in the middle.
- **Medial**—part nearer the median plane.
- **Lateral**—part further away from median plane.
- **Superficial**—part nearer the skin.
- **Deep**—structure away from the skin.
- **Proximal**—structure nearer to the trunk or root of the limb.
- **Distal**—structure away from the trunk or root of the limb.

TERMS OF MOVEMENT (TABLE 1.1)

- Movements of the trunk along the sagittal plane are known as **flexion** (surfaces coming closer to each other) and **extension** (straightening or surfaces moving away from each other).
- Movements of the trunk along the coronal plane are known as **lateral flexion**, in the limb they are called **abduction** (movements away from the median plane) and **adduction** (towards the median plane).
- **Rotation** is the term applied to the movement in which a part of the body is turned around its own longitudinal axis.
- **Flexion:** Bending the head forward towards the chest.
- **Extension:** Bending the head backward with the face towards the sky.
- **Rotation:** Turning the head to the left or the right.
- **Side-bending:** Tipping the head to the side or touching an ear to the ipsilateral shoulder.

Table 1.1: Terms of movement as per the plane.

Movements	*Sagittal plane*	*Coronal plane*	*Longitudinal plane*
Trunk	Flexion, extension	Side to side (lateral flexion)	—
Limbs	Flexion, extension	Adduction, abduction	Medial, lateral rotation
Thumb	Adduction, abduction	Flexion, extension	—

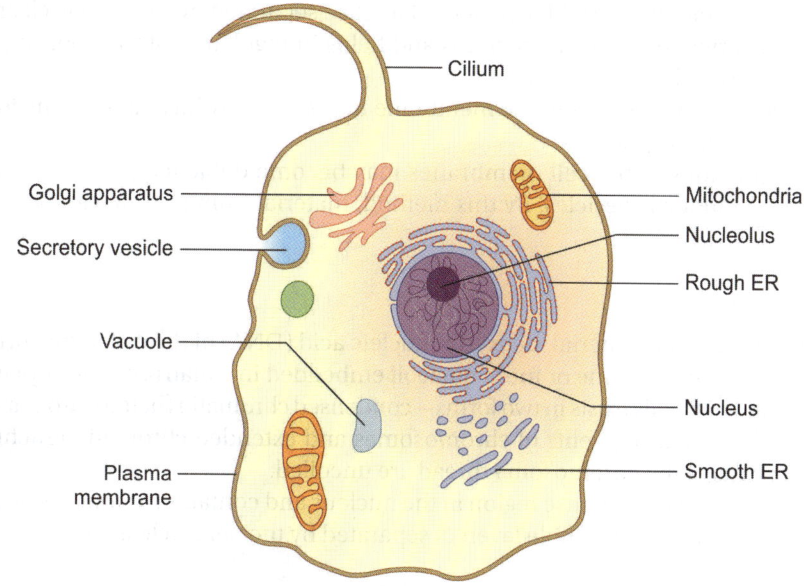

Fig. 1.1: Diagrammatic representation of a cell.

CELL AND ITS ORGANELLES

Introduction

- The basic structural unit of all tissues and organs of the body are formed by the cells.
- The shape of the cell differs in many ways. It may be flattened, cubical, columnar, fusiform, stellate, pyramidal or flask shaped.
- Each cell consists of cell membrane (plasma membrane), nucleus and cytoplasm with organelles **(Fig. 1.1)**.

Plasma Membrane (Fig. 1.2)

- It forms the outer boundary of the cell and separates it from adjacent cells and external environment.

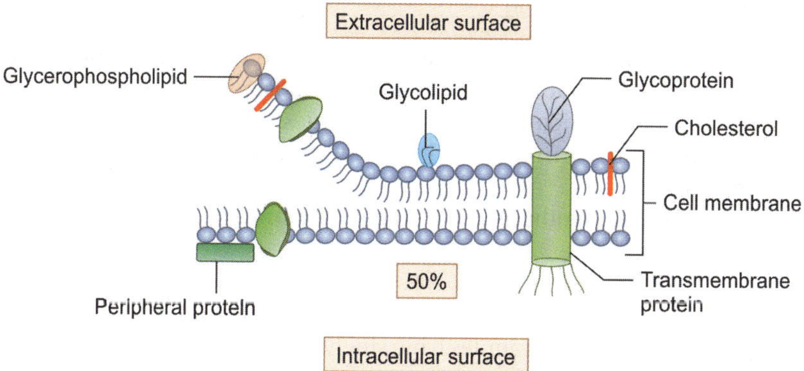

Fig. 1.2: Plasma membrane.

- It is a trilaminar membrane with two dense lamellae separated by a relatively clear layer.
- It forms a covering for the cell structures and helps in regulation of transporting selected substances into and out of the cell.
- In some cells the surface area of the membrane may be greatly increased by the formation of microvilli, for absorption.
- Small invaginations of the cell membranes may become detached to lie free within the cytoplasm as pinocytic vesicles. By this method, material from outside can be taken into the cell.

Nucleus (Fig. 1.3)

- It contains the genetic material, deoxyribonucleic acid (DNA) of the cell in the form of thin threads (chromatin) and one or more nucleoli embedded in a matrix of nucleoplasm.
- The chromatin normally exists in two forms—condensed chromatin (heterochromatin) which represents the coiled segments of chromosomes and extended chromatin (euchromatin) where segments of the chromosome thread are uncoiled.
- The nucleolus is seen as a dense region in the nucleus and contains ribonucleic acid (RNA).
- The nuclear membrane is double layered, separated by the perinuclear space.

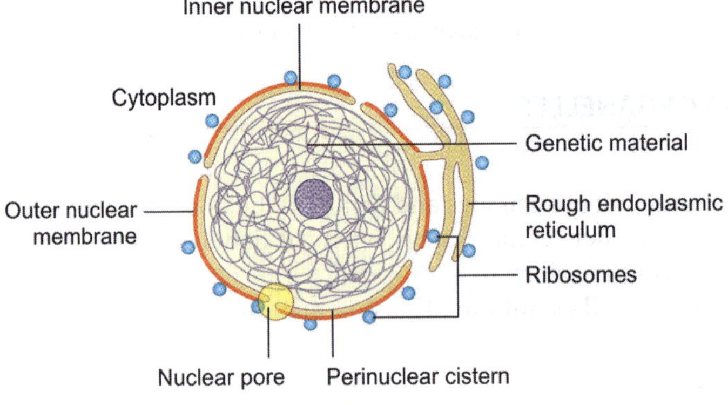

Fig. 1.3: Nucleus.

Organelles

Endoplasmic Reticulum (ER) (Fig. 1.4)

- It consists of a system of intercommunicating membranous sacs or channels and exists in two forms—rough endoplasmic reticulum which has ribosomes attached to the outer surface and smooth endoplasmic reticulum with no ribosomes.
- They are typically arranged in flattened parallel rows. It is prominent in cells that are manufacturing proteins.
- Rough ER helps in protein synthesis and storage while smooth ER helps in lipid and steroid synthesis.

Ribosomes

- They appear as dense rounded granules lying singly or in dense clusters in the cytoplasm in the form of rosettes or spirals (polysomes) or may be attached to ER.
- They are composed of ribonucleoproteins and are sites of protein synthesis.

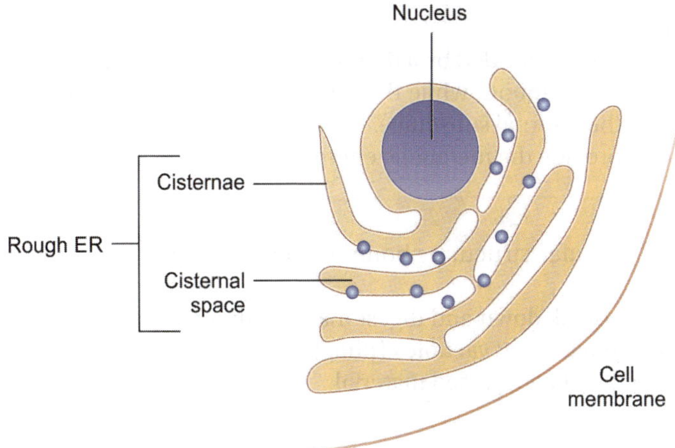

Fig. 1.4: Rough endoplasmic reticulum.

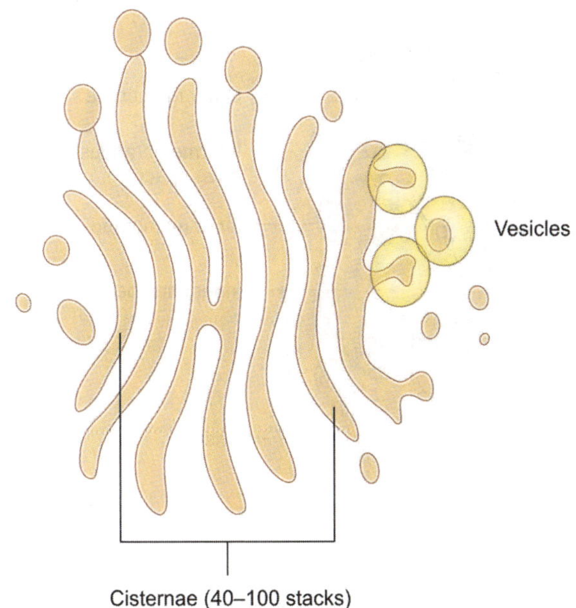

Fig. 1.5: Golgi apparatus.

Golgi Apparatus (Fig. 1.5)

- This is a system of sacs arranged like stacks of coins and vesicles like endoplasmic reticulum but with no ribosomes attached to it.
- It is also seen prominently in secretory cells.
- They transfer materials synthesized by the ribosomes at the endoplasmic reticulum to the cell surface.
- The part of the Golgi apparatus that contains newly manufactured material breaks away from the rest and pass towards the surface of the cell as secretion granules.

Mitochondria (Fig. 1.6)

- They are rod-like bodies bounded by a double layered membrane.
- The outer membrane is smooth while the inner membrane is thrown into folds or cristae which project into the internal substance.
- The mitochondria provide the metabolic energy for the cell by generating ATP.

Lysosomes (Fig. 1.7)

- These are dense granular structures bounded by membrane and containing hydrolytic enzymes.
- Their function is to break down and digest material that has been brought into the cell by phagocytosis. The phagocytic vacuoles (phagosomes) fuse with lysosomes to enable the enzymes to act on the phagocytosed material.

Fibrils

- They are present in many cells and help to maintain the cell shape.
- The fibrils present in the muscle fibers are responsible for their contractility.

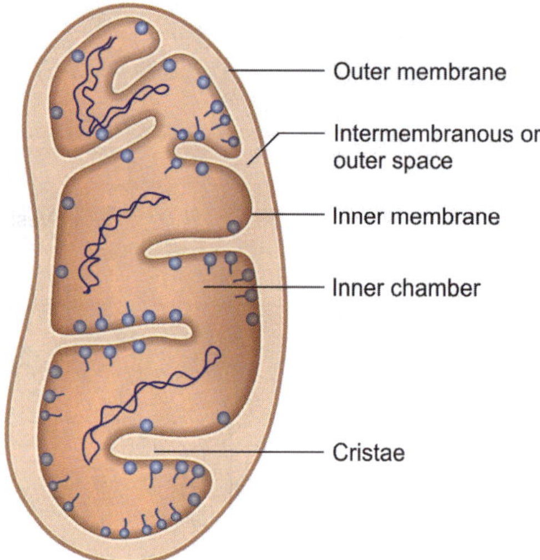

Fig. 1.6: Mitochondria.

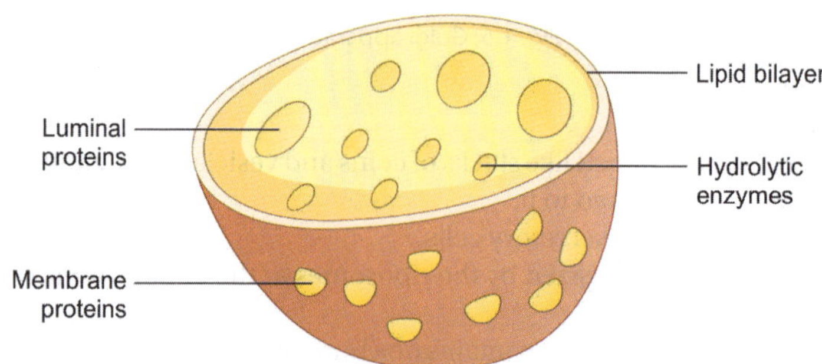

Fig. 1.7: Lysosome.

Microtubules

- They become part of mitotic spindles in dividing cells.
- In the resting cells, if they are seen (as in processes of the nerve cells), they act as stabilizing elements.

Centrioles

- These are a pair of short rod-shaped bodies found adjacent to the nucleus lying at right angles to each other.
- During mitosis they undergo replication and then each pair moves to opposite poles of the nucleus where they take part in the formation of mitotic spindle.
- Centrioles also give rise to cilia.

Inclusions

These are pigments like melanin or lipofuscin, storage granules such as glycogen and fat, and secretion granules.

APPLIED ANATOMY

Terms of movement: In general, the movements will be affected if the muscles are paralyzed. For example: extension at the elbow joint will be affected if the triceps brachii (action is extension at elbow joint) is paralyzed. Paralysis of triceps brachii may be due to injury to radial nerve which supplies it.

SUMMARY

- Terms of position: The relations of the parts or structures of the body depend on the position or location in relation to anatomical position. For example: Imagine part A is placed closer to the front of the body compared to part B. Hence part A is termed anterior to part B in comparison to each other.
- Terms of movement: Some of the movements are different in each region of the body.
- Trunk: Anterior flexion, lateral flexion, extension
  - Limbs—flexion, extension, adduction, abduction, medial rotation, lateral rotation, circumduction
  - Head and neck—anterior flexion, lateral flexion, extension, rotation
- Cell and its organelles: Cells vary in size and shape and are the functional and structural units of the body. It is surrounded by cell membrane and has nucleus (contains chromosomes and controls cell activities), cytoplasm (gel-like fluid with organelles) and organelles (endoplasmic reticulum, Golgi complex, mitochondrion, lysosomes, centrioles).

QUESTIONS

Long Essay

- Describe cell and its organelles.

Short Essays

- Draw a diagram of cell and label the parts.
- Cell membrane—structure and functions.
- Nucleus—structure and functions.
- Mitochondria—structure and functions.
- Endoplasmic reticulum—structure and functions.
- Golgi apparatus—structure and functions.

Epithelial Tissue and Glands

LEARNING OBJECTIVES

The student should be able to:

- Describe basic tissues with its classification with examples.
- Describe epithelium under definition, classification, description with examples, functions.
- Describe glands under classification, description with examples.

INTRODUCTION

- **Tissue (French:** Tissue-weave or texture) is a collection of cells embedded in intercellular substances which performs a similar function.
- **There are four basic types of tissues in the human body:** Epithelial tissue, connective tissue, muscular tissue, nervous tissue.

EPITHELIAL TISSUE (FLOWCHART 2.1)

- It is highly specialized to perform the function of protection, absorption and secretion.
- The epithelial cells are closely fitted together on a basement membrane to form epithelial membranes.
- The epithelial membranes are devoid of blood vessels.
- They obtain their nutrients through diffusion from the adjacent capillaries and tissue fluids.
- The epithelial tissue is found covering the body surfaces and lining the lumen of the hollow cavities like gut, respiratory system, blood vessels, etc.

Simple

Simple Squamous (Figs. 2.1 and 2.3A)

- A single layer of flattened cells rests on the basement membrane.
- The nucleus is flattened and causes a bulge in the cell.
- From the surface, the cells look like pavement.
- It is suitable to perform a dialyzing or a filtering function.

For example: Buccal smear, lung alveoli, lining of blood vessels (endothelium), lining of pleura, pericardium, peritoneum (mesothelium).

Flowchart 2.1: Classification of epithelial tissue.

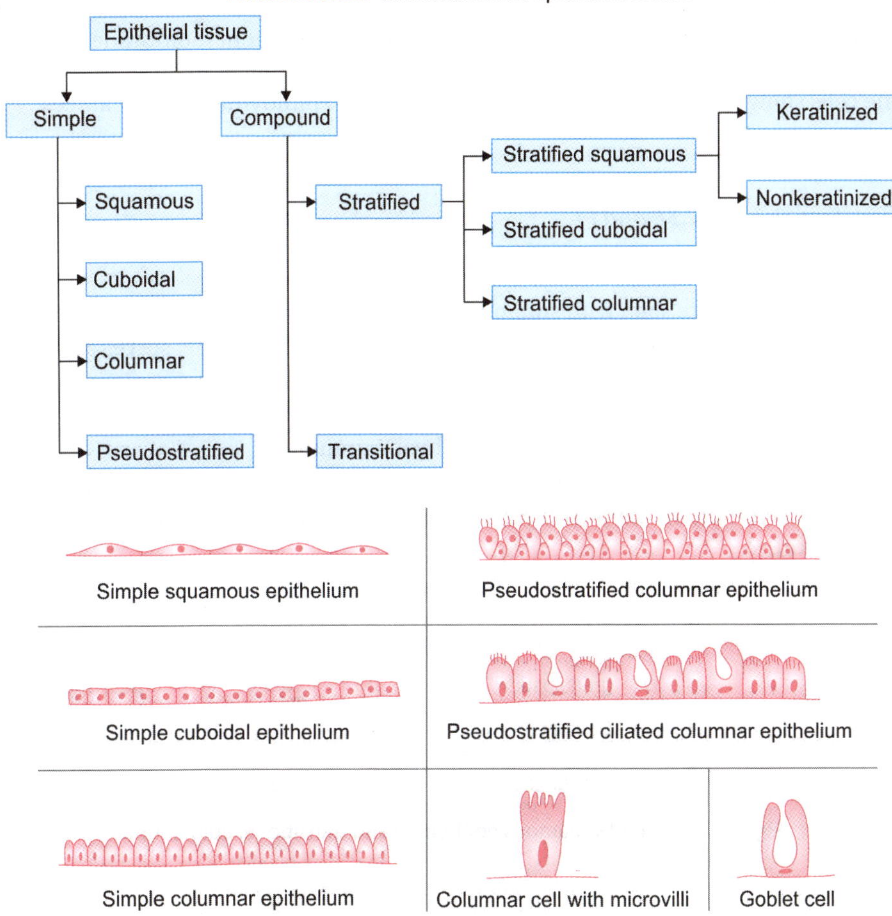

Fig. 2.1: Simple epithelium.

Simple Cuboidal (Figs. 2.1 and 2.3B)

- A single layer of cells, length and breadth are the same, rests on the basement membrane.
- The nucleus is spherical and centrally placed. For example: Thyroid follicle, ovary.

Simple Columnar (Figs. 2.1 and 2.3C)

- A single layer of cells, whose length is longer than the breadth, rests on the basement membrane.
- The nucleus is elongated and slightly below the center of the cell.
- They perform protective, absorptive and secretory functions.
- Some cells show surface modifications like villi (e.g., intestines), microvilli (e.g., gallbladder), or stereocilia (e.g., epididymis) at their apices.
- The specialized types of cells which secrete mucus are called goblet cells. They are so called because the supranuclear portion of these cells commonly gets so distended by accumulating secretion that the cell assumes the form of a goblet, e.g., epithelium of large intestine, trachea. For example: Stomach, intestines.

Pseudostratified Columnar (Figs. 2.1 and 2.3D)

- A single layer of cells with different heights rests on the basement membrane.
- The nuclei of these cells appear to be at different levels, so appear to be stratified.
- Some cells show cilia (e.g., trachea) or stereocilia (e.g., epididymis) at their apices.

Compound

Stratified (Figs. 2.2 and 2.3E and F)

Keratinized stratified squamous

- Many layers of cells are seen with squamous cells at the surface.
- *Stratum basale* with columnar cells present on basement membrane, serves as stem cells.
- *Stratum spinosum* with polyhedral cells present spine like surface projections, contain keratin filaments.
- *Stratum granulosum* with cells having keratohyalin granules.
- *Stratum lucidum* with cells having pyknotic or no nucleus, seen only in palm and sole.
- *Stratum corneum* or the keratin layer with dead squamous cells without nucleus. For example: Skin.

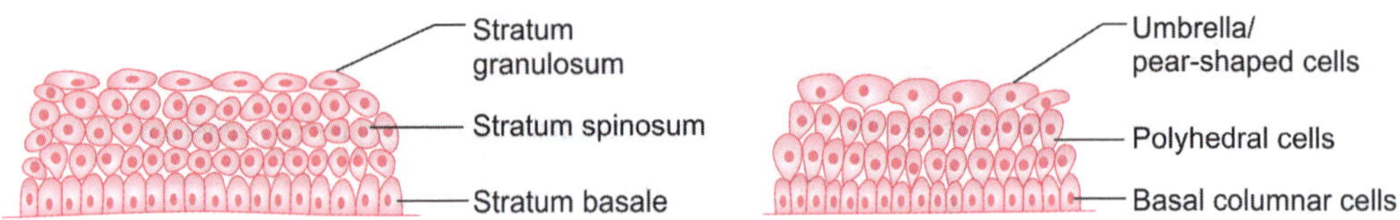

Fig. 2.2: Stratified squamous epithelium and transitional epithelium.

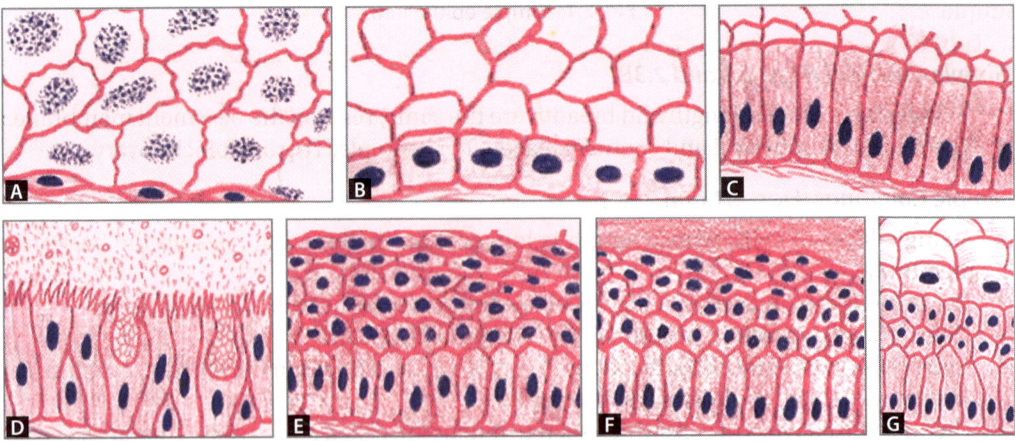

Figs. 2.3A to G: Epithelium: (A) Simple squamous epithelium; (B) Simple cuboidal epithelium; (C) Simple columnar epithelium; (D) Pseudostratified columnar with goblet cells; (E) Nonkeratinized stratified squamous epithelium; (F) Keratinized stratified squamous epithelium; (G) Transitional epithelium.

Nonkeratinized stratified squamous

- The basal three layers as above are present.
- Surface layers are squamous cells with nucleus.

For example: Mucous membrane of mouth, pharynx, esophagus, vagina.

Stratified cuboidal

Many layers of cells with cuboidal cells on the surface. For example: Ducts of salivary gland.

Stratified columnar

Many layers of cells with columnar cells on the surface. For example: Ducts of prostate gland.

Transitional (Figs. 2.2 and 2.3G)

Many layers of cells with basal columnar, over which there are polyhedral cells, pear-shaped cells and towards the surface, large umbrella-shaped cells. For example: Ureter, urinary bladder, urethra.

EPITHELIAL GLANDS

- The secretions provided by some of the lining epithelial cells on the surfaces and body cavities are not sufficient for the body needs.
- In places where more secretions are required, the epithelial cells of the membrane grow from the surface into the underlying supporting connective tissue to form highly specialized structures called glands.
- Glands have a secretory part (acinus) and a conducting part (duct) through which secretions are poured out.

Classification

According to Gross Structure (Figs. 2.4A to D)

Simple: Open through a single duct. Three types are seen.

1. **Tubular:** The duct is long and tube-like.
2. **Alveolar:** The ends of the duct are flask-shaped.
3. **Tubuloalveolar:** A mixture of tubular and alveolar type.

Compound: Open through more than one duct.

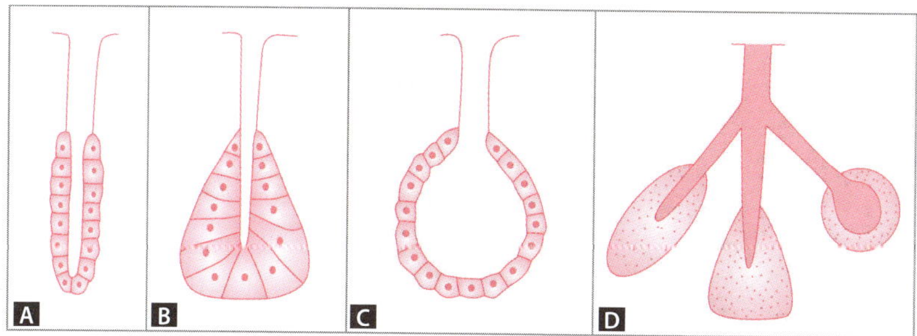

Figs. 2.4A to D: (A) Simple tubular; (B and C) Simple alveolar; (D) Tubuloalveolar glands.

According to Microscopic Structure and Type of Secretion

Serous salivary gland (Figs. 2.5A and B)

- Each lobule has got serous acini and many ducts.
- Serous acini lined by pyramidal cells, which are eosinophilic, granular, have microvilli at their tips, and have spherical nucleus.
- **Intralobular ducts:** There are two types: (1) intercalated ducts are lined by cuboidal cells and (2) striate ducts are lined by columnar cells which have basal indentations with mitochondria in between them.
- Interlobular ducts are lined by simple columnar epithelium.

For example: Parotid salivary gland.

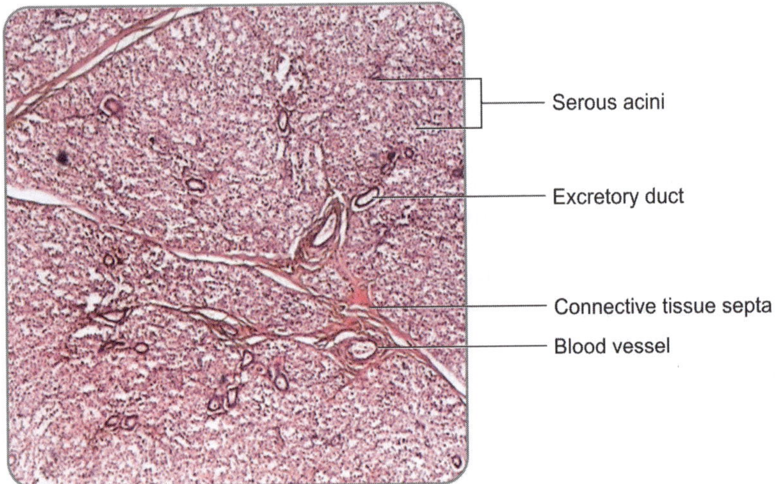

Fig. 2.5A: Photomicrograph of serous salivary gland.

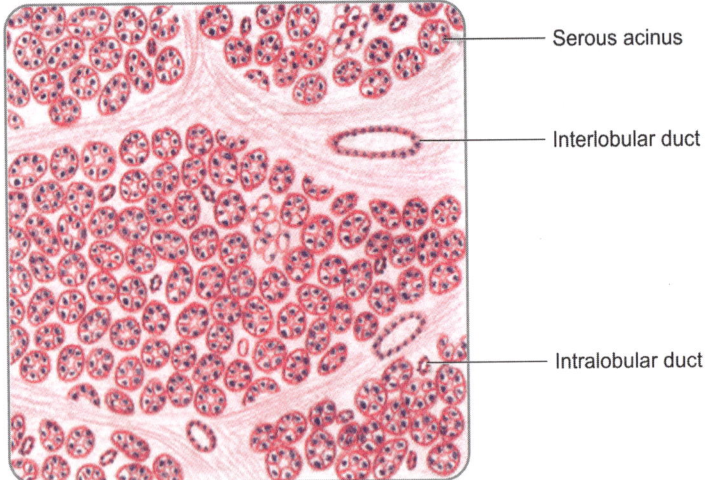

Fig. 2.5B: Diagrammatic representation of serous salivary gland.

Mucous salivary gland (Figs. 2.6A and B)

- Each lobule has got mucous acini and few ducts.
- Mucous acini lined by short columnar cells, which are basophilic, agranular, no microvilli, have flattened nuclei which are pushed to the base of the cell by the mucous above.
- **Intralobular ducts:** There are two types; intercalated ducts are lined by cuboidal cells and striate ducts are lined by columnar cells which have basal indentations with mitochondria in between them.
- Interlobular ducts are lined by simple columnar epithelium.

For example: Sublingual salivary gland.

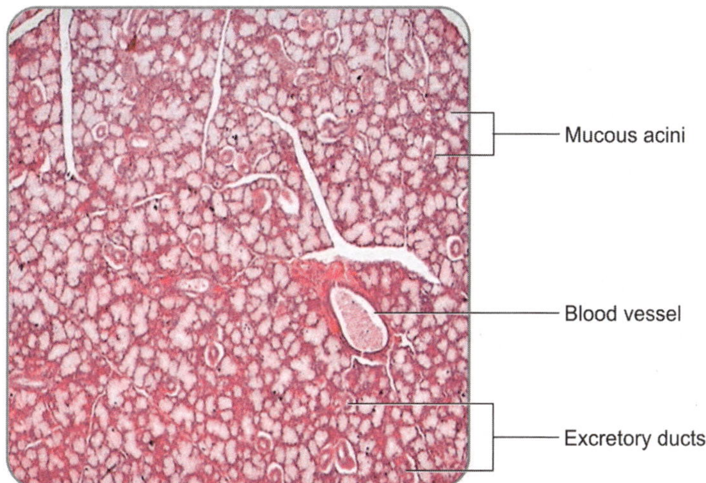

Fig. 2.6A: Photomicrograph of mucous salivary gland.

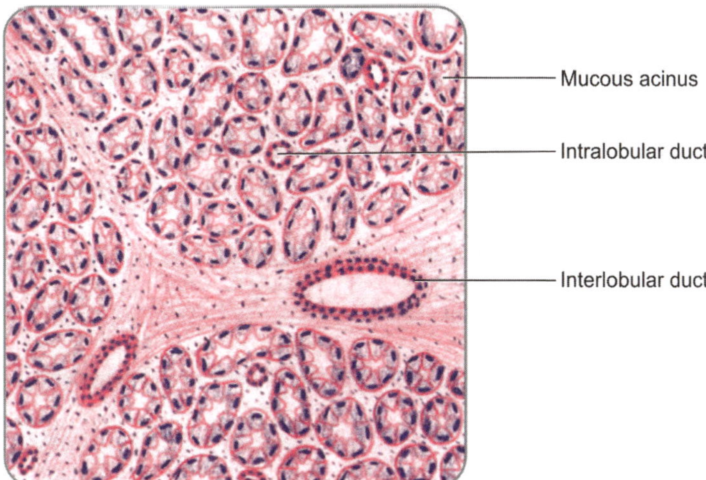

Fig. 2.6B: Diagrammatic representation of mucous salivary gland.

Mixed salivary gland (Figs. 2.7A and B)

- Both serous and mucous acini are present with many ducts.
- Mucous acini are capped by serous demilunes which by their serous secretions decrease the viscosity of the mucous in the mucous acini.

For example: Submandibular gland.

According to Function

Exocrine

The secretions called enzymes are transferred through the ducts. For example: Gastric glands, acinar part of pancreas, salivary glands.

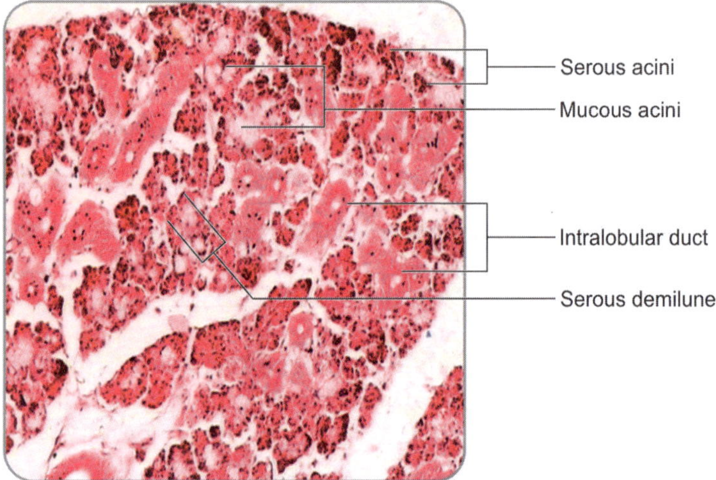

Fig. 2.7A: Photomicrograph of mixed salivary gland.

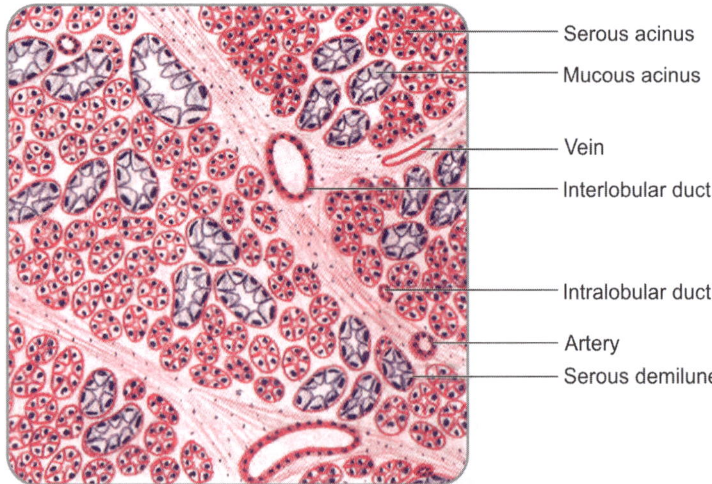

Fig. 2.7B: Diagrammatic representation of mixed salivary gland.

Endocrine

- There are no ducts.
- The secretions are poured directly into blood vessels.

For example: Thyroid, parathyroid, pituitary, islets of pancreas.

According to Mode of Secretion

The secretions are conveyed to the cell surface and are discharged in different ways:

Eccrine/Merocrine

- The cell is intact.
- Membranes of vesicles containing the secretions fuse with plasma membrane to release their contents to the exterior.

For example: Sweat glands.

Apocrine

The apex of the cytoplasm is pinched off with the contained secretions. For example: Mammary gland.

Holocrine

The whole cell disintegrates to liberate the accumulated mass of secretory vesicles. For example: Sebaceous gland.

APPLIED ANATOMY

- **Carcinoma:** Cancer developing in the epithelial tissue.
- Smoking leads to the death of cilia in respiratory epithelium and in turn may lead to lung cancer.

SUMMARY

Epithelial Tissue

- It is avascular, covers external and internal surfaces of the body, cells rest on basement membrane. It is classified as simple and compound epithelium.
- Simple epithelium (one layer) further classified into simple squamous (flat cells, diffusion, alveoli of lung), simple cuboidal (cuboidal cells, absorption/secretion/excretion, thyroid follicles), simple columnar (tall cells, absorption, secretion, stomach) and pseudostratified (one layer but appears more than one layer, propulsion of mucus).
- Compound epithelium (more than one layer) further classified into stratified-protection (stratified squamous keratinized-skin, stratified squamous nonkeratinized-esophagus, stratified cuboidal-ducts of salivary glands, stratified columnar-ducts of prostate gland) and transitional (urinary bladder, can stretch when full).

Epithelial Glands

- They have secretory part (acinus) and conducting part (duct).
- Classification according to: Structure-simple (tubular-long tube, stomach fundus; alveolar-end of duct dilated, sebaceous gland, tubuloalveolar-submandibular gland) and compound (branched).

- Type of secretion-mucous (viscous fluid, sublingual gland), serous (clear fluid, parotid gland), mixed (both, submandibular gland).
- Mode of secretion-exocrine/merocrine (cell intact, sweat gland), apocrine (apex of cell pinched off, mammary gland) and holocrine (whole cell disintegrates, sebaceous gland).

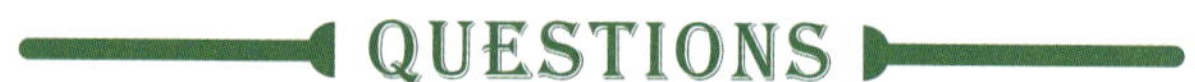

QUESTIONS

Long Essays

- Classify epithelium, explain giving examples.
- Classify glands, explain giving examples.

Short Essays

- Transitional epithelium.
- Differences between exocrine and endocrine glands.
- Histology of serous, mucous and mixed glands.

CHAPTER 3

Connective Tissue and Skeletal System

LEARNING OBJECTIVES

The student should be able to:

- Describe cartilage under classification, histology with examples.
- Describe bone under classification, sesamoid bones, names of bone cells, parts of long bone, blood supply, microscopy of compact bone, names of all bones including carpals, tarsals and skull, explanation of clavicle, scapula, humerus, femur, tibia, ribs, vertebrae, fetal skull, ossification.
- Describe joints under classification with examples, synovial joint in detail, explanation of shoulder, hip and temporomandibular joints.

CONNECTIVE TISSUE

- Connective tissue supports, binds and protects the special (well differentiated) tissues of the body.
- It has both cellular and extracellular components.
  - *Cellular:* Fibroblasts, macrophages, plasma cells, mast cells, fat cells, pigment cells or melanocytes.
  - *Extracellular matrix:* Consists of fibrous and nonfibrous element.
- Fibrous element includes three types of fibers—collagen, elastin and reticulin.
- Nonfibrous element is formed by ground substance.

Types of Connective Tissue

Loose Connective Tissue

- It is most extensively distributed in the body.
- It consists of network of thin collagen and elastin fibers embedded in a semifluid ground substance.

For example: Subcutaneous tissue in eyelids, penis, scrotum, labia minora; investing sheaths of muscles, vessels and nerves; internal support of compound glands (binding lobes and lobules), of hollow viscera, and fibers of muscles and nerves.

Dense Connective Tissue

Irregular connective tissue

- It is found in those parts of the body which are subjected to mechanical stress.
- It contains a high proportion of collagen fibers with a few fibroblasts.

For example: Reticular layer of dermis; connective tissue sheaths of muscles, vessels and nerves, adventitia of large vessels; capsules of various glands and organs; sclera of eye, periostea and perichondria.

Regular connective tissue

Regular arrangement of collagen fibers forms sheets—*fasciae and aponeurosis*, or thicker bundles—*tendons and ligaments.*

Tendons

- Muscles usually end in tendons which are then attached to a bone.
- It consists of type I collagen fibers in predominance because of response to tensile strain and the fibers run parallel to one another.
- Matrix or ground substance is less.
- Tendon cells are arranged in single rows on the surface of the fibers. The cells present wing-like processes between the bundles of fibers, giving stellate appearance in cross-section. For example: Biceps tendon, triceps tendon.

Ligaments

- Fibrous bands which connect adjacent bones, forming integral parts of the joints.
- Collagen fibers predominate because of response to tensile strain. For example: Glenohumeral ligament, tibial collateral ligament.

Raphe

A linear fibrous band formed by interdigitation of tendinous or aponeurotic ends of muscles. For example: Linea alba, mylohyoid raphe.

Adipose Tissue

It is made up of large groups of fat cells usually arranged in loculi formed by fibrous septa carrying blood vessels.

For example: Superficial fascia of buttocks, loins, nape of neck, breast; lower part of anterior abdominal wall and front of thighs; fatty capsules of kidney; mesenteries and omenta.

Pigmented Connective Tissue

Occurs in choroid and lamina fusca of sclera of the eye.

Mucoid Tissue

- It is an embryonic type of connective tissue, which forms Wharton's jelly of umbilical cord, and vitreous body of the eye.
- The tissue consists of a copious matrix carrying fine meshwork of collagen with fibroblasts.

SKELETAL SYSTEM

- Skeletal system forms the general framework of the body.
- It bears weight without bending and has considerable tensile strength.
- It consists of cartilage and bone.

CARTILAGE

It is a special connective tissue with the following properties:

- It possesses great tensile strength. It is made of dense network of collagen or elastic fibers which give tensile strength. These fibers lie embedded in a firm jelly-like amorphous substance which allows the cartilage to bear weight without bending.
- The surface of the cartilage can take polish. When lubricated, the cartilaginous surfaces can move against each other without friction and wear. They are well adapted to coat the articular ends of the movable joints.
- It is a nonvascular tissue. Invasion of cartilage by blood vessels results in calcification and death of cartilage. The chondrocytes receive nutrients by means of substances diffusing through the jelly-like intercellular matrix. In some regions as in epiphyseal plates, blood vessels pass through the cartilage in protected canals, hence no calcification or death occurs.
- Except at articular surfaces, each cartilage is surrounded by a connective tissue membrane called perichondrium. The outer part of this membrane is made of dense collagen fibers (fibrous) and the inner part shows cartilaginous characteristics (cellular).

Classification (Histological)

Hyaline Cartilage (Figs. 3.1A and B)

- Homogenous/translucent ground substance which is basophilic.
- Intercellular substance is a firm gel made of collagen fibers immersed in a large quantity of amorphous substance which contains proteoglycans.
- The ground substance has the same refractive index as the collagen fibers and hence fibers are not seen distinctly, hence called homogenous matrix.
- Cartilage cells called chondrocytes are seen in groups within lacunae; these are called cell nests.
- Matrix around the nests is called territorial matrix which is darker than the inter-territorial matrix.
- Perichondrium consisting of outer fibrous and inner cellular components. For example: Thyroid cartilage, cricoid cartilage, articular cartilage.

Elastic Cartilage (Figs. 3.2A and B)

- Cartilage cells are seen in lacunae.
- Ground substance contains yellow elastic fibers which branch and anastomose.
- Perichondrium consisting of outer fibrous and inner cellular components.
- Calcification does not occur.

For example: Auricle, auditory tube, epiglottis, corniculate and cuneiform cartilages of larynx.

Fibrocartilage (Figs. 3.3A and B)

- Absence of perichondrium.

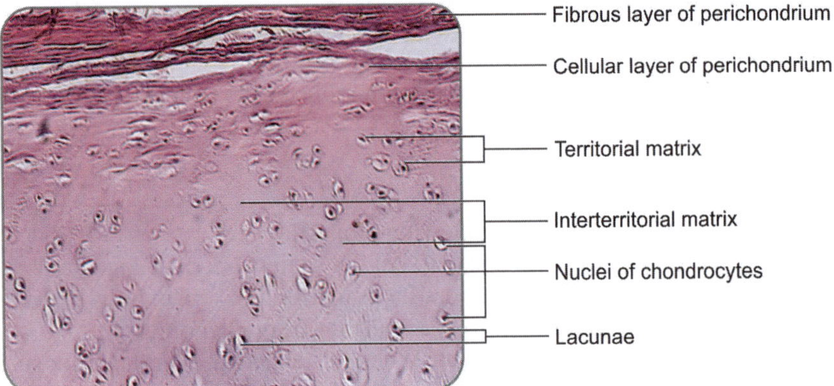

Fig. 3.1A: Photomicrograph of hyaline cartilage.

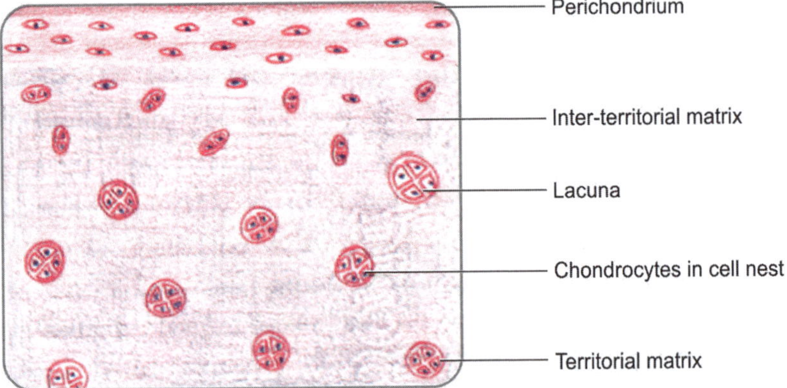

Fig. 3.1B: Diagrammatic representation of hyaline cartilage.

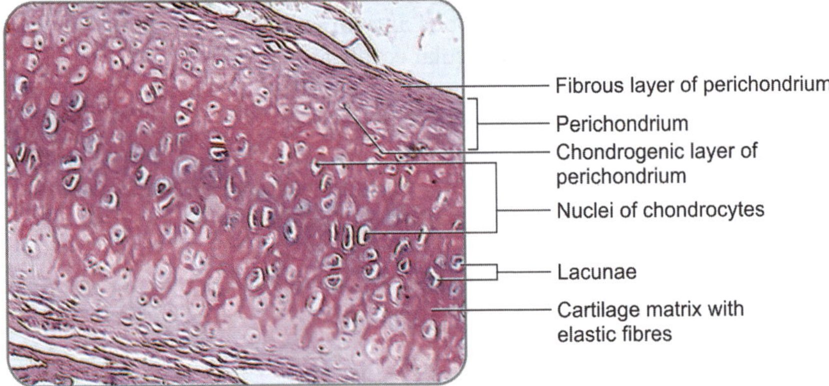

Fig. 3.2A: Photomicrograph of elastic cartilage.

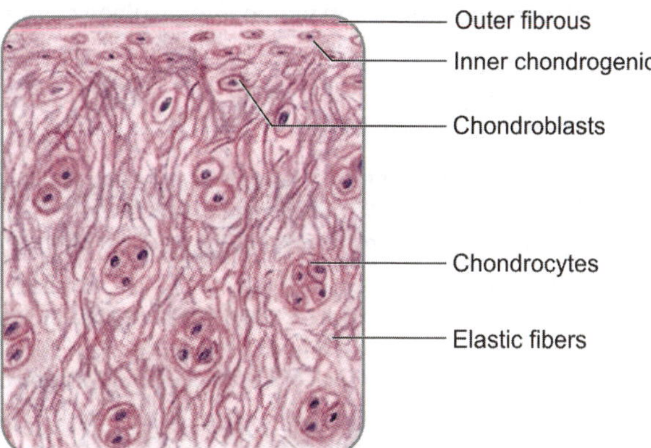

Fig. 3.2B: Diagrammatic representation of elastic cartilage.

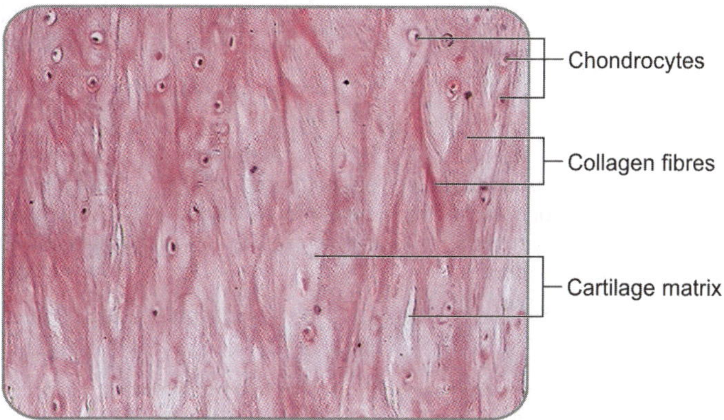

Fig. 3.3A: Photomicrograph of white fibrocartilage.

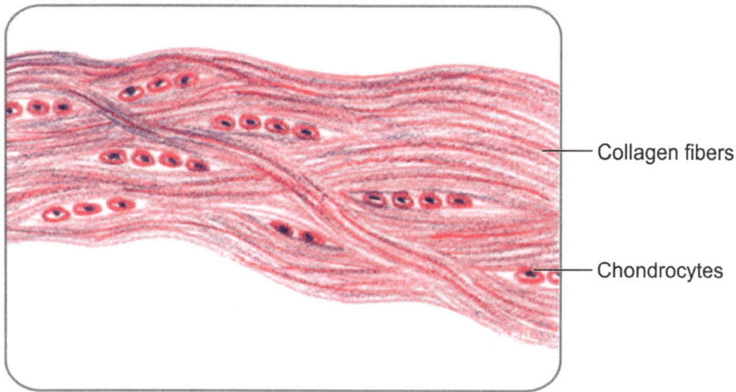

Fig. 3.3B: Diagrammatic representation of white fibrocartilage.

- Presence of thick bundles of collagen fibers between which few cartilage cells are sandwiched in rows.
  For example: Intervertebral discs, symphysis pubis.

Differences between the three cartilages are depicted in **Table 3.1**:

Table 3.1: Differences between the three cartilages.

Components	*Hyaline cartilage*	*Elastic cartilage*	*White fibrocartilage*
Matrix	Homogeneous glassy matrix	Structure similar to hyaline cartilage except that the matrix has dense network of elastic fibers	Alternating layers of hyaline cartilage matrix and bundles of dense collagen fibers
Ground substance	Collagen fibers embedded in glycosaminoglycans	Collagen fibers embedded in glycosaminoglycans	Collagen fibers embedded in glycosaminoglycans
Cells (chondrocytes)	Cells in spaces (lacunae), surrounded by territorial and interterritorial matrix	Cells in spaces (lacunae), surrounded by territorial and interterritorial matrix	Chondrocytes arranged in rows surrounded by less amount of ground substance, and fibroblasts scattered in collagen fibers
Perichondrium	Present	Present	Absent
For example	Articular surfaces of joints, costal cartilages, cartilages of nose, larynx, trachea and bronchi, precursor of bone in the developing skeleton	External ear (pinna), epiglottis, corniculate/ cuneiform cartilages, Eustachian tube	Intervertebral discs, symphysis pubis, articular discs, menisci, places where the tendons attach to the bones

BONE

- Bone is a hard type of connective tissue which is highly vascular, living, changing minerals and having a low metabolic rate.
- Apart from its mechanical function, it is a storehouse for calcium.
- Although hard, it is elastic and has characteristic growth mechanism and regenerative capacity.

Classification

Based on Development

Intramembranous/Membrane/Dermal

They are formed directly from the mesenchymal condensations.
For example: Bones of vault of the skull.

Intracartilaginous/Cartilaginous/Endochondral

They are formed by replacing the cartilaginous models.
For example: Bones of base of skull, long bones of limbs, etc.

Based on Histological Appearance

Compact bone (Fig. 3.4)

- **Transverse section (Figs. 3.4A and C):**
  - Made up of a number of cylindrical units called Haversian systems.
  - Each Haversian system consists of a Haversian canal containing nerves, blood vessels and lymphatics, surrounded by concentric bony lamellae.
  - Oval spaces between the lamellae are called lacunae which contains osteocytes.
  - Canaliculi are fine radiating channels which interconnect the lacunae and contain processes of osteocytes.
  - Interstitial lamellae occupy the angular intervals between the Haversian systems.
  - Circumferential lamellae are present adjacent to periosteum and endosteum.
- **Longitudinal section (Figs. 3.4B and C):**
  - Each Haversian canal is connected to one another by inter-Haversian canals.
  - Each canal is connected to the periosteum and endosteum by Volkmann's canals.

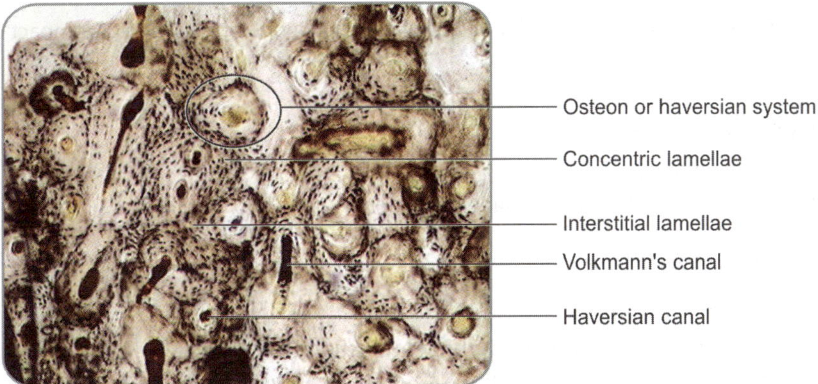

Fig. 3.4A: Photomicrograph of transverse section of compact bone.

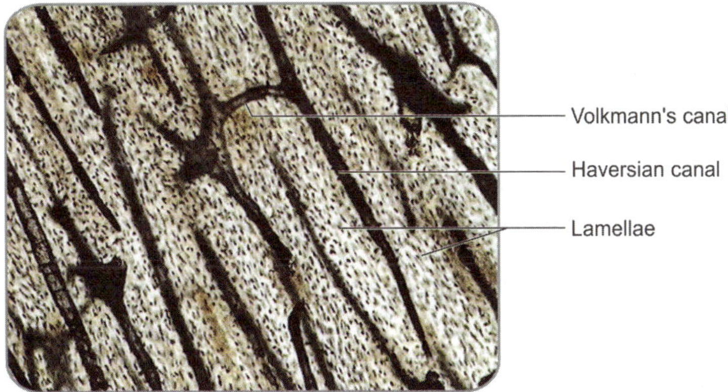

Fig. 3.4B: Photomicrograph of longitudinal section of compact bone.

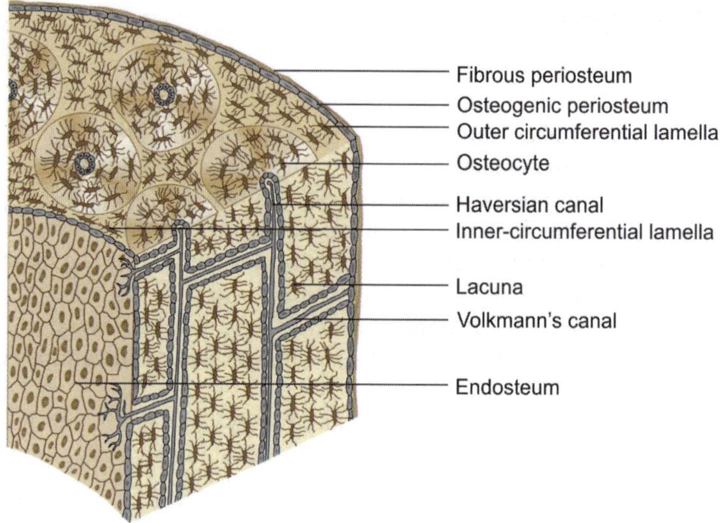

Fig. 3.4C: Diagrammatic representation of transverse and longitudinal section of compact bone.

Cancellous or spongy bone

- It has a spongy texture.
- Less of bony matter and more of spaces are seen.

Based on Shape and Structure

Long bones

- Each long bone has a shaft and ends which are usually expanded.
- The shaft has a cortex and a medulla. The cortex is made of compact bone whereas the medullary cavity is filled with marrow.
- The ends are covered by a thin layer of compact bone and enclosing in it a spongy bone containing red marrow.
  For example: Femur, humerus, metacarpals.

Parts of a long bone (Fig. 3.5)

- **Diaphysis:** It is the shaft of the bone which is developed from the primary center of ossification.
- **Epiphysis:** It is the part of the bone which is directly developed from the secondary center of ossification. They are at the ends of the bones. Every long bone has one or more epiphyseal centers.
- **Metaphysis:** It is the growing end of the diaphysis. They are partly intracapsular in certain regions like upper and lower ends of humerus, upper end of radius, lower end of ulna, upper and lower ends of femur.
- Metaphysis is an important region because (i) its vascularity is great, (ii) growth and metabolic activities are high, (iii) muscles are mostly inserted here, (iv) it is a place which is more prone to pathological conditions than the rest of the bone.

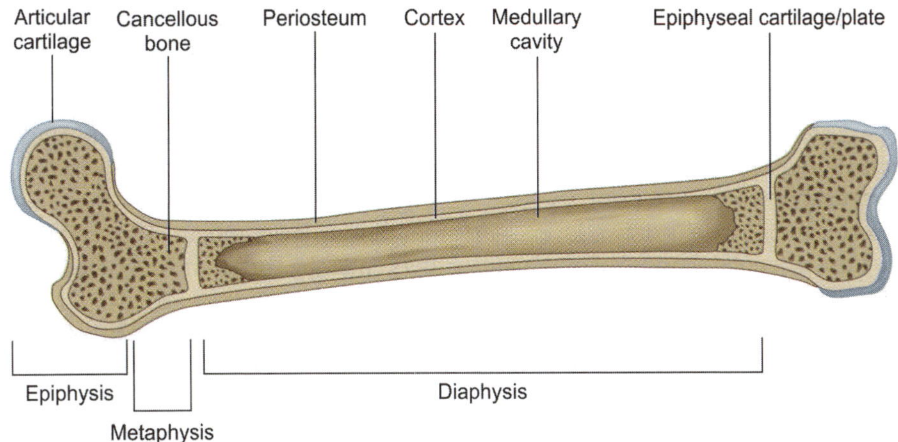

Fig. 3.5: Parts of a long bone.

Short bones

They are chiefly made of spongy bones covered by a thin layer of compact bone.
For example: Carpals and tarsals.

Flat bones

- They have thin cortex of compact bone with marrow inside.
- For example: Skull bones and ribs.

Irregular bones

They are irregular in shape and have a layer of compact bone on the exterior with spongy bone inside.
For example: Vertebrae and scapula.

Sesamoid bones

They are nodular, small bones or fibrocartilages developing in a tendon over a bony surface. They do not ossify.
For example: Patella, fabella.

Pneumatic bones

They have air-filled cavities to lighten the bone and help in phonation.
For example: Maxilla, sphenoid, frontal bones of skull.

Based on Position in the Body

Axial bone

Present in the median plane of the body.
For example: Vertebrae, sternum, ribs, skull bones.

Appendicular bone

Present in the limbs.
For example: Femur, humerus.

Periosteum

- The bones are covered by a membrane called periosteum during life.
- The tendons and muscles which insert into the bone blend with the periosteum.
- The periosteal blood vessels and nerves enter the periosteum where tendons and ligaments attach to the bone and periosteal vessels freely communicate with the vessels of the underlying bone.
- The periosteum consists of two layers—an outer fibrous layer and an inner cell rich layer (fibroblast, osteoblast). Some of the collagen fibers enter the cortex and are called Sharpey's fibers.
- In young bones, the periosteum is thick and vascular and beneath it is a layer of subperiosteal soft vascular osteogenic tissue containing osteoblasts (bone forming cells) and granular cells.
- In older bones the periosteum becomes thin and less vascular. In the subperiosteal tissue the cells are quiescent and potentially osteogenic.

Ossification

- The process of bone formation is called ossification.
- The first stage in the bone formation is the condensation of mesenchyme to form plates or membranes.
- In the *intramembranous bones*, the mesenchymal plates are gradually converted into bone by ossification.
- In the *endochondral bones* the mesenchymal plates become converted into cartilage models which are subsequently replaced by bones.
- Some of the mesenchymal cells differentiate into osteoblasts which actively form the bones.
- *Osteocytes* are mature bone cells, *osteoblasts* are bone forming cells and *osteoclasts* are bone destroying cells.
- The bone formation starts actively from certain constant areas and spreads to other parts of the bone. Such areas are referred to as *ossification centers.*
- Some specialized mesenchymal cells, osteogenic progenitor cells multiply and condense around dense capillary network in such ossific centers to lay down bone.
- The ossification centers which appear before birth are called *primary centers.*
- The *secondary centers* usually appear after birth, exceptions being lower end of femur and upper end of tibia.

Laws of Ossification

- The primary centers appear before birth. Multiple primary centers appear at the same time.
- The secondary centers appear after birth except the lower end of femur which appears before birth. Multiple secondary centers appear at different time intervals.
- The secondary center which appears first fuses last and that extremity of the bone is the growing end, except lower end of fibula. Growing end is away from the direction of the nutrient artery.
- In the upper limb bones the nutrient foramina of the shaft are directed towards the elbow.
- In the lower limb bones they are directed away from the knee joint. Fibula violates the law of ossification.

Blood Supply of Long Bone

- The shaft or diaphysis of long bones has, about its middle, 1 or 2 nutrient foramina which are directed away from the growing end.
- A nutrient artery with two veins is transmitted by these foramina.
- This diaphyseal artery reaches the medulla where it divides into ascending and descending branches which reach the ends of the bones where they again divide repeatedly and communicate with the terminal branches of the epiphyseal and metaphyseal arteries.
- They also send branches into the Haversian canals and communicate with the periosteal vessels on the surface of the bone.
- Thus the blood supply to the shaft is from inner to outer zones of the cortex although to some extent the blood flows in the reverse direction from the periosteal vessels especially to supply the peripheral parts of the cortex.
- The periosteal vessels are usually derived from the muscular branches of the arteries at the attachment of the muscles.
- The metaphyseal arteries directly enter the metaphysis through numerous foramina from the neighboring systemic vessels.
- The epiphyseal arteries are derived from the periarticular vascular arches which are found on the nonarticular parts of the ends of the bones.
- The veins come out through separate openings unlike in the diaphysis.
- There are free communications between the diaphyseal, epiphyseal and metaphyseal arteries in the mature adult bones.
- The latter two are much more in number and can easily replace the diaphyseal arteries.
- In the immature bones where the epiphyseal cartilages persist, there is no connection between metaphyseal and epiphyseal arteries.

Lymphatics

Lymphatics are seen in the periosteum close to the vessels, but they cannot be made out in the bones.

Nerve Supply

- Nerve fibers enter the bone along with the blood vessels.
- Some of these fibers are said to be concerned with pain and others have a trophic function, in some way governing the growth and repair of the bones.
- Nerve fibers are seen in plenty in the periosteum.

Bones of Upper Limb

Clavicle, scapula, humerus, radius, ulna, 8 carpal bones, 5 metacarpals and 14 phalanges.

Clavicle (Fig. 3.6)

- **Parts:** Two ends [lateral (acromial) and medial (sternal)] and a shaft.
- **Attachments:** Medial 2/3 of the shaft: Pectoralis major, sternocleidomastoid, sternohyoid, subclavius; lateral 1/3 of the shaft: Deltoid, trapezius.
- **Applied anatomy:** Commonly fractured at the junction of medial 2/3 and lateral third during fall on the shoulder on an outstretched hand.

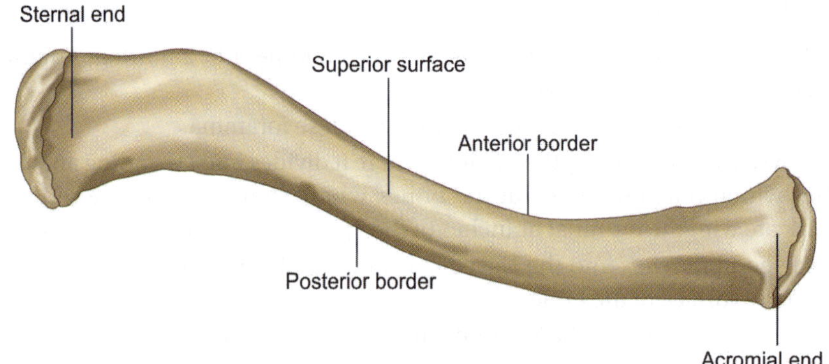

Fig. 3.6: Clavicle.

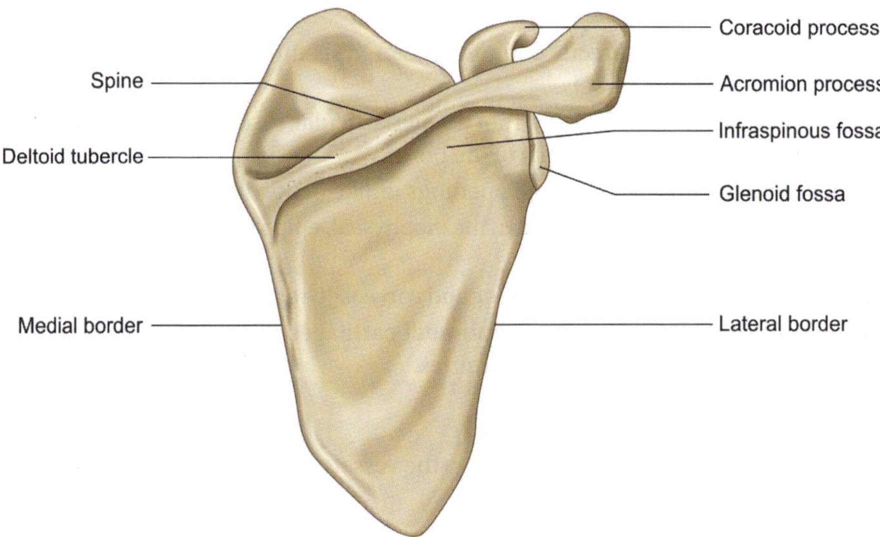

Fig. 3.7: Scapula.

- **Peculiarities:** No medullary cavity, only long bone placed horizontally, two primary centers for ossification and first bone to ossify.'

Scapula (Fig. 3.7)

- **Parts:** Body with two surfaces [costal (ventral) and dorsal], 3 borders (superior, lateral and medial), 3 angles (superior, inferior and lateral), 3 bony processes (spine, acromion and coracoid) and glenoid cavity which articulates with head of humerus to form shoulder joint.
- **Attachments:** Body: Serratus anterior, rhomboideus major, rhomboideus minor, levator scapulae, teres major, teres minor, supraspinatus, infraspinatus, subscapularis; glenoid process: Long head of biceps, long head of triceps; spine: Trapezius, deltoid; acromion process: Trapezius, deltoid, coracoid process: Short head of biceps, coracobrachialis, pectoralis minor.

- **Applied anatomy:** If muscles attached to scapula are paralyzed, the position of the bone is affected leading to dropped shoulder (by paralysis of trapezius) and winged scapula (by paralysis of serratus anterior).

Humerus (Fig. 3.8)

- **Parts:** Upper end (head, neck, greater and lesser tubercles), shaft and lower end (medial epicondyle, trochlea, capitulum and lateral epicondyles).
- **Attachments:** Upper end: Pectoralis major, teres major, latissimus dorsi, subscapularis, supraspinatus, infraspinatus, teres minor; shaft: Deltoid, coracobrachialis, brachialis; lower end: Flexors and extensors of forearm.

Applied anatomy

1. The humeral articular surface is about four times the area of the glenoid cavity of the scapula, so free movements of the shoulder joint is possible, but it is also prone for dislocations.
2. Three nerves are closely related to the bone, namely, axillary nerve winds round the surgical neck, radial nerve lies in the spiral groove and ulnar nerve curves behind the medial epicondyle. In fractures of humerus, these nerves may be involved.
3. Supracondylar fractures are common in children when they fall on the outstretched hands with the elbow slightly flexed. There is a danger of injury to the median nerve and brachial artery.

Radius (Fig. 3.9)

- **Parts:** Upper end (head, neck, tuberosity), shaft, lower end (styloid process).
- **Attachments:** Upper end: Biceps brachii; shaft: Flexor digitorum superficialis, flexor pollicis longus, pronator teres, pronator quadratus, abductor pollicis longus, extensor pollicis brevis, supinator; lower end: Brachioradialis.

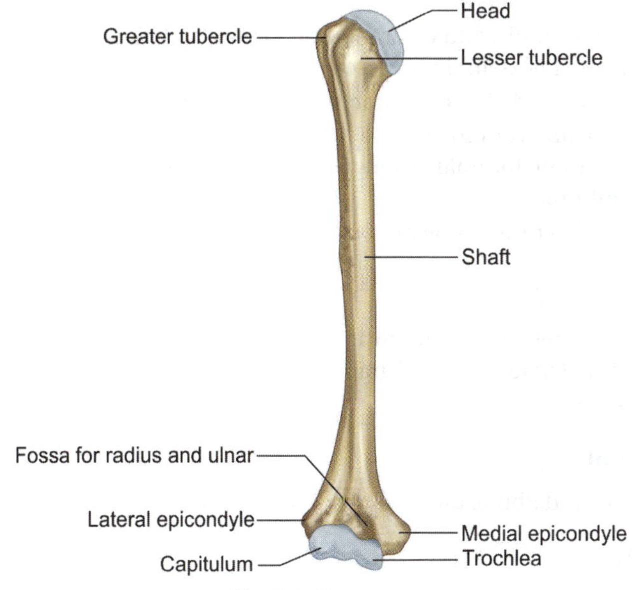

Fig. 3.8: Humerus.

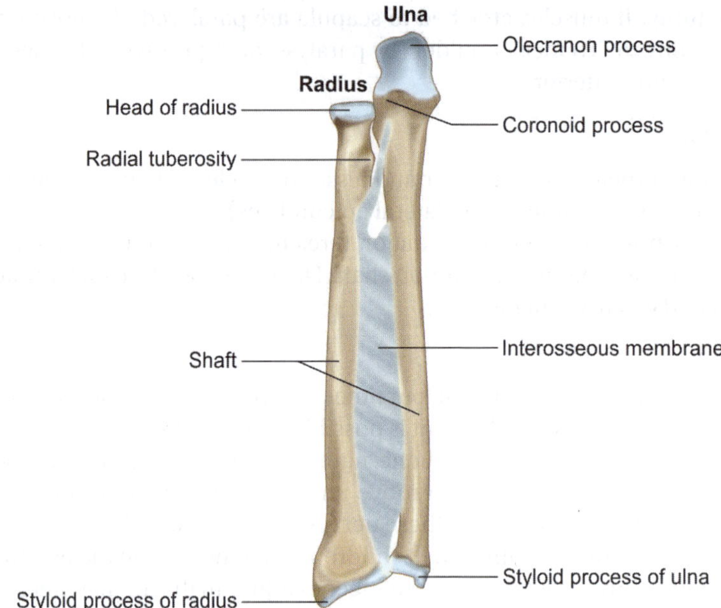

Fig. 3.9: Radius and ulna.

- **Applied anatomy:** Fractures (Colle's fracture-lower end of radius is displaced backwards and upwards, Smith's fracture-lower end is displaced forwards and styloid process is in level of styloid process of ulna), dislocation (subluxation) of head.

Ulna (Fig. 3.9)

- **Parts:** Upper end (coronoid and olecranon processes, trochlear and radial notches), shaft and lower end (head and styloid processes).
- **Attachments:** Upper end: Triceps, brachialis, supinator, flexor digitorum superficialis; shaft: Flexor digitorum profundus, flexor carpi ulnaris, pronator quadratus, extensor carpi ulnaris, anconeus, abductor pollicis longus, extensor pollicis longus, extensor indices, and interosseous membrane.
- **Applied anatomy:** Fracture, dislocations.

Articulated Hand (Fig. 3.10)

It consists of 8 carpal bones (proximal row from lateral to medial: scaphoid, lunate, triquetral, pisiform; distal row from lateral to medial: trapezium, trapezoid, capitate, hamate), 5 metacarpals and 14 phalanges.

Bones of Lower Limb

Hip bone, femur, tibia and fibula, tarsal bones, 5 metatarsals, 14 phalanges in the digits.

Hip Bone (Fig. 3.11)

Parts: Ilium, ischium and pubis united at the acetabulum.

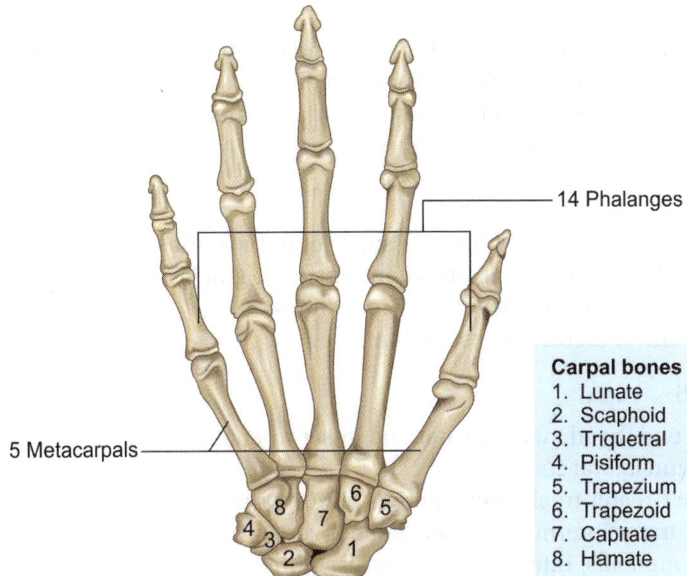

Fig. 3.10: Articulated hand.

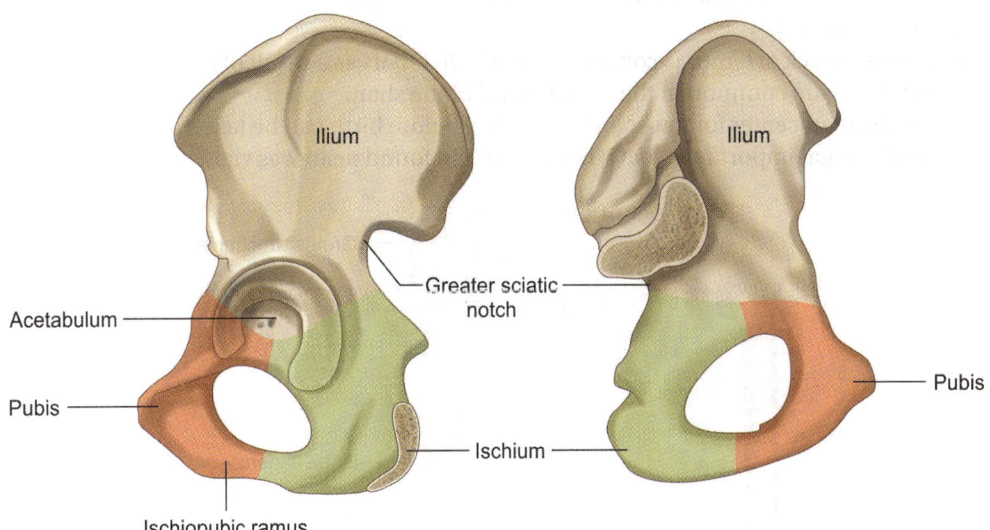

Fig. 3.11: Hip bone.

Ilium

- **Parts:** Iliac crest, iliac tubercle, anterior superior iliac spine, anterior inferior iliac spine, posterior superior iliac spine, posterior inferior iliac spine, gluteal surface, iliac surface, medial surface.
- **Attachments:** Sartorius, inguinal ligament, rectus femoris, external oblique, internal oblique muscles of abdomen, gluteus maximus, medius and minimus.

Ischium

- **Parts:** Body (ischial spine, ischial tuberosity) and ramus.
- **Attachments:** Hamstring muscles (semimembranosus, semitendinosus, long head of biceps femoris, adductor magnus), gemellus superior and inferior, coccygeus, posterior fibers of levator ani, obturator externus, quadratus femoris.

Pubis

- **Parts:** Pubic tubercle, pubic symphysis, superior pubic ramus and inferior pubic ramus.
- **Attachments:** Adductor longus, brevis and magnus, gracilis, inguinal ligament, obturator externus, obturator internus, levator ani, pectineus.
- **Applied anatomy:** Fracture of acetabulum.

Femur (Fig. 3.12)

- **Parts:** Upper end (head, neck, greater and lesser trochanter), shaft, linea aspera and lower end (medial and lateral condyles).
- **Attachments:** Greater trochanter: Gluteus minimus, gluteus medius, piriformis, obturator externus, obturator internus with the gemelli; lesser trochanter: Iliacus and psoas major; shaft: Vastus medialis, intermedius, lateralis, gluteus maximus, adductors, gastrocnemii, pectineus, short head of biceps femoris; linea aspera: Vastus lateralis, short head of biceps femoris, adductor longus, adductor brevis, adductor magnus, vastus medialis; lower end: Popliteus, lateral head of gastrocnemius, adductor magnus.
- **Applied anatomy:**
  - Fracture neck of femur is common in old individuals as a result of fall.
  - Fractures are common in the middle third of the shaft.
  - Ossification center for lower end appearing before birth can be taken as an evidence for medicolegal importance that a newborn child found dead was viable.

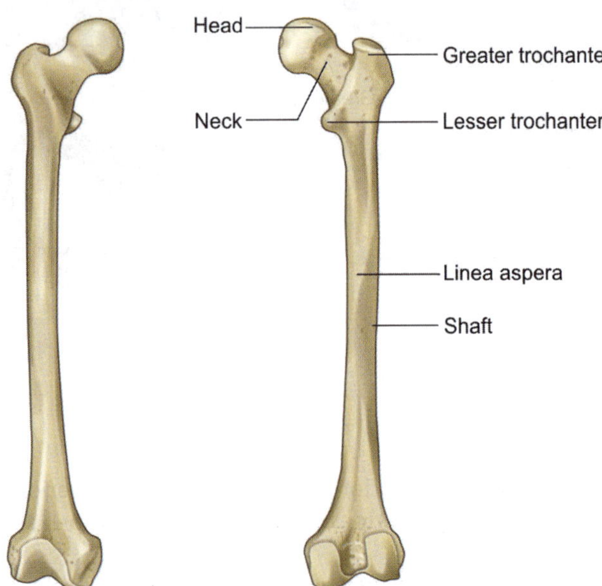

Fig. 3.12: Femur.

Tibia (Fig. 3.13)

- **Parts:** Upper end (medial and lateral condyles, intercondylar area), shaft and lower end (medial malleolus).
- **Attachments:** Upper end: Semimembranosus, extensor digitorum longus, anterior and posterior horns of medial and lateral menisci, anterior and posterior cruciate ligaments, ligamentum patella at tibial tuberosity; shaft: Tibialis anterior, sartorius, gracilis, semitendinosus; tibialis posterior, soleus, flexor digitorum longus, popliteus.
- **Applied anatomy:**
  - Upper end is one of the commonest sites for acute osteomyelitis.
  - Indirect violence can cause fracture at the junction of upper two thirds and lower one-third of the shaft.
  - Bone graft can be taken from the subcutaneous medial surface of tibia.
  - Pott's fracture (spiral fracture of lateral malleolus, avulsion of tibial collateral ligament, posterior margin of lower end of tibia shears off against the talus).

Fibula (Fig. 3.13)

- **Parts:** Upper end (head), shaft and lower end (lateral malleolus).
- **Attachments:** Upper end: Biceps femoris; shaft: Extensor digitorum longus, extensor hallucis longus, peroneus longus, brevis and tertius, soleus, flexor hallucis longus, tibialis posterior.
- **Applied anatomy:**
  - Fractures of the neck of fibula can cause injury to the common peroneal nerve.
  - Can be used for bone grafts since it does not take part in weight transmission.

Articulated Foot (Fig. 3.14)

It consists of tarsal bones (talus, calcaneus, navicular, three cuneiforms, cuboid), 5 metatarsals, 14 phalanges in the digits.

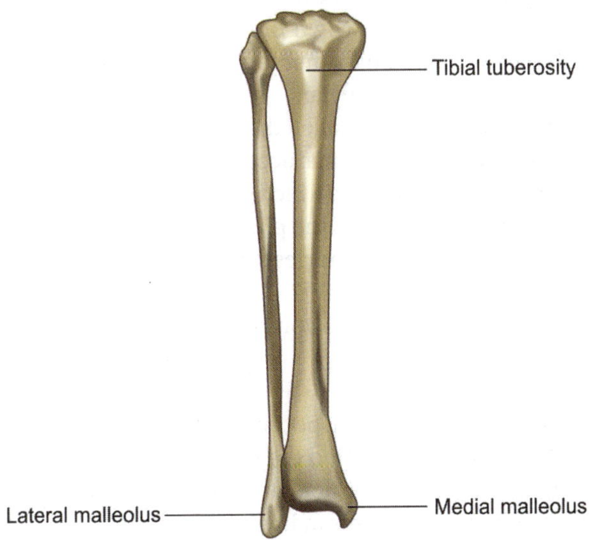

Fig. 3.13: Tibia and fibula.

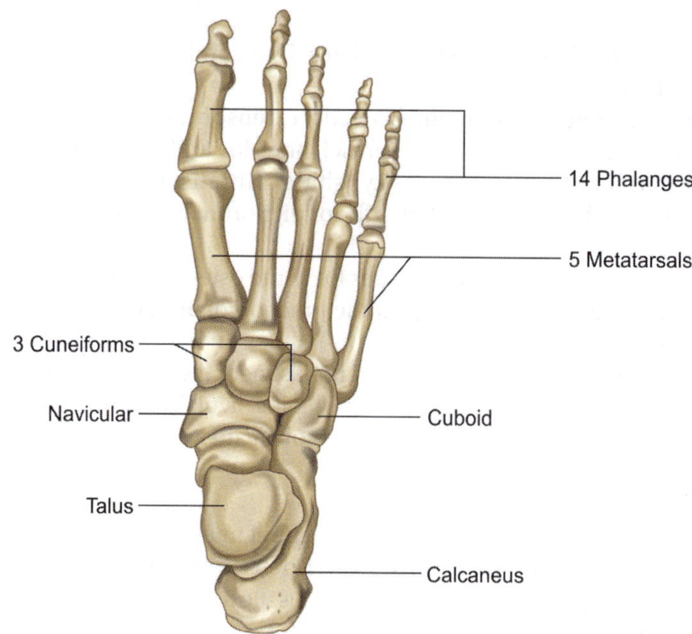

Fig. 3.14: Articulated foot.

Bones of Head and Neck

Bones of skull **(Fig. 3.15)** are: *Paired*: Parietal, temporal, maxilla, lacrimal, nasal, palatine, zygomatic bones. *Unpaired*: Frontal, occipital, sphenoid, ethmoid, vomer, mandible.

Occipital Bone

- It forms the posterior aspect and base of the skull.
- **Foramina:** Jugular foramen through which the 9th, 10th and 11th cranial nerves and the internal jugular vein passes. Hypoglossal nerve passes through hypoglossal canal.
- **Parts:** Squamous, basilar and two condylar.
- Squamous part shows a large foramen called the foramen magnum through which medulla oblongata, 4th part of vertebral artery, spinal accessory nerves pass. On the posterior aspect it shows the external occipital protuberance which gives attachment to the ligamentum nuchae.
- Basilar part on the inferior aspect shows the pharyngeal tubercle.
- The condylar part shows two occipital condyles that articulate with the atlas vertebrae forming the atlanto-occipital joint.
- **Attachments:** Trapezius, sternocleidomastoid and superior constrictor muscle.

Parietal Bones

- Two in number. They lie on the lateral aspect of the skull on either side. Each bone shows a protuberance on the outer surface called the parietal eminence and a foramen called the parietal foramen. The parietal bones articulate with the frontal bone anteriorly at coronal suture and the occipital bone posteriorly at lambdoid suture.
- The two parietal bones meet each other in the midline at the sagittal suture.

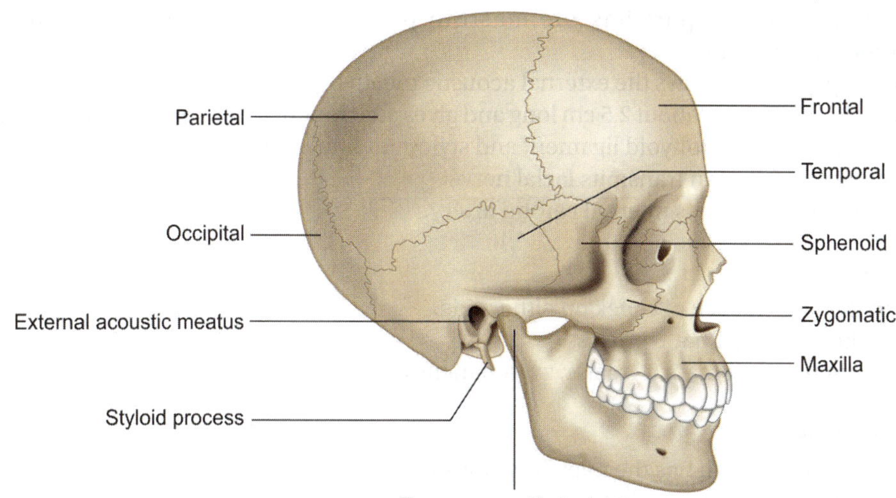

Fig. 3.15: Skull and temporomandibular joint.

Frontal Bone

- Lies on the anterior aspect of skull.
- **Parts:** Squamous part and orbital part.
- Squamous part is the upper vertical part that forms the forehead. This shows the supraorbital margins and supraorbital foramen.
- Orbital part is the lower horizontal part which forms the roof of the orbits.
- The frontal bone meets the two parietal bones at the coronal suture.

Sphenoid Bone

- Lies in the center of the base of the skull.
- It has a body that has the sphenoid air sinuses.
- **Parts:** Butterfly shaped bone with a central body, a pair of greater wings, lesser wings and pterygoid processes.
- The body on the superior surface shows the hypophyseal fossa that lodges the pituitary gland.
- **Attachments:** Medial pterygoid, lateral pterygoid.
- Foramina in sphenoid bone are foramen ovale through which mandibular nerve and lesser petrosal nerve pass, foramen rotundum through which maxillary nerve pass and foramen spinosum through which meningeal branch of the mandibular nerve passes. The optic nerve and ophthalmic artery pass through the optic canal. The branches of ophthalmic nerve, the 3rd, 4th and the 6th cranial nerves pass through superior orbital fissure.

Temporal Bones

- Two in number. Each has four parts.
- **Parts:** Squamous, petromastoid, tympanic and styloid process.
- The squamous part shows the superior and inferior temporal lines between which is the temporal fossa. This gives attachment to temporalis muscle.

- The petromastoid part has the mastoid process which has the attachment of sternocleidomastoid.
- The tympanic part shows the external acoustic meatus.
- The styloid process is about 2.5 cm long and gives attachment to the styloglossus, stylohyoid, stylopharyngeus, stylohyoid ligament and stylomandibular ligament.
- Stylomastoid foramen transmits facial nerve.
- Carotid canal transmits internal carotid artery.

Zygomatic Bones

- Form the prominence of cheek on either side.
- They show the zygomatic process.
- **Attachments:** Zygomaticus major, zygomaticus minor, masseter, temporalis.

Maxillary Bones

- Two in number. Each has the maxillary sinus in it.
- **Parts:** Alveolar processes that contain the upper teeth; horizontal process called palatine process projects posteriorly from the bone to form the anterior 2/3rd of the hard palate.
- **Attachments:** Orbicularis oris, orbicularis oculi, levator labii superioris alaeque nasi, levator labii superioris, levator anguli oris, nasalis, depressor septi, buccinator.
- Infraorbital nerve and vessels passes through infraorbital foramen.

Ethmoid Bone

- Single bone showing the cribriform plate of ethmoid and the labyrinths.
- The cribriform plate of ethmoid shows perforations that transmit olfactory nerves from the nasal cavity to the brain.

Lacrimal Bones

Show lacrimal fossa in which the lacrimal gland is present.

Nasal Bones

Form the bridge of nose.

Palatine Bones

Form posterior 1/3rd of hard palate.

Vomer

Forms the posteroinferior part of nasal septum.

Mandible (Fig. 3.16)

Lower jaw is the largest and strongest bone of the face.

- **Parts:** Body, ramus, condyloid process, coronoid process.
- Body lodges teeth.
- Pair of rami gives attachment to muscles. Each ramus has the condyloid and coronoid processes. Condyloid process takes part in the formation of the temporomandibular joint.
- The body shows the symphysis menti in the center where the two halves of body meet.
- There is a mental foramen through which passes the mental nerves and vessels.

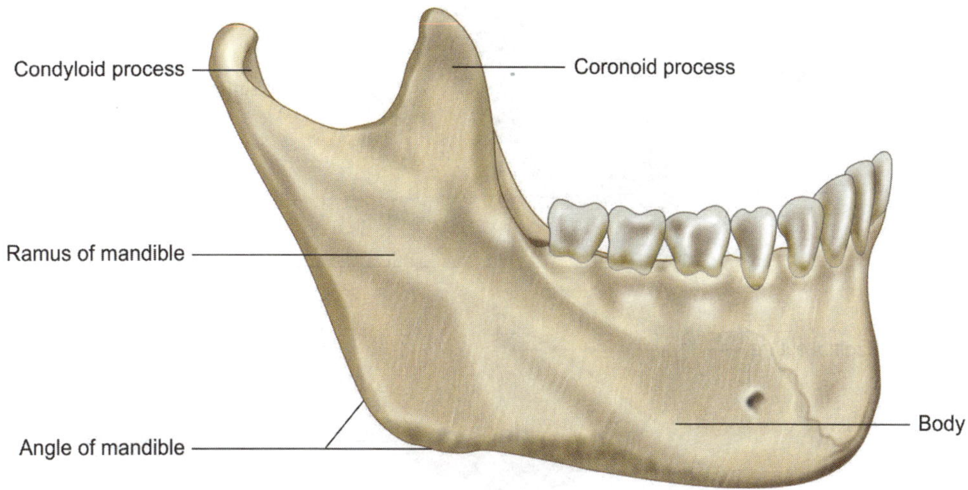

Fig. 3.16: Mandible.

- The mandible is related to the parotid and submandibular glands.
- **Attachments:** Muscles of mastication (medial pterygoid, lateral pterygoid, masseter, temporalis), buccinator, geniohyoid, genioglossus, superior constrictor, depressor labii inferioris, depressor anguli oris, mentalis, orbicularis oris, mylohyoid, anterior belly of digastric, platysma.

Fontanelles of Fetal Skull (Fig. 3.17)

- They are gaps in some sites of the bony vault of skull, which are bridged by membranes formed by fusion of periosteum of the bones and underlying dura mater.
- There are 6 fontanelles: Anterior, posterior, 2 anterolateral (pterion) and 2 posterolateral (asterion).
- The anterior fontanelle is the largest of all fontanelles and lies between the frontal bone anteriorly and the two parietal bones posteriorly in the sagittal and coronal sutures.
- It closes by the age of 18 months.
- Importance of anterior fontanelles:
  - Giving intravenous injections and fluids
  - Drawing of blood for diagnostic purposes
  - Determining age of the infant
  - Determining lie of the fetus during labor
- The posterior fontanelle lies between the parietal bones and the occipital bones posteriorly. It lies in the lambdoid suture.

Hyoid Bone

- U shaped bone. Situated in the anterior midline of the neck between chin and the thyroid cartilage.
- It is kept suspended in position by muscles and ligaments.
- It provides attachment to the floor of mouth, tongue, larynx, epiglottis and pharynx.

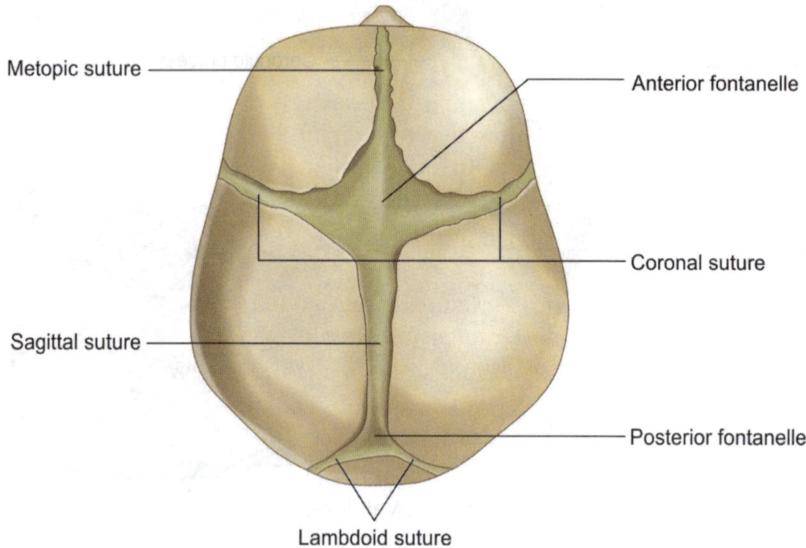

Fig. 3.17: Fontanelles of fetal skull.

- **Parts:** Body, pair of cornua/horns (greater cornu, lesser cornu).
- **Attachments:** Geniohyoid, mylohyoid, hyoglossus, genioglossus, sternohyoid, omohyoid, thyrohyoid, middle constrictor.

Bones of Thorax

Ribs (Fig. 3.18)

- There are 12 pairs of ribs.
- **Parts:** Each rib has an anterior end that articulates with costal cartilage and a posterior end that articulates with the corresponding vertebra. The posterior end shows head, neck and tubercle.
- The shaft of each rib is flattened such that it shows a superior border, inferior border, inner surface and outer surface.

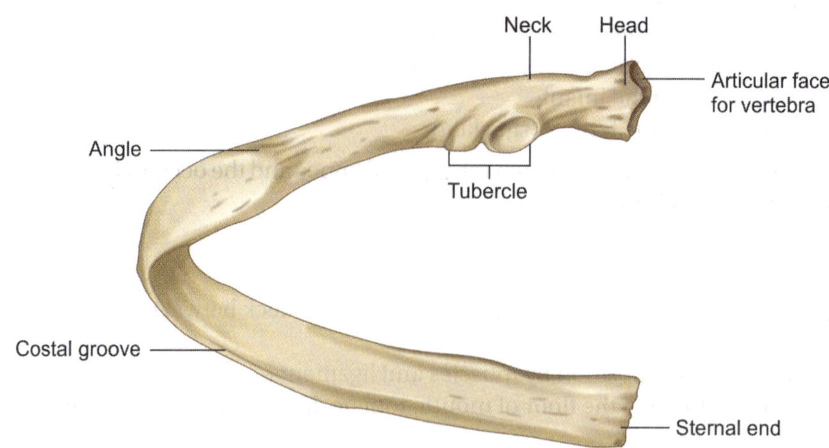

Fig. 3.18: Typical rib.

- The inner surface is smooth and covered by pleura and shows the costal groove which lodges intercostal artery, vein and nerve.
- **Classification:**
  - True ribs (1 to 7)—Directly articulate with sternum.
  - False ribs (8 to 10)—Indirectly join the sternum through 7th costal cartilage.
  - Floating ribs (11 and 12)—Short and do not articulate with sternum.
  - Typical ribs—3rd to 9th ribs are typical ribs.
  - Atypical ribs—1st, 2nd, 10th, 11th, 12th ribs are atypical ribs.
- **Attachments:**
  - *Typical ribs:* Iliocostalis thoracis, levatores costarum, serratus anterior, external intercostal, internal intercostal, innermost intercostal, external oblique.
  - *First rib:* Scalenus anterior, subclavius, scalenus medius, 1st digitation of serratus anterior.
  - *Second rib:* 1st and 2nd digitations of serratus anterior, scalenus posterior, serratus posterior.
  - *12th rib:* Internal intercostal, quadratus lumborum, diaphragm, external intercostal, internal intercostal, levator costae, erector spinae, latissimus dorsi, longissimus thoracis, iliocostalis, latissimus dorsi, external oblique, serratus posterior inferior.
- **Applied anatomy:**
  1. *Cervical rib*: The costal element of the 7th cervical vertebra may elongate and form cervical rib in 5% of individuals. It may cause compression on lower trunk of brachial plexus and subclavian artery leading to pain along the medial side of forearm and hand, wasting of small muscles of the hand and disturbances in the circulation of upper limb.
  2. Fracture of rib is rare in children. In adults, the middle ribs are usually involved near the angle which is the weakest part of rib.

Sternum (Fig. 3.19)

- **Parts:** Manubrium, body and xiphoid process.
- **Attachments:** Sternocleidomastoid, sternohyoid, sternothyroid, pectoralis major, sternocostalis, rectus abdominis, diaphragm.

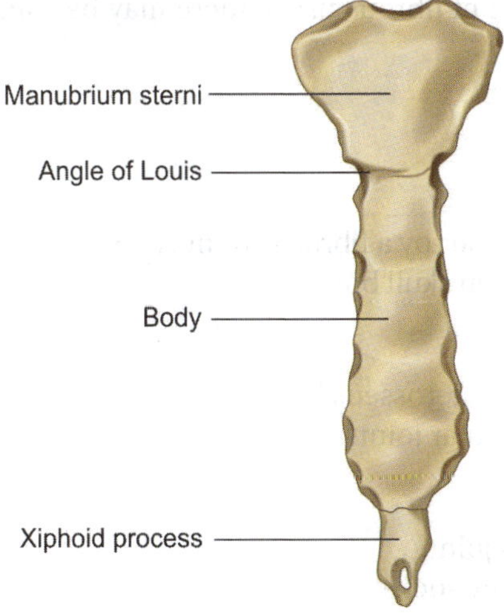

Fig. 3.19: Sternum.

- **Applied anatomy:**
  1. Sternal puncture is made through the manubrium for examining the bone marrow.
  2. It may be split for approaching the heart, great vessels and thymus.

Vertebrae (Figs. 3.20 to 3.23)

There are 33 vertebrae: 7 cervical, 12 thoracic, 5 lumbar, 5 sacral and 4 coccygeal.

- **Parts:** Body, dorsal vertebral or neural arch with vertebral foramen in between. Vertebral arch has 2 pedicles, 2 laminae, 2 transverse processes, 2 superior and 2 inferior articular processes, 1 spinous process.
- In articulated vertebral column, vertebral foramina together form a canal called vertebral canal which lodges spinal cord, meninges and blood vessels.
- Intervertebral foramina are in between the pedicles and vertebral notches.

Intervertebral discs

- They are fibrocartilaginous discs interposed between adjacent surfaces of vertebral bodies from 2nd cervical vertebra to sacrum.
- They constitute a symphyseal type of joint between adjoining vertebral bodies.
- Each disc has a peripheral part called annulus fibrosus and a central part nucleus pulposus.
- **Applied anatomy:** Herniation of nucleus pulposus or slipped disc, kyphosis (curvature of vertebral column with backward convexity), lordosis (exaggeration of lumbar curvature with forward convexity), scoliosis (lateral deviation of column).

JOINTS

- A joint is formed where two or more bones come together whether or not there is movement between them.
- The joints can be classified as follows according to the tissues that unite the bone ends—fibrous, cartilaginous and synovial joints.

Fibrous Joints

- In this type the articulating surfaces are connected by fibrous tissue.
- Depending on the length of fibrous tissue there may be some degree of movement or no movement at all.

Types of Fibrous Joints

Sutural joints

The two bones are held together by a fibrous connective tissue called sutural ligaments.
For example: Joints in between skull bones.

Syndesmosis

The bones are connected by interosseus ligament.
For example: Inferior tibiofibular joints.

Gomphosis

It is a peg and socket type of joint.
For example: Tooth in its bony socket.

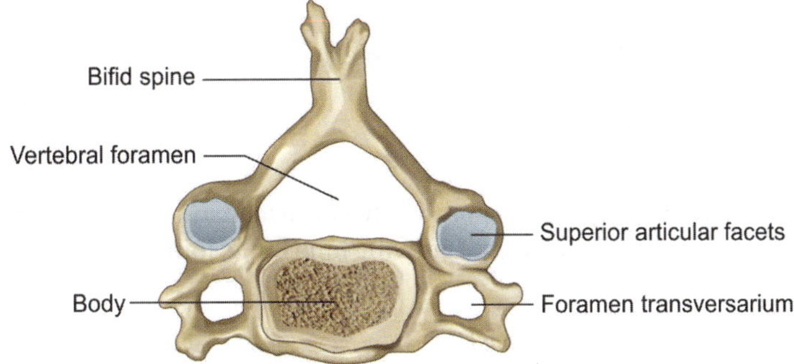

Fig. 3.20: Cervical vertebra.

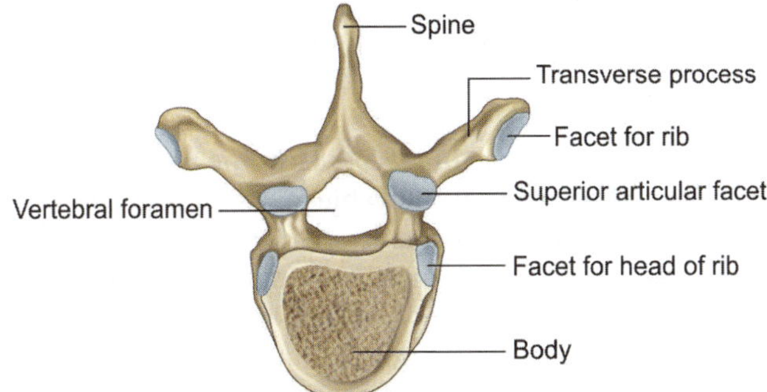

Fig. 3.21: Thoracic vertebra.

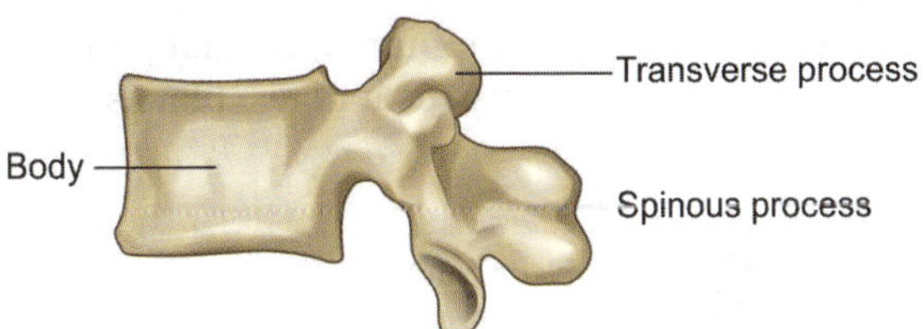

Fig. 3.22: Lumbar vertebra.

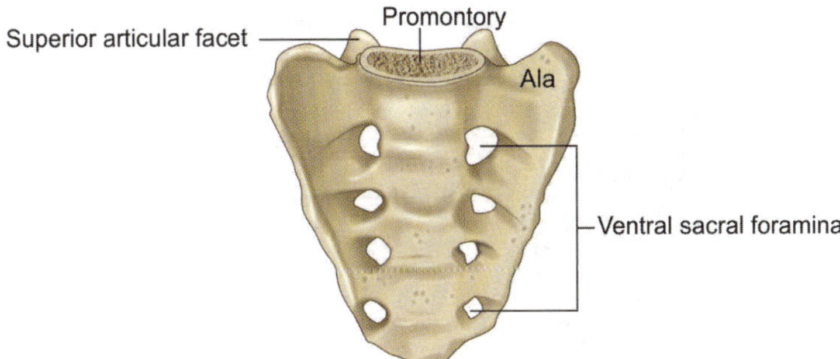

Fig. 3.23: Sacrum.

Cartilaginous Joints

Articular ends are connected by a piece of cartilage.

Types of Cartilaginous Joints

Primary cartilaginous joint (synchondrosis)

A piece of bar of hyaline cartilage is interposed between articulating ends of bones. For example: Union between diaphysis and epiphysis of growing long bone, joint between basisphenoid and basiocciput.

Secondary cartilaginous joint (symphysis)

- Articulating ends are covered by a thin layer of hyaline cartilage and connected by a plate of fibrous cartilage.
- These joints are slightly movable.
  For example: Symphysis pubis, intervertebral joints.

Synovial Joints (Fig. 3.24)

- Articulating surfaces are covered by a thin layer of hyaline articular cartilage and separated by a synovial joint cavity. They are freely movable joints.
- The cavity is enclosed within a fibrous capsule.
- The inner surface of capsule and the nonarticular parts of the articulating ends of bones which are inside the capsule are lined by synovial membrane.
- The articular surfaces are lubricated by synovial fluid.
- The fluid has a property of having a variable viscosity. It is thick in slow movements and thin in rapid movements, which is due to hyaluronic acid.
- The synovial fluid is produced and absorbed by synovial membrane.
- In certain joints an articular disc made of fibrocartilage may be interposed into the joint to divide its cavity into two (For example: Temporomandibular joint).
- Discs are found in joints where movements occur in two planes.

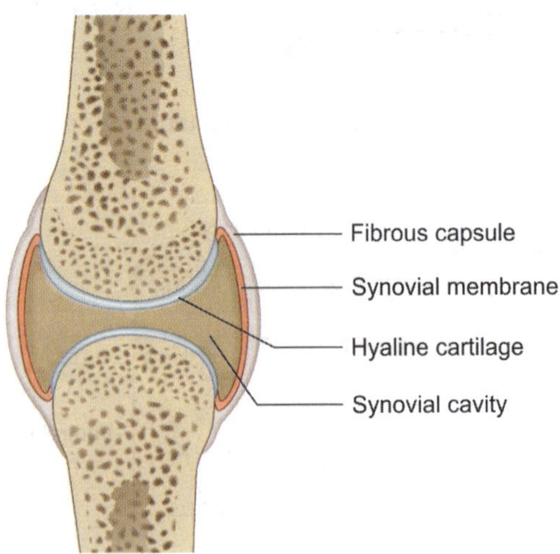

Fig. 3.24: Parts of a synovial joint.

- Functions of discs are:
  1. To make the relatively incongruent surfaces more congruent.
  2. To act as spreaders of the synovial fluid between the joint surfaces.
  3. To act as shock absorbers.
  4. To help fill the dead spaces created within the joint during its movement.
- Intracapsular fatty pads are found in some synovial joints, but they are outside the synovial membrane (For example: Knee joint).

Classification of Synovial Joints

Ball and socket joint

- One of the articular surfaces is spherical and ball-like and the other end presents a concave cup-like cavity.
- Movements can take place around many axes (poly-axial).
  For example: Shoulder joint, hip joint.

Hinge joint

Movements occur in one plane only (uniaxial) around a transverse axis. For example: Ankle joint, elbow joint, interphalangeal joints.

Pivot joint

Movements occur in one plane only (uniaxial) around a longitudinal axis. For example: Proximal radioulnar joint, atlantoaxial joint.

Condyloid joint

- These are modified hinge joints.
- One of the articular ends is convex and condyle like and the other end is reciprocally concave.
- Movements occur around two axes (biaxial) causing adduction, abduction, extension, flexion, circumduction, but no rotation.
  For example: Knee joint, temporomandibular joint.

Ellipsoid joint

- An elliptical convex surface fits into an elliptical concave surface.
- Movements occur around two axes causing adduction, abduction, extension, and flexion.
  For example: Wrist joint, metacarpophalangeal joint.

Saddle joint

Articular surfaces are reciprocally concavo-convex and movements can occur in all planes. For example: Carpometacarpal joint of thumb, calcaneocuboid joint.

Plane joint

Articular surfaces are flat and movements are restricted to slight gliding, tilting and rotation. For example: Joints between articular processes of adjacent vertebrae, intercarpal joints.

Hilton's Law

A nerve supplying a joint also supplies the muscles moving the joint and the skin overlying the insertions of the muscles.

Temporomandibular Joint (See Fig. 3.15)

Type of Joint

Condyloid variety of synovial joint.

Articular Ends

Above: Mandibular fossa of temporal bone; *below*: Condyle or head of mandible. There is a meniscus or fibrocartilaginous disc interposed between the articular ends.

Ligaments

Capsule

- Inner surface is lined by synovial membrane.
- It is *attached above* to the articular tubercle, circumference of mandibular fossa, squamotympanic fissure and *below* to the neck of mandible.

Lateral temporomandibular ligament

It is *attached above* to the auricular tubercle and *below* to posterolateral aspect of the neck of mandible.

Sphenomandibular ligament

It is *attached superiorly* to the spine of sphenoid and *inferiorly* to the lingula of mandibular foramen.

Stylomandibular ligament

It is *attached above* to the lateral surface of the styloid process and *below* to the angle and posterior border of ramus of mandible.

Blood Supply

Maxillary and superficial temporal artery.

Nerve Supply

Auriculotemporal, masseteric nerve.

Movements and Muscles Causing Them

- **Depression:** Lateral pterygoid, digastric, mylohyoid, geniohyoid
- **Elevation:** Medial pterygoids, masseter, temporalis
- **Protrusion:** Medial and lateral pterygoids, masseter
- **Retraction:** Posterior fibers of temporalis of both sides
- **Side-to-side movement:** Medial and lateral pterygoids of both sides acting alternately.

Shoulder Joint (Fig. 3.25)

Shoulder joint is a polyaxial synovial joint belonging to the ball and socket variety.

Articular Ends

- Proximally, glenoid fossa of scapula and distally, head of humerus.

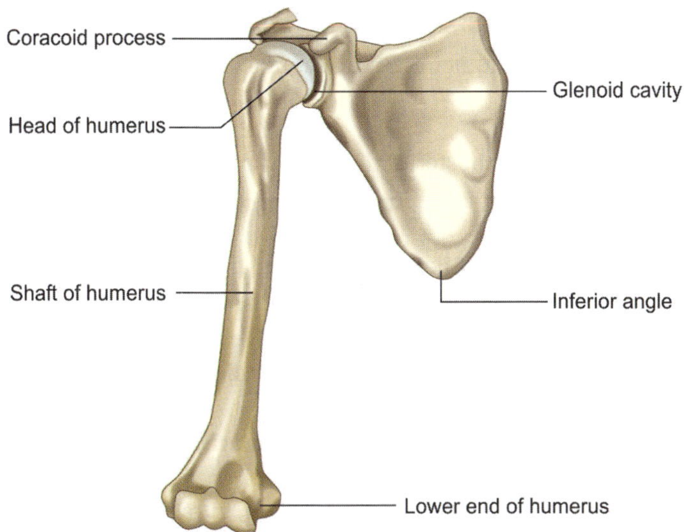

Fig. 3.25: Shoulder joint.

- Glenoid fossa is slightly depressed in the center. Its area and concavity are increased by a fibrocartilaginous ribbon-like structure, glenoidal labrum which is attached to its margins. It is covered by a layer of hyaline cartilage, which is thinner in the center than at the periphery.
- The head of humerus is covered with hyaline cartilage which is thicker in the center than at the periphery.

Ligaments

Capsule

- It is a loose fibrous covering for the joint and its inner surface is lined by synovial membrane.
- It is lax, weak and is compensated by the expansions derived from the adjoining tendons of subscapularis, supraspinatus, infraspinatus and teres minor forming rotator cuff.
- **Attachments:** Medial: Scapula beyond supraglenoid tubercle and margins of glenoidal labrum; lateral: Anatomical neck of humerus except superiorly which is deficient for passage of tendon of long head of biceps.

Accessory ligaments

- **Glenohumeral ligaments:** They are *attached above* to the upper end of the anterior border of the glenoid fossa and *below* to the lesser tuberosity.
- **Transverse humeral ligament:** It is *attached* between greater and lesser tuberosities of the humerus.
- **Coracohumeral ligament:** It is *attached* from coracoid process to the greater tuberosity of humerus.

Coracoacromial arch

Coracoid process, coracoacromial ligament, acromian process together is called coracoacromial arch which prevents upward dislocation of the humerus.

Blood Supply

Anterior and posterior circumflex humeral, suprascapular and subscapular arteries.

Nerve Supply

Lateral pectoral, suprascapular and posterior division of axillary nerve.

Movements and Muscles Causing Them

- **Flexion:** Pectoralis major, anterior fibers of deltoid.
- **Extension:** Posterior fibers of deltoid, teres major, latissimus dorsi.
- **Abduction:** Supraspinatus, lateral fibers of deltoid, trapezius, serratus anterior.
- **Adduction:** Latissimus dorsi, pectoralis major, teres major, coracobrachialis, long head of triceps.
- **Medial rotation:** Anterior fibers of deltoid, subscapularis, pectoralis major, teres major, latissimus dorsi.
- **Lateral rotation:** Posterior fibers of deltoid, teres minor, infraspinatus.
- **Circumduction:** Combination of all the movements occurring successively.

Hip Joint (Fig. 3.26)

Type

Synovial joint, ball and socket variety.

Articular Ends

- Proximally acetabulum of hip bone; distally head of femur.

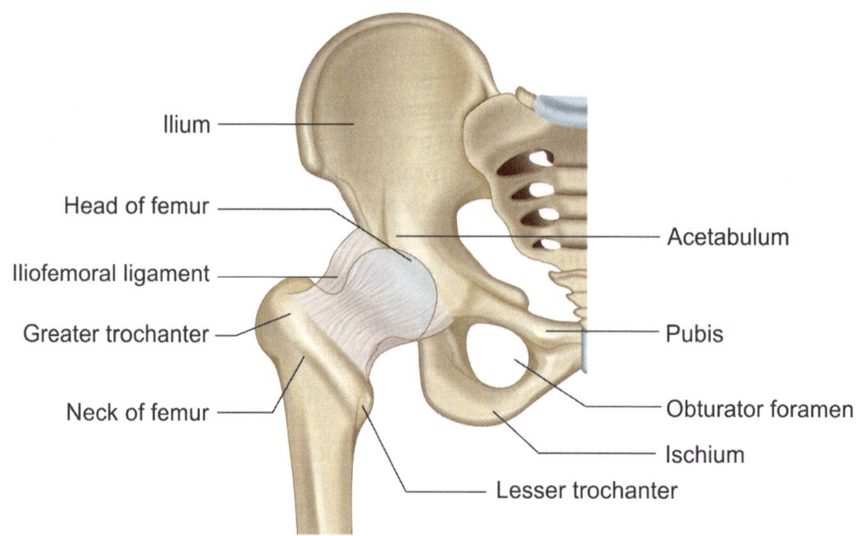

Fig. 3.26: Hip joint.

- Within the acetabulum, there is a horse-shoe shaped surface covered with articular cartilage called lunate surface.
- Below the lunate surface is a nonarticular area filled with a pad of fat ensheathed in the synovial membrane.
- A fibrocartilaginous ribbon-like structure called acetabular labrum is attached to the margins of the acetabulum.

Ligaments

Capsule

- It is a loose thick fibrous sac enclosing the joint cavity. Its inner surface and nonarticular parts inside the capsule are lined by synovial membrane.
- **Attachments:** On the *hip bone*: To acetabular labrum, transverse acetabular ligament, above and behind the acetabulum and on the *femur*: To intertrochanteric line and 1 cm behind intertrochanteric crest.

Transverse ligament

It *bridges* across the acetabular notch which is a gap in the lower part of the acetabular rim.

Round ligament of head of femur

It is triangular in shape. Its apex is *attached* to the pit on the femoral head and the base to the margins of the acetabular notch.

Iliofemoral ligament

It is the strongest ligament in the body, triangular in shape; apex is *attached* to anterior inferior iliac spine, base to intertrochanteric line.

Pubofemoral ligament

It is *attached* to iliopubic eminence, obturator crest, obturator membrane superiorly and merges with capsule, lower band of iliofemoral ligament inferiorly.

Ischiofemoral ligament

The fibers *extend* from ischium to acetabulum.

Blood Supply

Medial and lateral circumflex femoral (branch of profunda femoris artery), superior gluteal, inferior gluteal, acetabular branch of obturator (branches of internal iliac) artery.

Nerve Supply

Femoral and obturator nerves.

Movements and Muscles Causing Them

- **Flexion:** Iliacus, psoas major
- **Extension:** Gluteus maximus
- **Abduction:** Gluteus medius and minimus
- **Adduction:** Adductor longus, brevis and magnus

- **Medial rotation:** Psoas major
- **Lateral rotation:** Piriformis, gemelli, obturator internus and externus, quadratus femoris.

Knee Joint

- Condylar joint
- Condyles of femur above, condyles of tibia below and patella in front.

Ligaments

- Capsule
- Ligamentum patellae
- Tibial collateral ligament
- Fibular collateral ligament
- Anterior and posterior cruciate ligaments
- Medial and lateral menisci.

Blood Supply

Genicular branches of popliteal artery, femoral artery, anterior and posterior tibial arteries.

Nerve Supply

Femoral, sciatic and obturator nerves.

Movements and Muscles Causing Them

- **Flexion:** Biceps femoris, semimembranosus, semitendinosus
- **Extension:** Quadriceps femoris
- **Medial rotation:** Popliteus (unlocking)
- **Lateral rotation:** Biceps femoris.

APPLIED ANATOMY

Bones

- **Clavicle:** Commonly fractured at the junction of medial 2/3rd and lateral 1/3rd during fall on the shoulder or on an outstretched hand.
- **Scapula:** Paralysis of trapezius leads to drooped shoulder, paralysis of serratus anterior leads to winging of scapula.
- **Humerus:** Dislocations in fractures three nerves (axillary, radial, ulnar) closely related to humerus may be injured, and in children when they fall on outstretched hand with elbow flexed supracondylar fractures are common.
- **Radius:** Dislocations, fractures (Colle's fracture-lower end of radius is displaced backwards and upwards, Smith's fracture-lower end is displaced forwards and styloid process is in level of styloid process of ulna).
- **Ulna:** Dislocations, fractures.
- **Hip bone:** Fracture of acetabulum.
- **Femur:** Fracture neck is common in old individuals and also common in middle third of shaft, and secondary ossification center for lower end appearing before birth can be taken as evidence for medicolegal importance of a newborn child found dead.

- **Tibia:** Upper end common for osteomyelitis, bone graft can be done from subcutaneous medial surface and Pott's fracture (spiral fracture of lateral malleolus, evulsion of tibial collateral ligament, shearing off of posterior margin of lower end of tibia).
- **Fibula:** Fracture neck can cause injury to common peroneal nerve; can be used for bone grafts.
- **Ribs:** Cervical rib (rib develops from 7th cervical vertebra causing compression on lower trunk of brachial plexus and subclavian artery); usually fracture occurs at the angle of rib.
- **Sternum:** Sternal puncture made to withdraw bone marrow; sternum split into two during heart surgeries.
- **Vertebrae:** Slip disc (herniation of nucleus pulposus); kyphosis (curvature of vertebral column with backward convexity); lordosis (exaggeration of lumbar curvature with forward convexity); scoliosis (lateral deviation of vertebral column).

Joints

- **Osteoarthritis:** Most common of all joint diseases, also known as degenerative joint disease. It is a slow, progressive thinning of the joint cartilage that exposes underlying bone to pressure, abrasion and erosion.
- **Rheumatoid arthritis:** Chronic progressive disease that affects the cartilage surface of the joints and other collagen tissues throughout the body. It is characterized by recurrent inflammation of the lining of joints (synovitis).

SUMMARY

- Connective tissue (CT)
  - Adult CT
    - CT proper
      - General CT
        - Loose CT
        - Dense CT
          - Regular
          - Irregular
      - Special CT
        - Adipose
        - Reticular
        - Pigmented
    - Supporting CT
      - Cartilage
        - Hyaline
        - Elastic
        - White fibrous
      - Bone
  - Embryonic CT

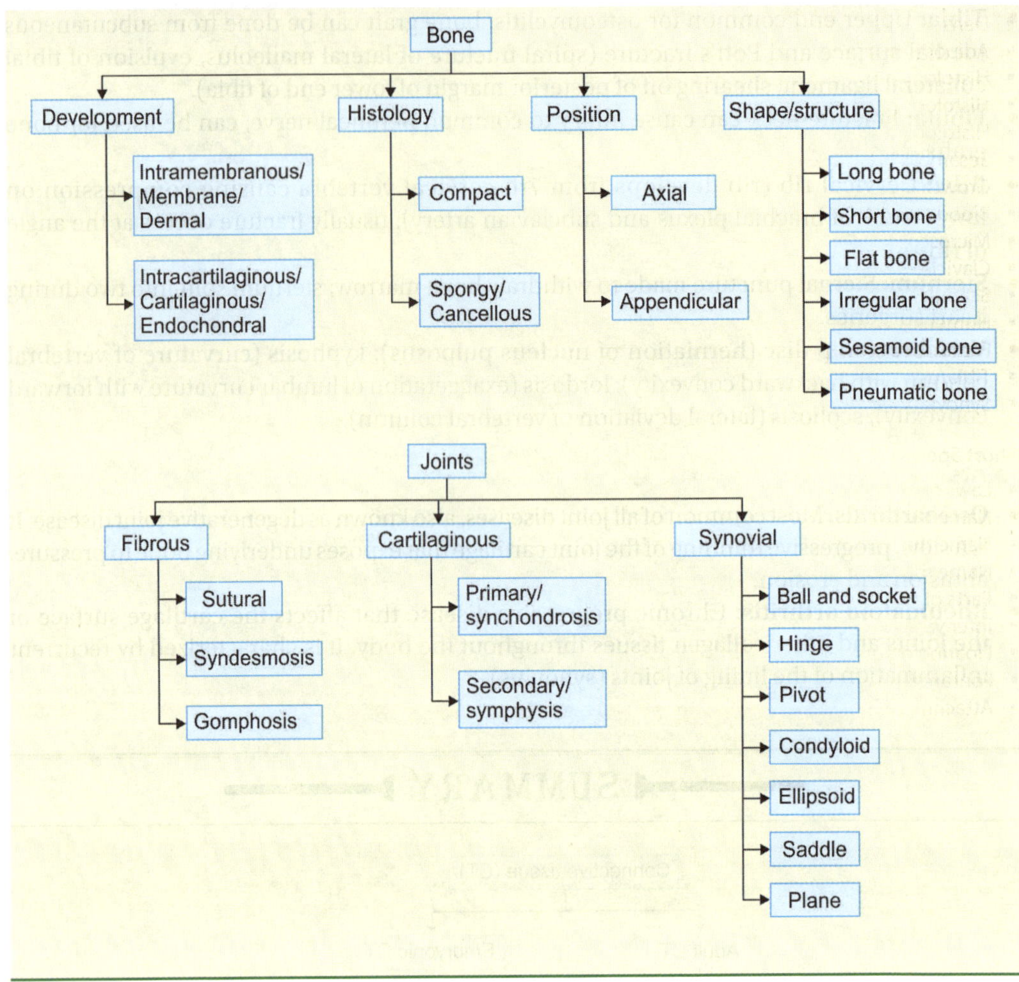

QUESTIONS

Long Essays

- Define cartilage, classify and explain giving examples.
- Classify bone, explain giving examples.
- Classify joints, explain giving examples. Explain synovial joint in detail.
- Describe temporomandibular joint in detail.
- Describe shoulder joint in detail.
- Describe hip joint in detail.
- Describe knee joint in detail.

Short Essays

- Connective tissue
- Cells of CT.
- Fibers of CT.

- Dense CT.
- Adipose tissue
- Histology of hyaline cartilage, give examples.
- Histology of elastic cartilage, give examples.
- Histology of fibrocartilage, give examples.
- Sesamoid bone.
- Growth of long bone.
- Blood supply of long bone.
- Microscopy of compact bone.
- Clavicle.
- Scapula.
- Humerus/upper end of humerus/lower end of humerus.
- Femur/upper end of femur/lower end of femur.
- Tibia/upper end of tibia.
- Synovial joint.

Short Specific Answers

- Laws of ossification.
- Name the cartilage cells.
- Name the bone cells.
- Name the carpal/tarsal/skull bones.
- Parts of long bone.
- Inter vertebral disc.
- Floating ribs.
- Fontanelles of fetal skull.
- Attachments of coracoid/acromion/spine of scapula.

CHAPTER 4

Muscular System

LEARNING OBJECTIVES

The student should be able to:

Muscle: Classification of muscular tissue and histology, names of muscles of upper limb, lower limb, intercostals, abdomen, neck, mastication, pharynx, larynx, soft palate, tongue, explain biceps brachii, triceps brachii, deltoid, trapezius, gluteus maximus, hamstrings, layers of scalp.

INTRODUCTION

- Muscle cells are the contractile elements in the muscle tissue and are called muscle fibers since they are elongated.
- They are designed for movements, which is due to contractility of muscle fibers.
- **Details of important muscles in the body are summarized in Table 4.1.**

Classification

- Skeletal muscle
- Smooth muscle
- Cardiac muscle.

SKELETAL MUSCLES

- They are called so because they produce movements to the skeleton.
- It has two attachments called origin and insertion.
- The middle fleshy portion is called belly.
- Its ends are attached to bones, cartilages or ligaments by cords of fibrous tissue called tendons.
- Flat muscles end in expanded strong sheet of fibrous tissue called aponeurosis.
- They are called voluntary muscles as they are controlled by will.

Types Based on Direction of Fibers (Fig. 4.1)

Parallel or Strap Muscles (Figs. 4.1A to C)

- Muscle fibers are arranged parallel to the long axis of the muscle.
- They cause greater range of movements.
  For example: Sartorius.

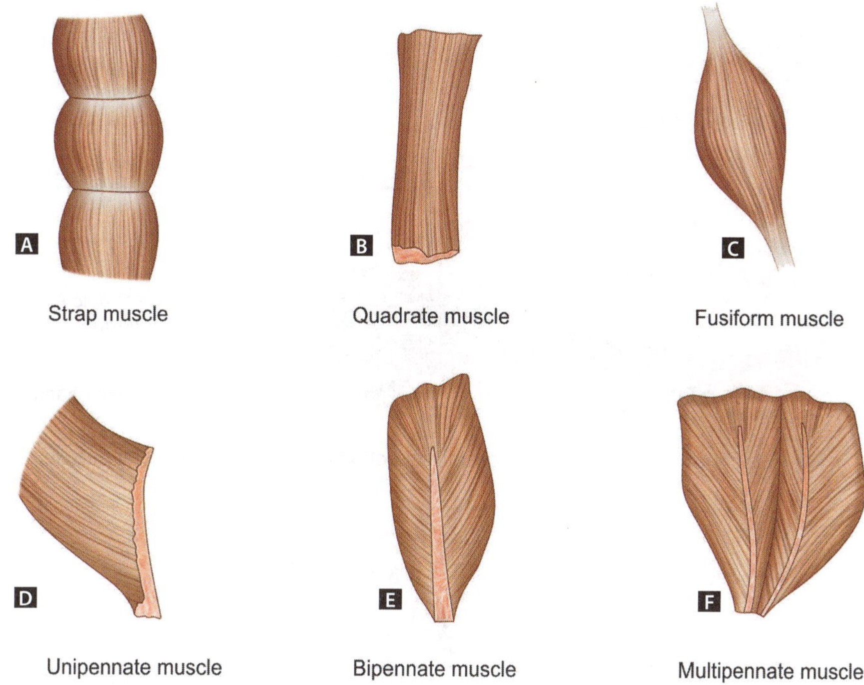

Figs. 4.1A to F: Classification of muscle based on direction of fibers.

Pennate Muscles

- Muscle fibers are arranged obliquely to the long axis of the muscle. They have more fibers and are more powerful. There are three types:
  1. *Unipennate* ***(Fig. 4.1D):*** The tendon lies along one side of the muscle and the muscle fibers pass obliquely to it, e.g., extensor digitorum longus, flexor pollicis longus.
  2. *Bipennate* ***(Fig. 4.1E):*** The tendon lies in the center of the muscle and muscle fibers pass to it from two sides, e.g., rectus femoris.
  3. *Multipennate* ***(Fig. 4.1F):*** Tendon may lie in the center and the muscle fibers pass to it from all sides, e.g., tibialis anterior or the muscle may have several pennate groups lying side-by-side, e.g., middle part of deltoid.

Histological Structure

Longitudinal Section (LS) (Figs. 4.2A and B)

- Each muscle fiber is cylindrical and long, enclosed in a membrane called sarcolemma, supported by connective tissue.
- Cytoplasm is called sarcoplasm.
- Muscle fibers show fine longitudinal striations due to myofibrils and prominent transverse striations alternating dark and light bands due to cytoplasm containing actin and myosin filaments.
- Fibers do not divide and do not anastomose with neighboring fibers.
- Fibers are multinucleated; nuclei are flattened and pushed to the periphery.

For example: Muscles of limbs.

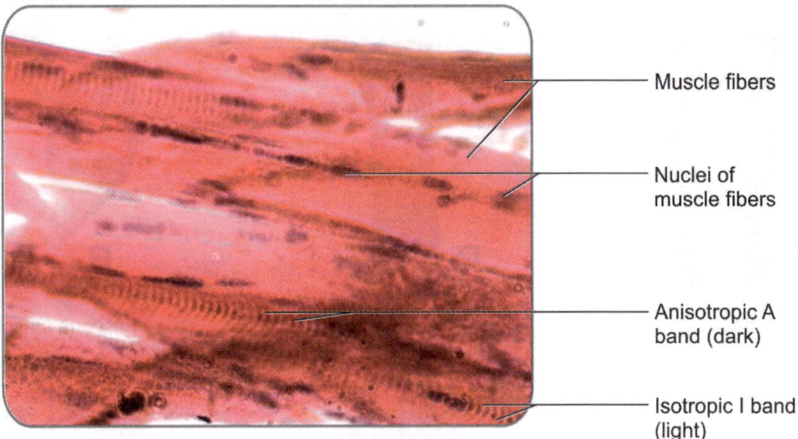

Fig. 4.2A: Photomicrograph of longitudinal section of histology of skeletal muscle.

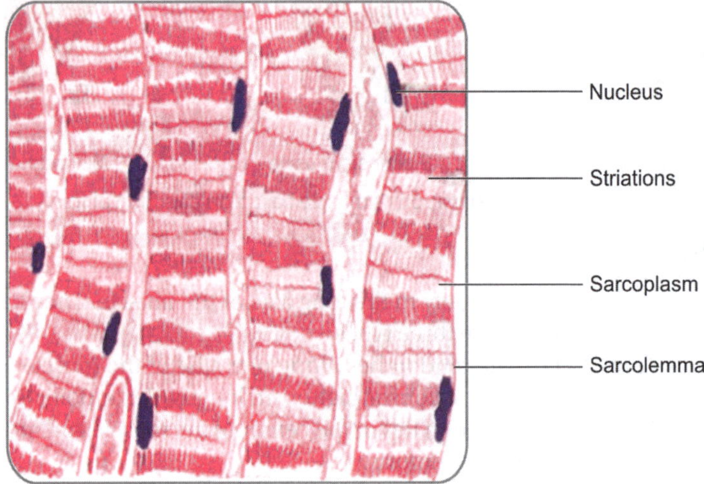

Fig. 4.2B: Diagrammatic representation of longitudinal section of histology of skeletal muscle.

Transverse Section (TS) (Fig. 4.3)

- Each fiber is surrounded by fine connective tissue called endomysium.
- Fibers are aggregated into groups or bundles or fascicles by coarser connective tissue called perimysium.
- Group of bundles together form muscle which is surrounded by epimysium.
- Nuclei are seen in the periphery of each muscle fiber.

SMOOTH MUSCLE

It is involuntary in action. It is elongated and spindle-shaped with tapering ends.

Histological Structure (Figs. 4.4A and B)

- Cytoplasm consists of myofibrils and sarcoplasm.

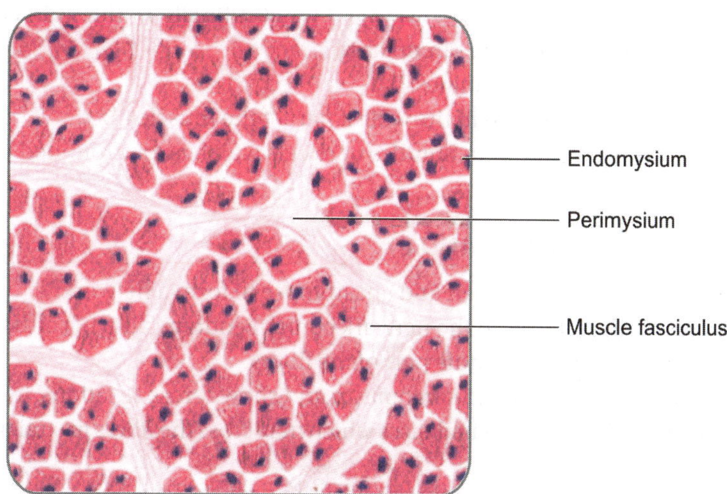

Fig. 4.3: Diagrammatic representation of transverse section of histology of skeletal muscle.

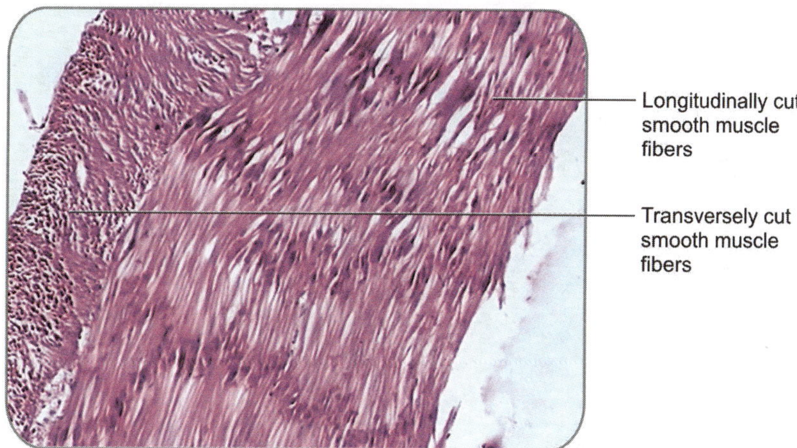

Fig. 4.4A: Photomicrograph of histology of smooth muscle.

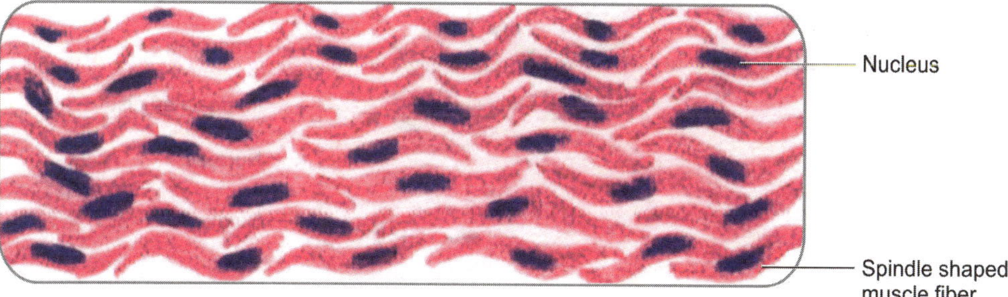

Fig. 4.4B: Diagrammatic representation of histology of smooth muscle.

- Myofibrils are thread-like structures arranged longitudinally in the fluid component of cytoplasm of the muscle fiber, e.g., sarcoplasm.
- Sarcoplasm contains glycogen granules.
- Nucleus is cylindrical and is seen in the widest part of the muscle fiber.
- Fibers may be arranged singly or in bundles or sheets which are surrounded by elastic type of connective tissue.

CARDIAC MUSCLE (FIGS. 4.5A AND B)

- Muscle fibers are cylindrical, branch and anastomose to form a network.
- Interstices between the strands in the network contain endomysium of cardiac muscle.
- Nuclei are ovoid and lie in the middle part of the fibers.
- Cytoplasm contains myofibrils and sarcoplasm and shows cross striations.
- Fibers are crossed by dark intercalated discs which may cross the fibers in straight or stepwise lines.
- Under EM, they are seen as cell membrane of cardiac muscle cell.

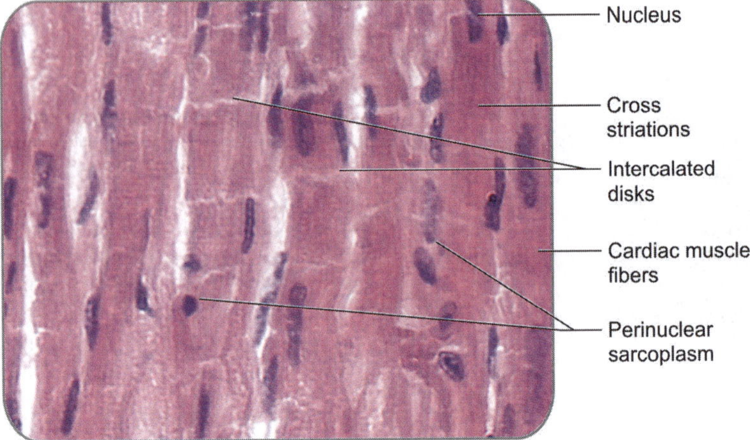

Fig. 4.5A: Photomicrograph of histology of cardiac muscle.

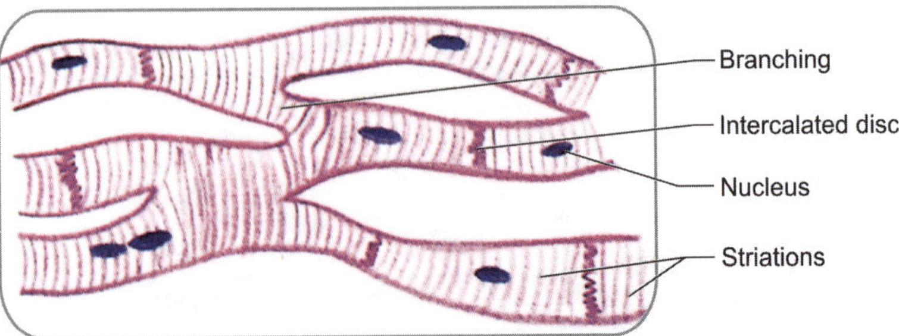

Fig. 4.5B: Diagrammatic representation of histology of cardiac muscle.

Muscles of Upper Limb (Figs. 4.6 and 4.7A to C)

Muscles of Pectoral Region

Pectoralis major and minor (supplied by medial and lateral pectoral nerve).

Muscles of Back

Latissimus dorsi, teres major and minor, supraspinatus, infraspinatus, subscapularis, levator scapulae, rhomboideus major and minor, serratus anterior and posterior.

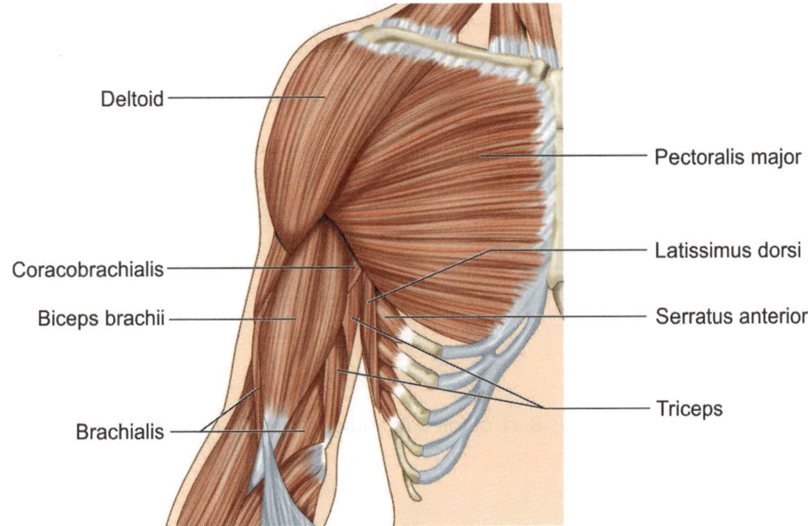

Fig. 4.6: Muscles of pectoral region and front of arm.

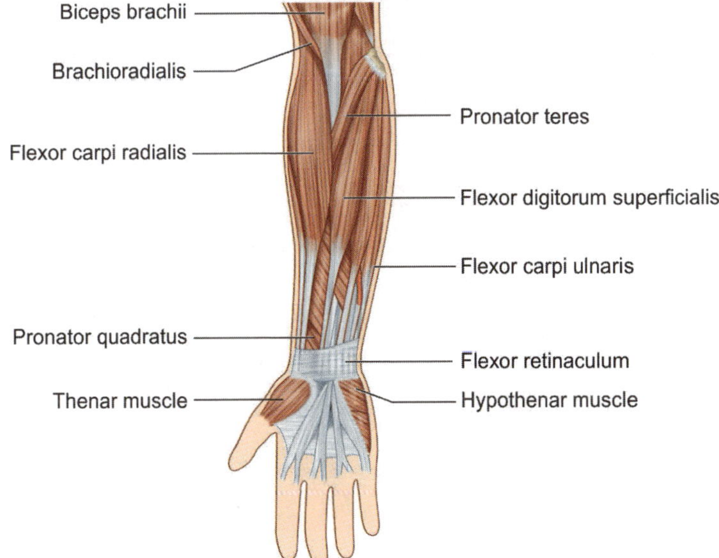

Fig. 4.7A: Muscles of front of forearm and palm.

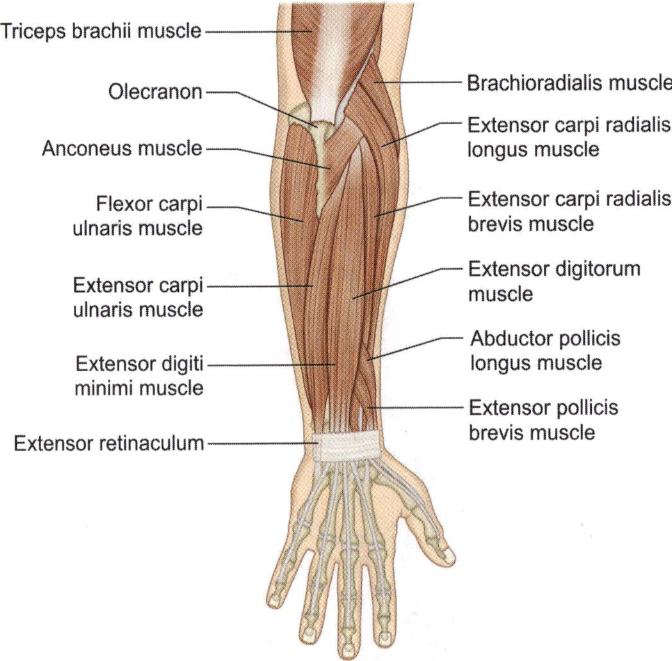

Fig. 4.7B: Back of forearm and dorsum of hand.

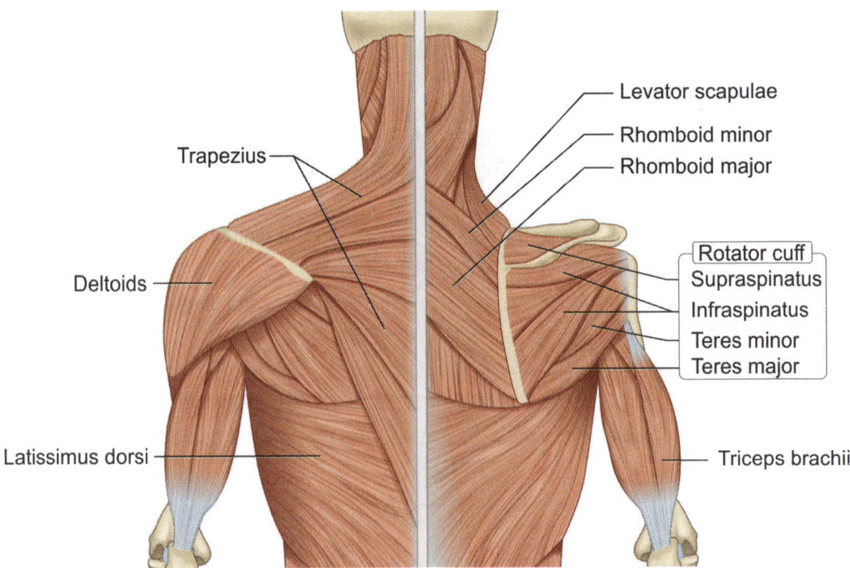

Fig. 4.7C: Muscles of back of arm and scapular region.

Muscles of Front of Arm

Biceps brachii, brachialis, coracobrachialis (supplied by musculocutaneous nerve).

Muscles of Back of Arm

Triceps brachii (supplied by radial nerve).

Muscles of Front of Forearm

- **Superficial:** Pronator teres, flexor carpi radialis, palmaris longus, flexor digitorum superficialis (supplied by median nerve), flexor carpi ulnaris (ulnar nerve).
- **Deep:** Pronator quadratus, flexor digitorum profundus, flexor pollicis longus (supplied by anterior interosseous nerve). Flexor digitorum profundus also supplied by ulnar nerve.

Muscles of Back of Forearm

- **Superficial:** Brachioradialis, extensor carpi radialis longus, extensor carpi radialis brevis, anconeus (supplied by radial nerve), extensor digitorum, extensor digiti minimi, extensor carpi ulnaris (posterior interosseous nerve).
- **Deep:** Supinator, abductor pollicis longus, extensor pollicis brevis, extensor pollicis longus, extensor indicis (posterior interosseous nerve).

Muscles of the Hand

- **Thenar muscles:** Abductor pollicis brevis, flexor pollicis brevis, opponens pollicis (supplied by median nerve), adductor pollicis (ulnar nerve).
- **Hypothenar muscles:** Palmaris brevis, abductor digiti minimi, flexor digiti minimi, opponens digiti minimi (ulnar nerve).
- **Lumbricals and interossei muscles:** 4 lumbricals attached to the tendons of flexor digitorum profundus (first two are supplied by median nerve 3rd and 4th supplied by ulnar nerve), four palmar interossei and four dorsal interossei (all supplied by ulnar nerve).

Muscles of Lower Limb (Figs. 4.8 to 4.10)

Muscles of Front of Thigh

Sartorius, quadriceps femoris (supplied by femoral nerve).

Muscles of Back of Thigh/Hamstrings

Semitendinosus, semimembranosus, biceps femoris, adductor magnus (supplied by sciatic nerve).

Muscles of Medial Compartment of Thigh

Gracilis, adductor longus, brevis and magnus (supplied by obturator nerve).

Muscles of Gluteal Region

Gluteus maximus (supplied by inferior gluteal), medius and minimus (supplied by superior gluteal nerve).

Structures deep to gluteus maximus

- **Bony structures:** Greater trochanter of femur, ischial tuberosity, ischial spine.
- **Bursae:** Trochanteric, ischial, gluteofemoral bursae.

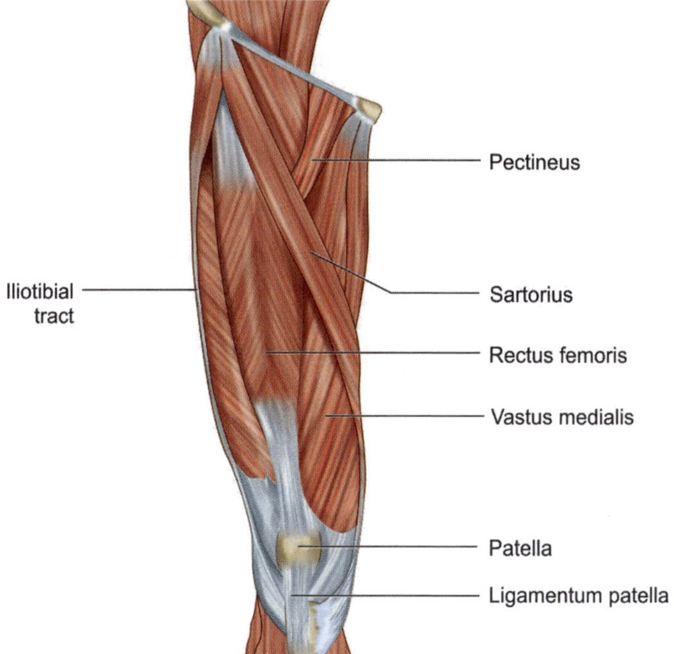

Fig. 4.8: Muscles of front of thigh.

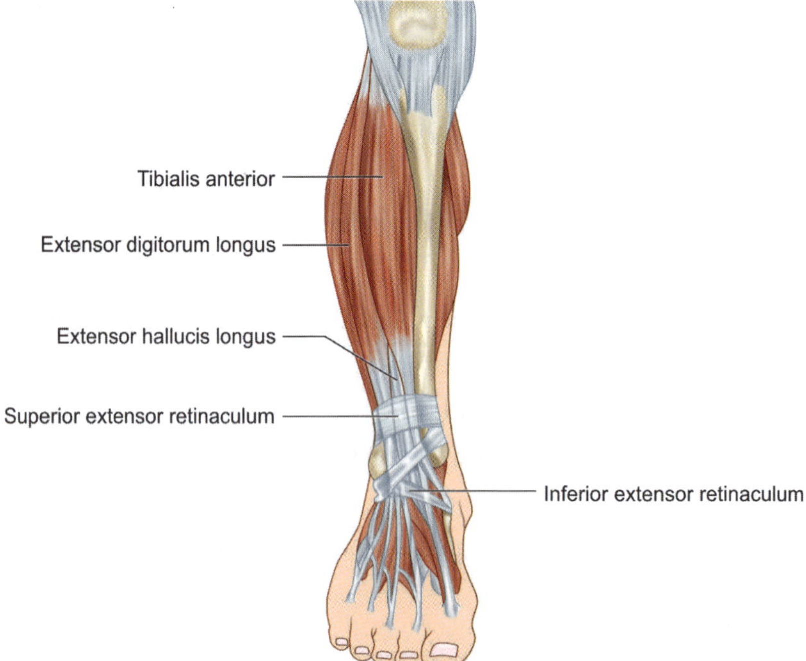

Fig. 4.9: Muscles of anterior compartment of leg and dorsum of foot.

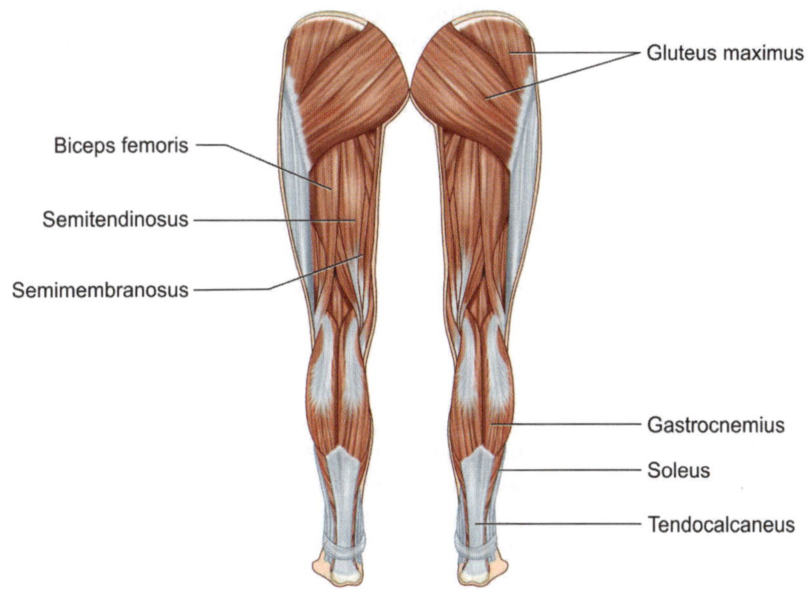

Fig. 4.10: Muscles of gluteal region, posterior compartment of thigh and leg.

- **Ligaments:** Sacrotuberous, sacrospinous ligaments.
- **Muscles:** Lower part of gluteus medius, gluteus minimus, piriformis, superior and inferior gemellus, quadratus femoris, upper part of adductor magnus, origin of hamstrings.
- **Nerves:** Sciatic, nerve to quadratus femoris, posterior cutaneous nerve of thigh, inferior gluteal nerve, pudendal nerve, nerve to obturator internus, superior gluteal nerve.
- **Blood vessels:** Superior gluteal, inferior gluteal, internal pudendal.

Muscles of Front of Leg

Tibialis anterior, extensor hallucis longus, extensor digitorum longus, peroneus tertius (supplied by deep peroneal nerve).

Muscles of Lateral Compartment of Leg

Peroneus longus and brevis (supplied by superficial peroneal nerve).

Muscles of Calf (Posterior Compartment of Leg)

- **Superficial:** Soleus and gastrocnemius (medial and lateral heads) form Achilles tendon (tendocalcaneus) (supplied by tibial nerve).
- **Deep:** Flexor hallucis longus, flexor digitorum longus, tibialis posterior (supplied by tibial nerve).

Muscles of Sole

First layer

Flexor digitorum brevis, abductor hallucis, abductor digiti minimi 2nd layer, flexor digitorum accessorius, 4 lumbricals, tendons of flexor digitorum longus, tendon of flexor hallucis longus 3rd layer, flexor hallucis brevis, flexor digiti minimi, adductor hallucis, 4th layer plantar interossei, 4 dorsal interossei and tendons of tibialis posterior and peroneus longus (supplied by medial and lateral plantar nerves).

Muscles of Head and Neck (Fig. 4.11)

Layers of Scalp

- Skin
- Connective tissue (subcutaneous) or superficial fascia
- Aponeurosis of occipitofrontalis or epicranial aponeurosis
- Loose areolar tissue
- Pericranium.

Muscles of Face (Supplied by Facial Nerve)

- **Palpebral fissure:** Orbicularis oculi, levator palpebrae superioris, occipitofrontalis.
- **Oral fissure:** Orbicularis oris, levator labii superioris, levator labii superioris alaeque nasi, levator anguli oris, zygomaticus minor, zygomaticus major, depressor anguli oris, depressor labii inferioris, mentalis, risorius, buccinator.
- **Nostrils:** Compressor naris, dilator naris.

Muscles of Mastication

Temporalis, masseter, medial and lateral pterygoid (supplied by mandibular nerve).

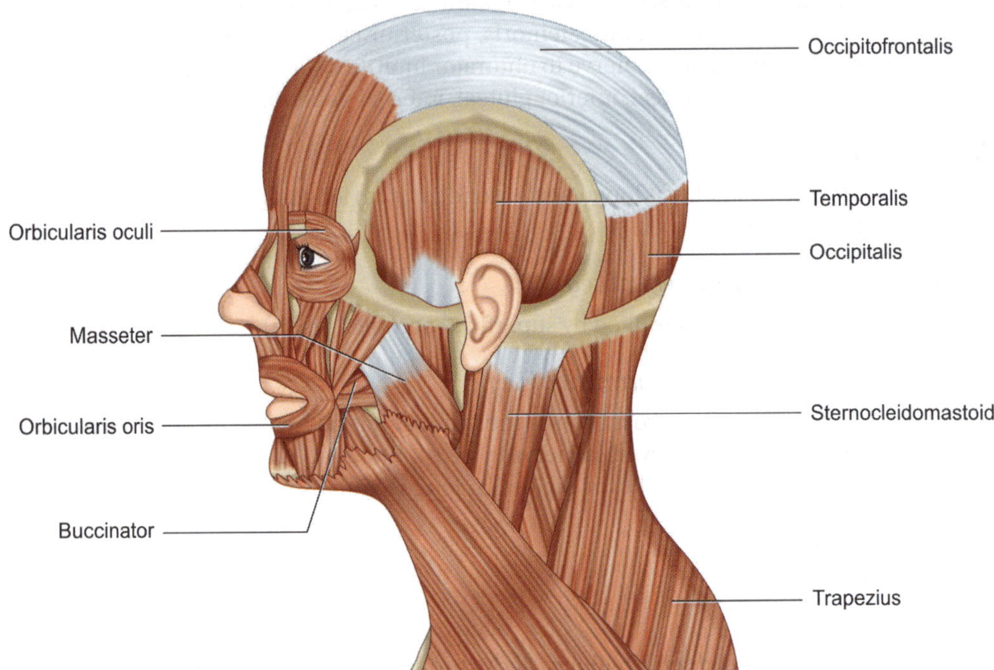

Fig. 4.11: Muscles of head and neck.

Muscles of Tongue (Supplied by Hypoglossal Nerve)

- **Intrinsic muscles:** Superior longitudinal, inferior longitudinal, transverse and vertical.
- **Extrinsic muscles:** Genioglossus, hyoglossus, styloglossus, palatoglossus (supplied by cranial accessory nerve).

Muscles of Eyeball

Medial, lateral, superior and inferior rectus, superior and inferior oblique.

Lateral rectus supplied by abducent nerve, superior oblique by trochlear nerves rest by oculomotor nerve.

Muscles of Soft Palate

Tensor veli palatini (supplied by mandibular nerve), levator veli palatini, musculus uvulae, palatoglossus, palatopharyngeus (supplied by cranial accessory nerve).

Muscles of Pharynx

Superior, middle and inferior constrictors, salpingopharyngeus, palatopharyngeus (by cranial accessory nerve), stylopharyngeus (by glossopharyngeal nerve).

Muscles of Larynx

Cricothyroid (supplied by external laryngeal nerve), posterior and lateral cricoarytenoid, transverse and oblique arytenoid, aryepiglotticus, thyroarytenoid, vocalis, thyroepiglotticus (supplied by recurrent laryngeal nerve).

Muscles of Neck

Sternocleidomastoid, suprahyoid muscles (mylohyoid, digastric, stylohyoid), infrahyoid muscles (sternothyroid, thyrohyoid, omohyoid).

Muscles of Abdomen (Fig. 4.12)

Muscles of Anterior Abdominal Wall

External and internal oblique, transversus abdominis, rectus abdominis.

Muscles of Posterior Abdominal Wall

Psoas major, quadratus lumborum, erector spinae.

Muscles of Thorax

Muscles of Intercostal Space

External, internal and innermost intercostal muscles.

Details of important muscles in the body are shown in **Table 4.1**.

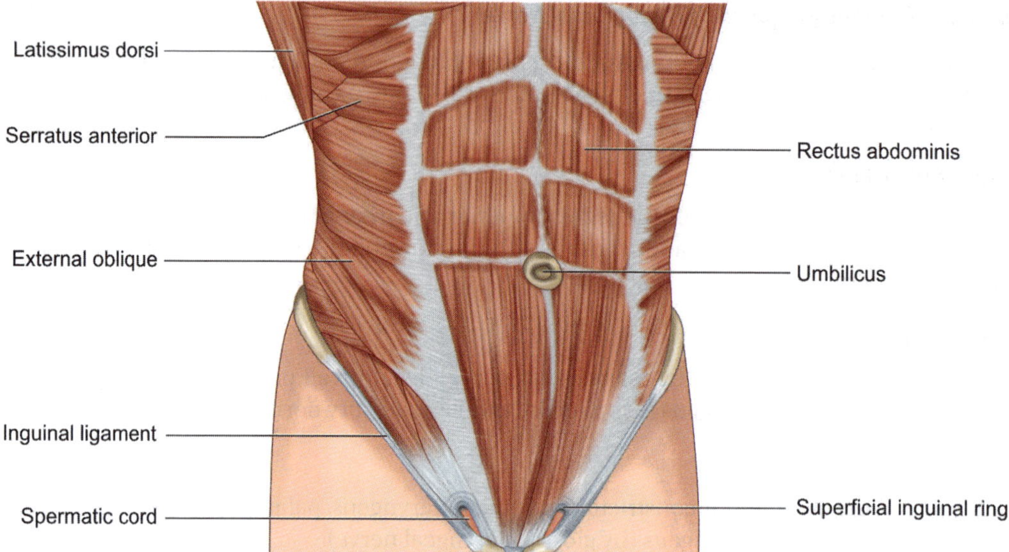

Fig. 4.12: Muscles of abdomen.

Table 4.1: Details of important muscles in the body.

Muscle	*Origin*	*Insertion*	*Nerve supply*	*Action*
Muscles of upper limb (Figs. 4.6 and 4.7)				
Pectoralis major	Anterior surface of the medial half of clavicle; lateral part of anterior surface of sternum; 2nd to 6th costal cartilages	Lateral lip of intertubercular sulcus of humerus	Medial and lateral pectoral nerves	Medial rotation, adduction, flexion
Serratus anterior	8 fleshy digitations from outer surfaces of upper 8 ribs	Medial border of scapula	Nerve to serratus anterior (C5,6,7)	Protracts the scapula around the chest wall in pushing and punching movements
Trapezius	Medial 1/3 of superior nuchal line of occipital bone; external occipital protuberance; ligamentum nuchae; 7th cervical and all thoracic spines; supraspinous ligaments	Lateral 1/3 of clavicle, acromion and spine of scapula	Spinal accessory, 3rd and 4th cervical nerves (proprioceptive).	Elevation of clavicle, drawing the head and neck backwards towards shoulder, lateral rotation of scapula

Contd...

Contd...

Muscle	*Origin*	*Insertion*	*Nerve supply*	*Action*
Latissimus dorsi	Lower 6 thoracic spines and their supraspinous ligaments; spines of all the lumbar and sacral vertebrae through the posterior layer of thoracolumbar fascia; outer lip of the iliac crest; lower 4 ribs; inferior angle of scapula	Floor of the intertubercular sulcus of humerus	Nerve to latissimus dorsi	Extension, medial rotation, adduction at the shoulder joint and helps in lifting up the trunk while climbing
Deltoid	Lateral 1/3 of clavicle; acromion and spine of scapula	Deltoid tuberosity of humerus	Axillary nerve	Flexion and medial rotation of arm (by anterior fibers), extension and lateral rotation of arm (by posterior fibers), abduction of arm (by middle fibers)
Biceps brachii	Long head from supraglenoid tubercle of scapula; short head from coracoid process	Radial tuberosity, bicipital aponeurosis to ulna	Musculo-cutaneous nerve	Supination of forearm when elbow is flexed; flexion of elbow and shoulder
Triceps brachii	Long head from infraglenoid tubercle of scapula; lateral head from an oblique ridge on the upper 1/3 of posterior surface of shaft of humerus above spiral groove; medial head from lower 2/3 of posterior surface of shaft of humerus below spiral groove	Olecranon process of ulna	Radial nerve	Extensor of elbow joint
Flexor digitorum superficialis	Medial epicondyle of humerus from the common flexor origin; coronoid process of ulna	The muscle ends in four tendons for the medial four fingers. At the proximal phalanx each tendon splits into two slips that get inserted in the middle phalanx	Median nerve	Flexion of proximal interphalangeal joint

Contd...

Contd…

Muscle	*Origin*	*Insertion*	*Nerve supply*	*Action*
Flexor digitorum profundus	Upper 3/4th of the anterior and medial surfaces of ulna and adjoining interosseous membrane	The muscle end in four tendons for the medial four fingers. At the proximal phalanx each tendon splits into two slips that rejoin as a single slip that gets inserted in the distal phalanx	Medial half by ulnar nerve. Lateral half by anterior interosseous nerve	Flexion of distal interphalangeal joint
Muscles of lower limb (Figs. 4.8 to 4.10)				
Quadriceps femoris: Consists of rectus femoris, vastus lateralis, vastus medialis, vastus intermedius	• **Rectus femoris:** Straight head from upper half of anterior inferior iliac spine; reflected head from a groove above acetabulum on outer surface of ilium • **Vastus lateralis:** Upper part of trochanteric line; base of greater trochanter; lateral lip of gluteal tuberosity and upper part of lateral lip of linea aspera of femur	Upper border of patella continuous with ligamentum patellae to tibial tuberosity	Femoral nerve	Extension of knee joint; rectus femoris flexes hip joint; vastus medialis prevents lateral displacement of patella while standing or extending knee joint
	• **Vastus medialis:** Lower part of trochanteric line; base of lesser trochanter; spiral line; medial lip of linea aspera and upper part of medial supracondylar ridge of femur • **Vastus intermedius:** Front and lateral surfaces of upper 2/3 of shaft of femur			

Contd…

Contd…

Muscle	*Origin*	*Insertion*	*Nerve supply*	*Action*
Adductor magnus	Inferior ramus of pubis; ramus of ischium; ischial tuberosity	Medial margin of gluteal tuberosity, medial lip of linea aspera, upper part of supracondylar line, adductor tubercle of femur	Posterior division of obturator nerve and tibial part of sciatic nerve	Adduction of thigh, extension of hip joint
Gluteus maximus: It is a thick quadrilateral muscle responsible for the gluteal prominence in man	Posterior gluteal line of ilium; area above and below it; outer sloping surface of dorsal 1/3 segment of iliac crest; sacrotuberous ligament; dorsal aspect of lower and lateral part of sacrum and sides of coccyx; fascia covering the muscle	Iliotibial tract and gluteal tuberosity of femur	Inferior gluteal nerve	Extension of hip joint, lateral rotation of thigh, steadies tibia on lower end of femur to maintain erect posture while standing
Semimembranosus	Superolateral part of ischial tuberosity	Groove on the posterior surface of medial condyle of tibia	Tibial part of sciatic nerve	Flexion at knee and extension at hip joint
Semitendinosus	Inferomedial part of ischial tuberosity	Upper part of medial surface of tibia.	Tibial part of sciatic nerve	Flexion at knee and extension at hip joint
Biceps femoris	**Long head:** Inferomedial part of ischial tuberosity; short head: Lower part of the lateral lip of the linea aspera and upper part of lateral supracondylar line of femur	Head of fibula in front of styloid process	Tibial part of sciatic nerve	Flexion at knee and extension at hip joint
Tibialis anterior	Lateral condyle of tibia; upper 2/3rd of less of the lateral surface of shaft of tibia; adjoining part of interosseous membrane	Inferomedial surface of medial cuneiform and adjoining part of base of 1st metatarsal bone	Deep peroneal nerve	Dorsiflexor and invertor of foot, maintains medial longitudinal arch of foot
Tibialis posterior	Upper 2/3rd of lateral part of posterior surface of tibia below soleal line; posterior surface of fibula in front of medial crest; posterior surface of interosseous membrane	Tuberosity of navicular bone. It also gives slips to all tarsal bones except talus and 2nd, 3rd and 4th metatarsal bones	Tibial nerve	Invertor and plantar flexor of foot, maintains medial and transverse arches of foot

Contd…

Contd...

Muscle	*Origin*	*Insertion*	*Nerve supply*	*Action*
Gastrocnemius	**Medial head:** Postero-superior depression on the medial condyle of the femur, adjoining raised area on the popliteal surface of femur, capsule of knee joint; lateral head: Lateral surface of lateral condyle of femur, lateral supra condylar line, capsule of knee joint	The two heads fuses with the tendon of soleus to form Achilles tendon (tendocalcaneus) which is inserted into middle 1/3rd of posterior surface of calcaneum	Tibial nerve	Flexors of knee and plantar flexors of foot which is important in walking and running
Soleus	Back of head and upper 1/4th of the posterior surface of shaft of fibula; soleal line and middle 1/3rd of the medial border of the shaft of tibia; tendinous arch stretching between tibia and fibula	Same as gastrocnemius	Tibial nerve	Plantar flexor of foot
Popliteus	Anterior part of popliteal groove on lateral surface of lateral condyle of femur; arcuate popliteal ligament; outer margin of lateral meniscus of knee joint. The tendon is intracapsular	Medial 2/3rd of triangular area above the soleal line on posterior surface of tibia	Tibial nerve	Flexes the knee joint, retract lateral meniscus, rotates femur laterally during initial stages of flexion of knee joint (unlocking of knee)
Muscles of head and neck (Fig. 4.11)				
Temporalis	Temporal fossa of skull	Coronoid process and anterior border of ramus of mandible	Mandibular nerve	Elevates and retracts the protruded mandible
Masseter	Zygomatic arch	Outer surface of ramus of mandible	Mandibular nerve	Elevates mandible
Medial pterygoid	**Superficial head:** Maxillary tuberosity; deep head: Medial surface of lateral pterygoid plate	Inner surface of the angle of mandible	Mandibular nerve	Elevates mandible
Lateral pterygoid	**Upper head:** Crest and infratemporal surface of greater wing of sphenoid bone; lower head: Lateral surface of lateral pterygoid plate	Pterygoid fovea of mandible and capsule and articular disc of temporomandibular joint	Mandibular nerve	Depresses the mandible

Contd...

Contd…

Muscle	*Origin*	*Insertion*	*Nerve supply*	*Action*
Buccinator	Upper fibers from maxilla and lower fibers from mandible	Upper fibers into upper lip and lower fibers into lower lip	Facial nerve	Flattens teeth against gums and teeth
Orbicularis oculi	• **Orbital part:** Around the orbital margins from the medial part of medial palpebral ligament. • **Palpebral part:** In the lids from the lateral part of medial palpebral ligament	• Orbital part winds as concentric rings around the orbital margins. • Palpebral part in palpebral raphe. Lacrimal part in the upper and lower tarsi	Facial nerve	• Closure of eyelid and blinking. • Lacrimal part dilates lacrimal sac and helps in flow of tears
Orbicularis oris	From the maxilla adjacent to upper teeth, mandible adjacent to lower teeth and the buccinator	Lips and angles of mouth	Facial nerve	Closure of mouth
Sternocleido-mastoid	**Sternal head:** Upper part of anterior surface of manubrium sterni; clavicular head: Upper border of anterior surface of medial 1/3 of clavicle	Mastoid process of temporal bone and superior nuchal line in occipital bone	Spinal accessory nerve (motor), anterior primary rami of C1, C2 (sensory)	Tilts head towards shoulder of same side; muscles of two sides draw the head forwards. If the head is fixed, they help to elevate the thorax as in forced inspiration. Applied anatomy: Wry neck or torticollis
Muscles of thorax				
External intercostals: 11 pairs extending from tubercle of rib behind to level of costal cartilage in front	Lower border of the rib above	Upper border of rib below	Intercostal nerves	Strong support for ribs preventing their separation. Elevate ribs during inspiration and help respiration. Act during inspiration
Internal intercostals: 11 pairs extending from lateral margin of sternum to level of angle of rib	Above to costal groove of upper rib	Below to upper border of succeeding rib	Intercostal nerves	Act during expiration

Contd…

Contd...

Muscle	*Origin*	*Insertion*	*Nerve supply*	*Action*
Innermost intercostals				
Intercostalis intimus: 11 pairs occupying middle 2/4 of each intercostal space	Inner surface of lower border of the rib above	Inner surface of the upper border of the rib below	Intercostal nerves	Strong support for ribs preventing their separation. Elevate ribs during expiration and help respiration. Act during expiration
Subcostal is muscle: In posterior part of intercostal space	Inner surface of one rib near the angle	Inner surface of 2nd or 3rd rib below	Intercostal nerves	Depression of ribs.
Sternocostalisone on each side, on inner surface of front wall of the chest	Lower 1/3 of posterior surface of the body and xiphoid process of sternum	Lower border and inner surface of costal cartilages of 2nd, 3rd, 4th, 5th and 6th ribs	Intercostal nerves	Draw down the cartilages to which they are attached
Muscles of abdomen and pelvis (Fig. 4.12)				
External oblique	Outer surface of lower eight ribs. Lower 34 slips interdigitate with latissimus dorsi and upper 45 with serratus anterior	Lower 1/3 fleshy fibers to outer lip of anterior 2/3 of ventral segment of iliac crest; aponeurosis of upper 2/3 to anterior superior iliac spine, pubic tubercle, pubic crest, pubic symphysis, linea alba, xiphoid process	Lower 5 intercostal, subcostal, iliohypogastric and ilioinguinal nerves	• **Protective:** For abdomen • **Respiratory:** By contracting alternately with diaphragm • **Expulsive:** Increase abdominal pressure by contracting with diaphragm and pelvic floor • **Movements of vertebral** • **Column:** Depress thorax, produce lateral flexion and rotation of vertebral column. Support for inguinal region

Contd...

Contd...

Muscle	*Origin*	*Insertion*	*Nerve supply*	*Action*
Internal oblique	Upper grooved surface of lateral 2/3 of inguinal ligament, anterior 2/3 of intermediate area of ventral segment of iliac crest, posterior and middle layers of lumbar fascia	Lower borders of 10th, 11th, 12th ribs. Upper edge of aponeurosis to xiphoid process, 7th, 8th, 9th ribs and linea alba. Forms conjoint tendon with transverses abdominis		
Transversus abdominis	• **Pelvic part:** Lateral 1/3 of upper grooved surface of inguinal ligament and anterior 2/3 of inner lip of ventral segment of iliac crest • **Vertebral part:** Transverse processes of lumbar vertebrae • **Costal part:** Inner surface of lower 6 ribs	Linea alba. Forms conjoint tendon with internal oblique.		
Rectus abdominis	• **Lateral head:** Pubic crest • **Medial head:** Anterior pubic ligament in front of pubic symphysis	5th, 6th, 7th costal cartilages and xiphoid process of sternum	Lower 5 intercostal and subcostal nerves	Flexion of trunk on pelvis
Diaphragm Openings: Vena-caval (T8): Inferior vena cava, right phrenic nerve. Esophageal (T10): Esophagus, right and left vagi, esophageal branch of left gastric artery. Aortic (T12): Abdominal aorta, thoracic duct, azygos vein	• **Sternal part:** Posterior aspect of xiphoid process. Costal part: Inner surfaces of lower six ribs and adjoining costal cartilages. • **Lumbar part:** By a pair of crura from the lumbar vertebral bodies and by two lumbocostal ligaments (arcuate ligaments)	Central tendon situated in the median depressed part close to the sternum	Motor: Phrenic; proprioceptive: Phrenic and lower intercostal nerves	Helps in respiration and expulsive phenomena like vomiting, defecation, etc

Contd...

Contd…

Muscle	*Origin*	*Insertion*	*Nerve supply*	*Action*
Psoas major	5 tendinous arches bridging over lumbar vessels at the sides of 5 lumbar vertebral bodies; 5 intervertebral discs from between T12-L1 to L4-L5; medial parts of anterior surfaces of 5 lumbar transverse processes	Lesser trochanter of femur with iliacus	L1-L4	Flexion, medial and lateral rotation of thigh
Quadratus lumborum	Iliolumbar ligament; adjoining part of iliac crest for 5 cm length	Lower border of medial half of last rib, Small tendons into apices of transverse process of upper 2 or 3 lumbar vertebrae	L1-L4	• Fixes last ribs for contraction of diaphragm during respiration. • Contraction of both muscles extends lumbar vertebrae. • Action of one muscle when pelvis is fixed cause flexion of vertebral column to same side
Levator ani	• **Pubococcygeus:** Pelvic surface of body to pubis and anterior part of white line of obturator fascia as far behind as obturator canal • **Iliococcygeus:** Posterior part of arcus tendineus, behind obturator canal	• **Pubococcygeus:** Tip of coccyx 7 anococcygeal raphe (pubococcygeus proper); U-shaped sling winding round anorectal junction to become continuous with fibers of opposite side (puborectalis); prostatic capsule (puboprostatic part in male); perineal body and vaginal wall (pubovaginalis in female • **Iliococcygeus:** Sides of coccyx and anococcygeal raphe, rectal wall	Perineal branch of S4 (pelvic surface), inferior rectal and deep branch of perineal nerve (perineal surface)	Support pelvic viscera

Contd…

Contd...

Muscle	Origin	Insertion	Nerve supply	Action
Coccygeus	Pelvic surface of ischial spine	• Sides of coccyx and lower sacrum. • Superficial fibers atrophy and remain as sacrospinous ligament		

APPLIED ANATOMY

- **Paralysis:** Muscle cannot contract due to the damage of the motor pathways or inherent disease of muscle. The damage of motor pathways can be either at the level of central nervous system or at the level of peripheral nervous system.
- **Disuse atrophy:** The muscles which are not used for long times become thin and weak. Muscular 'wasting' (reduction in size) is a feature of lower motor neuron paralysis and generalized debility.
- **Overuse hypertrophy:** Adequate or excessive use of particular muscles leads to better development or hypertrophy.

SUMMARY

Region	Major important muscles
Upper limb	• Pectoral region: Pectoralis major, pectoralis minor • **Back:** Latissimus dorsi, teres major, teres minor, supraspinatus, infraspinatus, subscapularis, levator scapulae, rhomboideus major, rhomboideus minor, serratus anterior and posterior • **Arm:** Biceps brachii, brachialis, coracobrachialis, triceps brachii • **Forearm:** Pronator teres, flexor digitorum superficialis and profundus, extensor digitorum, supinator
Lower limb	• **Thigh:** Sartorius, quadriceps femoris, hamstrings, adductors (longus, brevis, magnus) • **Gluteal region:** Gluteal muscles (maximus, medius, minimus), piriformis, obturator internus • **Leg:** Tibialis anterior, extensor digitorum longus, peroneus longus, soleus, gastrocnemius, flexor digitorum longus, tibialis posterior
Head and neck	Orbicularis oculi, orbicularis oris, buccinator, muscles of mastication, genioglossus, hyoglossus, sternocleidomastoid
Abdomen	External oblique, internal oblique, transversus abdominis, rectus abdominis, psoas major, quadratus lumborum, erector spinae
Thorax	External intercostal, internal intercostal, innermost intercostal

QUESTIONS

Long Essay

- Classify muscles (gross) giving examples.

Short Essays

- Classify muscles (gross) giving examples.
- Classify muscular tissue (microscopic) giving examples.
- Histological differences between skeletal, smooth and cardiac muscle.
- Biceps brachii muscle/triceps brachii muscle/deltoid muscle/trapezius muscle.

Short Specific Answers

- Name muscles of front of arm.
- Name muscles of back of arm.
- Name muscles of front of forearm.
- Name muscles of back of forearm.
- Name muscles of front of thigh/name the muscles forming quadriceps femoris.
- Name muscles of back of thigh/name the hamstring muscles.
- Name muscles of lateral compartment of leg.
- Name the muscles in the gluteal region.
- Name muscles of back of leg.
- Achilles tendon.
- Name muscles of anterior abdominal wall.
- Name muscles of posterior abdominal wall.
- Name the intercostal muscles.
- Name muscles of neck.
- Name the layers of scalp.
- Name the muscles of palate, pharynx, mastication, larynx.

CHAPTER 5

Lymphatic System

LEARNING OBJECTIVES

The student should be able to:
- Describe cisterna chyli and thoracic duct.
- Give the names of regional lymphatics and lymphatic circulation.
- Describe histology of lymphatic tissues—lymph node, thymus, tonsil and spleen.

INTRODUCTION

- About 80–90% of the tissue fluid formed at the arterial end of the capillary bed returns to the blood circulation through the venous ends of capillaries and the precapillary venules.
- The remaining fluid is transported to the venous system through lymphatic system which consists of closed system of vessels which ramify in the tissue spaces in and around the blood capillaries.
- It comprises of lymphatics, lymphatic organs (lymph node, thymus, spleen, tonsil) and other collection of lymphoid tissues in the walls of alimentary tract, respiratory tract.

LYMPHATICS OR LYMPH VESSELS

- They are larger in size but less regular than the adjoining blood capillaries.
- The lymph is normally a clear fluid, except that from the alimentary tract, which is milky white in color due to the presence of absorbed fat and this is called chyle. The vessels which drain the chyle are referred to as lacteals.
- They start in the tissue spaces at blind bulbous ends as lymphatic capillaries.
- The lymph capillaries join together and form larger vessels.
- The superficial lymph vessels run along the veins or they run independently, while deep ones course along the deep veins and arteries.
- Along their course the lymph vessels pass through one or more lymph nodes.
- They finally unite and end in two major lymph trunks, the *thoracic duct* on the left side and the *right lymphatic trunk* on the right side, which in turn empty into the left and right brachiocephalic veins respectively.
- The lymph capillaries are absent in avascular structures like epidermis, cornea, hair, nails and cartilages, also absent in CNS, splenic pulp and bone marrow.

- They have valves which are paired and formed by reduplication of endothelium with fibrous tissue in between.
- Due to stagnation, the parts of the vessel proximal to the valves are dilated and the lymph vessel gives a beaded appearance.
- The incompetence of the valves gives rise to retrograde flow of the lymph and this explains the retrograde spread of cancer in certain instances.
- In lymphatic obstructions, as in filariasis where microfilarial worms form ova obstruct lymph vessels, the tissue becomes edematous and distended with fluid containing protein due to back pressure.

Structure

- It has three coats, tunica intima, tunica media and tunica adventitia.
- They are lined by a single layer of endothelium with no basement membrane.
- The endothelium is permeable to colloid and particulate matter, like foreign bodies and bacteria.
- The absorption of tissue fluid into lymphatic capillaries takes place through fenestra between endothelial linings of capillaries or by micropinocytosis across the cell.

THORACIC DUCT (FIGS. 5.1A AND B)

- It is a great lymph channel which conveys the chyle and greater part of the lymph into the venous system.
- It drains all parts of the body excepting: (i) right side of head and neck, (ii) right side of chest wall, (iii) right lung, (iv) right side of heart, (v) right surface of liver, (vi) upper limb which drains into the right lymphatic duct.
- It starts from cisterna *chyli* and enters the diaphragm through the aortic opening and ends in the root of the neck by joining left subclavian vein near its junction with internal jugular vein.
- It is a tubular beaded structure 45 cm in length.

CISTERNA CHYLI

- This is an elongated lymphatic sac about 5–7 cm long.
- It is situated in front of L1 and L2 to the right of abdominal aorta.
- It is joined by the right and left lumbar and lymphatic trunks.
- The lumbar trunk carries lymph from the lower limb, pelvic walls and viscera, kidneys, suprarenal glands, testes, ovaries and abdominal walls.
- The intestinal trunks carry lymph from stomach, intestine, pancreas, spleen and liver.

LYMPHATIC ORGANS

Lymph Node (Figs. 5.2A and B)

- They are small oval bodies with a slight depression on one side called hilum.
- Blood vessels enter and leave the node through the hilum.
- Several afferent vessels enter different parts of the periphery of the lymph node, while a single efferent lymph vessel emerges out of the hilum.
- Each lymph node has an outer cellular, dense cortex and an inner lighter, less dense medulla.
- Cortex is deficient at the hilum where the medulla reaches the surface of the node.

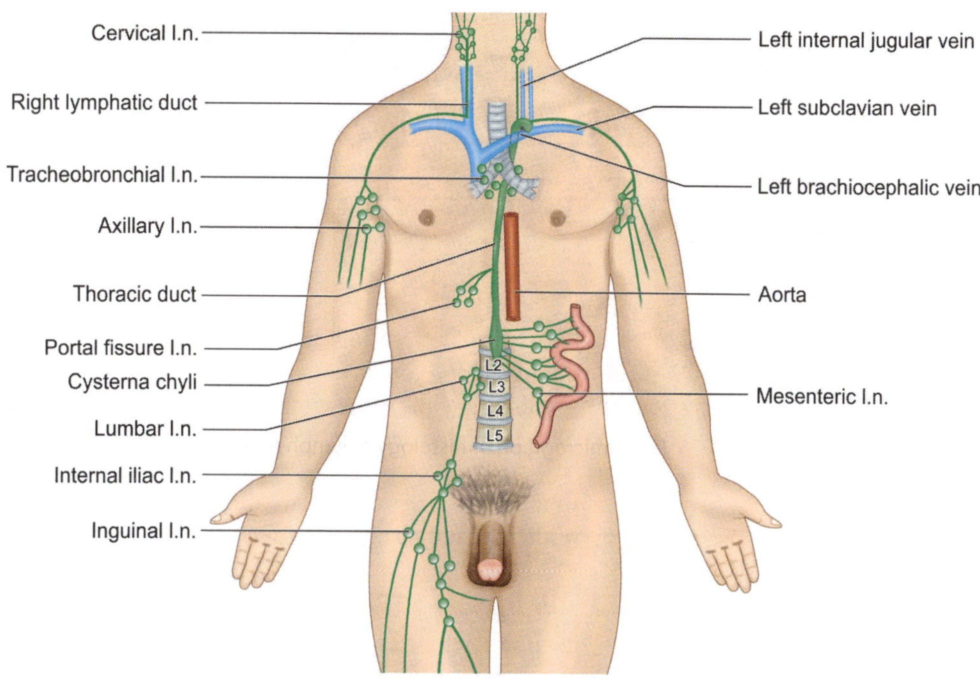

Fig. 5.1A: Thoracic duct.

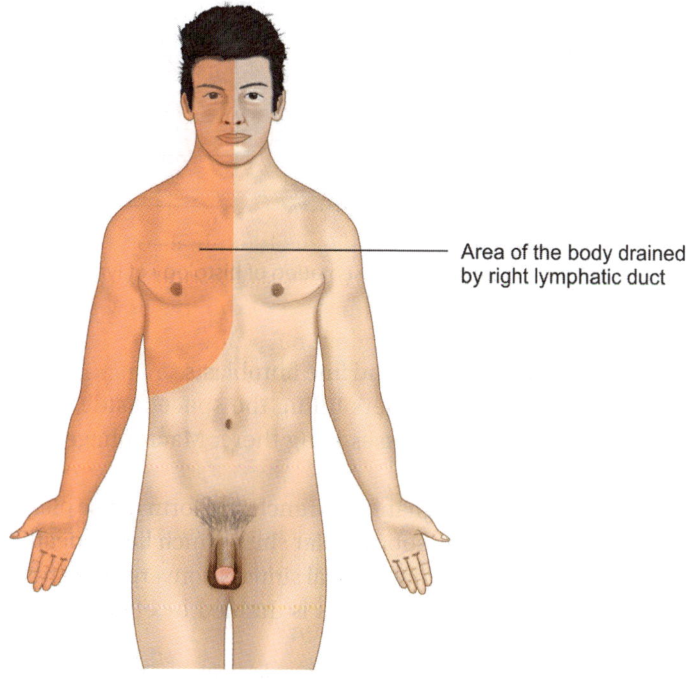

Fig. 5.1B: Thoracic duct.

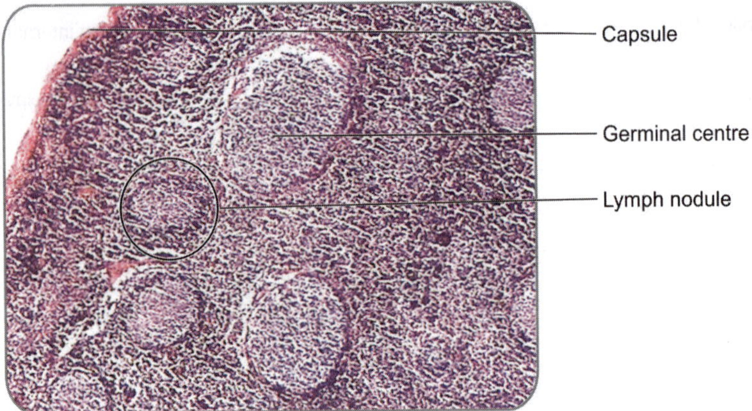

Fig. 5.2A: Photomicrograph of histology of lymph node.

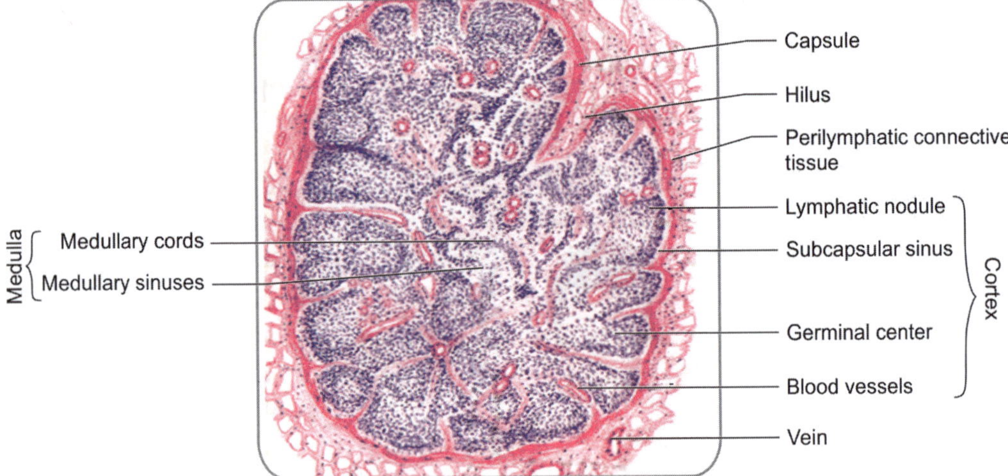

Fig. 5.2B: Diagrammatic representation of histology of lymph node.

- Thin capsule made of collagen fibers and fine fibroblasts.
- There is a meshwork of reticulin fibers filling the space inside the capsule, providing mechanical support for the cell masses lying there. Macrophages and lymphocytes lie entangled in the mesh
- **Lymph channels:** Afferent lymph channels branch and form dense plexus on the substance of the capsule. They open into the subcapsular sinus which lies beneath the capsule except at the hilum. From here several radial cortical sinuses converge towards the medulla where they fuse and form medullary sinuses. This is drained by efferent vessel emerging out of hilum. The trabeculae cross the sinuses.
- **Entangled cells:** (B and T lymphocytes and macrophages): Only a few lymphocytes are seen in lymph sinuses. In the cortex, the lymphocytes are densely packed and form lymphatic

follicles or nodules. In the central part of the nodule, the cells are larger, less deeply stained and dividing more rapidly (germinal center). Cells in the germinal center are mainly lymphoblasts. The newly-formed small lymphocytes get into lymph sinuses and leave the nodes.

- In medulla, lymphocytes are more loosely packed and form branching medullary cords between which reticulum of medullary sinuses are seen.
- T cells are seen between germinal centers and medulla, i.e., paracortex or thymus dependent zone. Immature B cells are seen on the outer parts of the follicles while mature B cells are seen mainly in medullary cords.

Thymus (Figs. 5.3A and B)

- Important lymphatic organ situated in the anterior and superior mediastina of thorax.
- There is a fibrous capsule on the periphery. A number of septa arise from the deep surface of the capsule and pass into the peripheral cortex of the gland dividing it into lobules. The septa do not extend into the medulla.

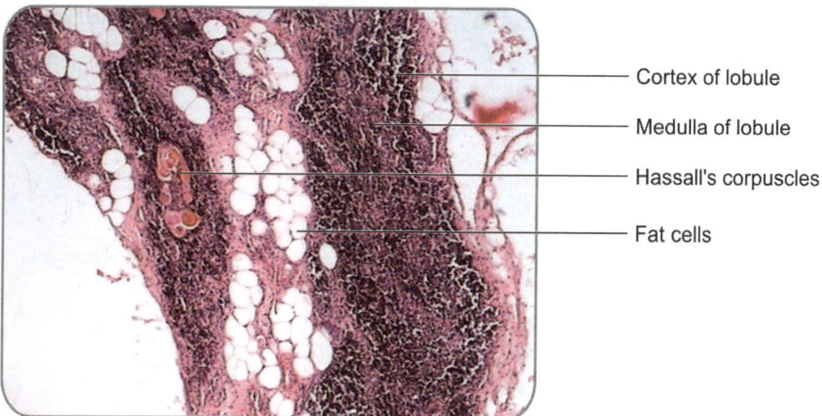

Fig. 5.3A: Photomicrograph of histology of thymus.

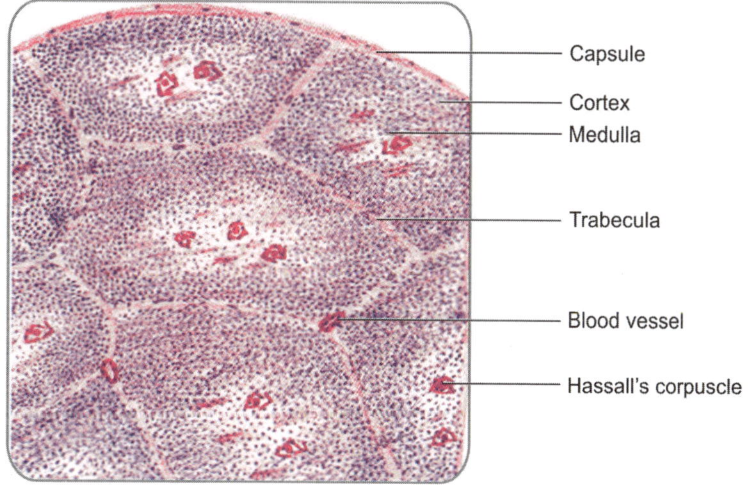

Fig. 5.3B: Diagrammatic representation of histology of thymus.

- In the cortex there are dense collections of lymphocytes supported by branching network of reticular cells.
- In the medulla, lymphocytes are less in number. The reticular cells are large branching cells with pale staining nuclei. Concentric Hassall's corpuscles are seen which has a central homogeneous hyaline material surrounded by concentric layers of flattened reticuloepithelial cells. The center of the corpuscles may contain broken up nuclei, cysts and calcium deposits.
- **Applied anatomy:** Thymic hyperplasia or tumor is associated with myasthenia gravis. The tumors may press on the trachea, esophagus, large veins of neck and brain through its branches.

Palatine Tonsil (Figs. 5.4A and B)

- It occupies the tonsillar sinus. Medial surface is free and covered by stratified squamous epithelium and lateral surface is attached and covered by a sheet of fascia forming capsule.

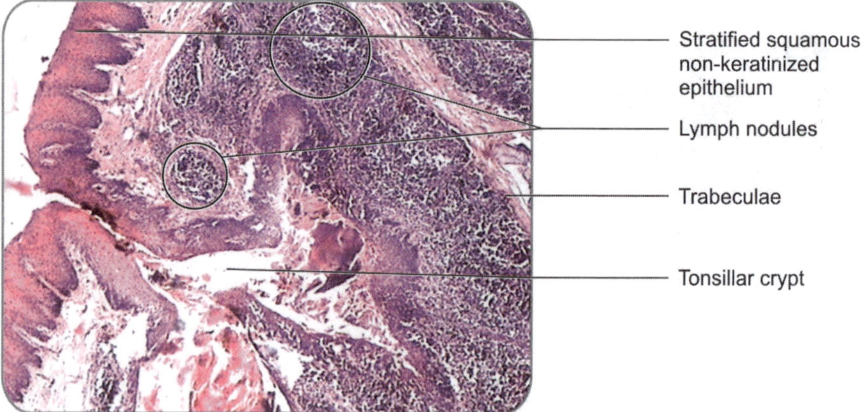

Fig. 5.4A: Photomicrograph of histology of tonsil.

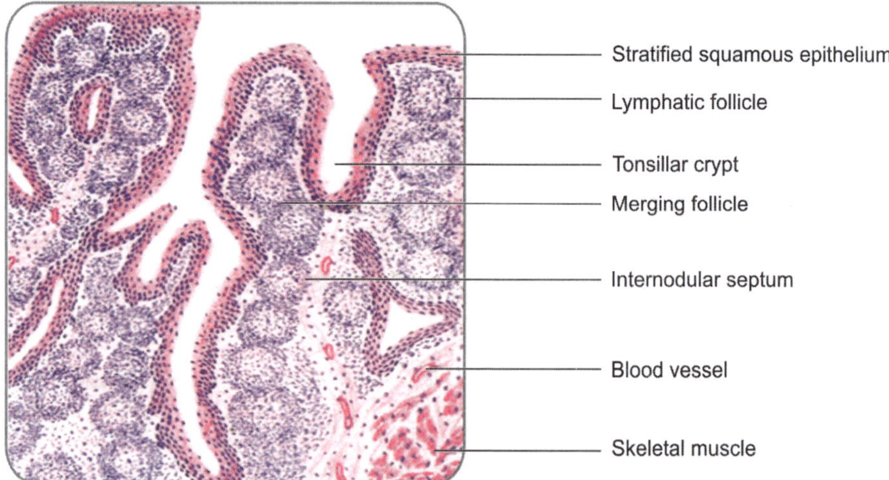

Fig. 5.4B: Diagrammatic representation of histology of tonsil.

- Tonsillar crypts can be made out in the section as cleft-like spaces.
- The main part of tonsil is made of dense collections of lymphatic tissue.
- Beneath the epithelium of the mucosa, in the connective tissue, mucous secreting acini are also seen.
- **Applied anatomy:** They are frequent sites of infection, enlarged infected tonsils need surgical removal called tonsillectomy.

Spleen (Figs. 5.5A and B)

- Spleen has a thick fibromuscular capsule. Smooth muscle fibers are plenty.
- From inner surface of capsule, thick trabeculae of similar structure pass deep into the organ dividing it incompletely.
- **White pulp** is made up of lymphatic tissue which densely collects as insulation around arteries. The collection of lymphoid tissue shows nodular swellings at regular

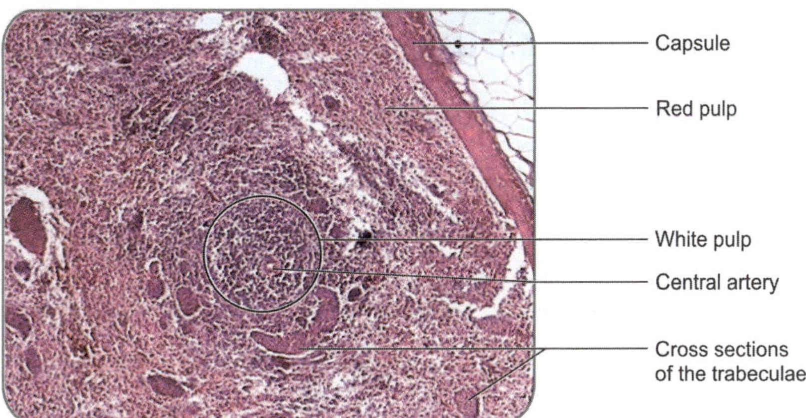

Fig. 5.5A: Photomicrograph of histology of spleen.

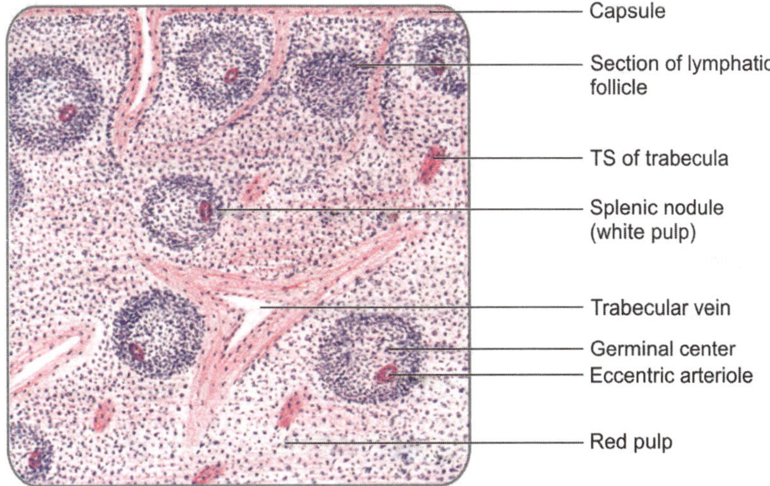

Fig. 5.5B: Diagrammatic representation of histology of spleen.

intervals. These swellings are called Malpighian or splenic corpuscle. Each corpuscle, in a section is seen as a circular area of dense collection of lymphatic tissue with an eccentric arteriole.

- **Red pulp** fills the rest of the spleen. It contains blood, erythrocytes, phagocytic reticuloendothelial cells (macrophages), lymphocytes and monocytes.
- There are sinusoids in the spleen lined by reticuloendothelial cells.

APPLIED ANATOMY

- **Cancer:** Spreads mainly through the lymphatic vessels from one part of the body to other part.
- **Thymic hyperplasia:** It is nothing but thymic tumor. It may compress trachea, esophagus, large veins of neck and brain.
- **Tonsillitis:** Frequent infection of tonsil, needs surgical removal called tonsillectomy.

SUMMARY

Parts	*Lymph node*	*Thymus*	*Tonsil*	*Spleen*
Capsule	Connective tissue	Connective tissue	Epithelium	Connective tissue
Connective tissue trabeculae	Incomplete	Incomplete, but divide into lobules	–	Incomplete
Components	Cortex-lymphatic follicles Medulla Medullary cords Medullary sinuses	Each lobule: Cortex-dense aggregation of lymphocytes Medulla-Few lymphocytes, Hassall's corpuscles	Crypts with surrounding lymphatic follicles	Red pulp-blood, erythrocytes, lymphocytes, monocytes, reticuloendothelial cells, white pulp-lymphocytes
Function	Filter lymph, immunity	Production of T-lymphocytes, immunity	Immunity, first line of defense	Filter blood, destruction of RBCs, store WBCs and platelets

QUESTIONS

Short Essays

- Histology of lymph node.
- Histology of thymus.
- Histology of spleen.
- Histology of tonsil.

Short Answers

- Cisterna chyli.
- Thoracic duct.

CHAPTER

Cardiovascular System

LEARNING OBJECTIVES

The student should be able to:

- Describe microscopic appearance of large artery, medium sized artery and vein, large vein.
- Describe mediastinum, its classification, boundaries and contents and applied aspects.
- Describe pericardium, its attachments, sinuses and applied aspects.
- Describe heart under size, location, chambers, exterior and interior, interatrial and interventricular septa, valves, systemic and pulmonary circulation.
- Describe coronary vessels: arteries and coronary sinus.
- Name the arteries of the body, main branches of aorta, common carotid artery, external carotid, subclavian artery, axillary artery, brachial artery, superficial palmar arch, femoral artery, popliteal, dorsalis pedis artery.
- Name the veins of the body, main veins (superior and inferior vena cava, internal jugular, portal, great saphenous vein, median cubital, cephalic, dural venous sinuses).

INTRODUCTION

- The thoracic cavity lodges the heart covered with pericardium in the center and lungs with pleura on each side. The midline, narrow space with structures in between the two pleural sacs is called mediastinum.
- The blood vascular system consists of the heart and blood vessels through which blood circulates.
- **Blood circulation:** Heart → large artery → medium sized artery → arteriole → capillary or sinusoid depending on structure and function → venule → vein → heart.

MEDIASTINUM

- It is the median septum of thorax between two lungs.
- **Boundaries:** Anterior: Sternum; Posterior: Vertebral column; Superior: Inlet of thorax; Inferior: Diaphragm; On each side: Mediastinal pleura.
- **Divisions:** It is divided into superior and inferior mediastina. Inferior mediastinum further subdivides into anterior, middle and posterior mediastina (**Table 6.1**).

Table 6.1: Boundaries and contents of the mediastina.

	Superior mediastinum	*Middle mediastinum*	*Anterior mediastinum*	*Posterior mediastinum*
Boundaries				
Anterior	Manubrium sterni	Bounded by pericardium on all the sides	Body of sternum	Pericardium, bifurcation of trachea, pulmonary vessels, posterior part of upper surface of diaphragm
Posterior	Upper four thoracic vertebrae		Pericardium	Lower eight thoracic vertebrae, intervening discs
Superior	Inlet of thorax		Imaginary line drawn from sternal angle to lower border of 4th thoracic vertebra	Imaginary line drawn from sternal angle to lower border of 4th thoracic vertebra
Inferior	Imaginary line passing from sternal angle to lower border of 4th thoracic vertebra		Diaphragm	Diaphragm
On each side	Mediastinal pleura		Mediastinal pleura	Mediastinal pleura
Contents				
Muscles	Sternohyoid, sternothyroid, longus colli	–	–	–
Arteries	Arch of aorta, brachiocephalic trunk, left common carotid artery, left subclavian artery	Ascending aorta, pulmonary trunk, two pulmonary arteries	Small mediastinal branches of internal thoracic artery	Descending thoracic aorta and branches
Veins	Right and left brachiocephalic veins, upper half of the superior vena cava, left superior intercostal vein	Lower half of superior vena cava, terminal part of azygos vein, right and left pulmonary veins	–	Azygos, hemiazygos, accessory hemiazygos
Nerves	Vagus, phrenic, cardiac, left recurrent laryngeal	Phrenic, deep cardiac plexus	–	Vagi, three splanchnic nerves (greater, lesser, least)
Lymph nodes	Paratracheal, brachiocephalic, tracheobronchial	Tracheobronchial	Lymph nodes with lymphatics	Posterior mediastinal lymph nodes
Others	Trachea, esophagus, thymus, thoracic duct	Heart, bifurcation of trachea, right and left principal bronchi	Sternopericardial ligaments, lowest part of thymus, areolar tissue	Esophagus, thoracic duct

Applied Anatomy

- Infection in retropharyngeal space, spaces on each side of trachea and esophagus, between trachea and esophagus, between tubes and carotid sheath may spread to superior and posterior mediastina since all are continuous with each other.
- **Mediastinal syndrome:** Compression of structures by tumor (bronchogenic carcinoma, Hodgkin's disease, aneurysm of aorta) may lead to pressure on the structures in mediastinum. Pressure on the following structures may lead to the following symptoms.
  - *Trachea:* Dyspnea.
  - *Esophagus:* Dysphagia.
  - *Left recurrent laryngeal nerve:* Hoarseness of voice.
  - *Phrenic nerve:* Paralysis of diaphragm.
  - *Vertebral column:* Erosion of vertebral bodies.

PERICARDIUM

- Pericardium is a fibroserous sac which invests and protects the heart and the roots of the great vessels.
- **Situation:** In the middle mediastinum behind the body of the sternum and the 2nd to 6th costal cartilages opposite the levels of 5th to 8th thoracic vertebral bodies.
- **Subdivisions:** Outer fibrous and inner serous which in turn has outer parietal and inner visceral layers.
- Between the parietal and visceral layers is a thin space called pericardial cavity filled with a thin film of fluid called pericardial fluid which prevents friction.
- **Oblique sinus:** It is a recess in the pericardial cavity situated behind the left atrium bounded by four pulmonary veins, superior vena cava and inferior vena cava.
- **Transverse sinus:** It is a passage in the pericardial space between the two sheaths of reflection of serous pericardium between the arterial and venous tubes.

HEART (FIG. 6.1)

- Heart is a hollow, conical, muscular organ situated in middle mediastinum covered by pericardium.
- Average size of the heart is that of a closed fist and weighs 300–350 g.
- There are four chambers, two atria and two ventricles in the heart. Atria are above and behind the ventricles.
- **Surfaces and borders:** Apex, base, three surfaces (anterior, inferior, left lateral) and four borders/margins (right, inferior, left, superior).
- **Apex:** It is formed by left ventricle. It is present in the left 5th intercostal space 8.7 cm from the midline.
- **Base (posterior surface):** It is formed by posterior wall of left atrium and a small part of right atrium.
- **Anterior or sternocostal surface:** It consists of an atrial and a ventricular part separated by the anterior part of coronary/atrioventricular sulcus. The right coronary artery runs downwards in this part of the coronary sulcus.
- The atrial part is formed chiefly by right atrium as the greater part of the left atrium is hidden by the ascending aorta and the pulmonary trunk and only a small part of its auricle projects forwards on the left side of the pulmonary trunk.

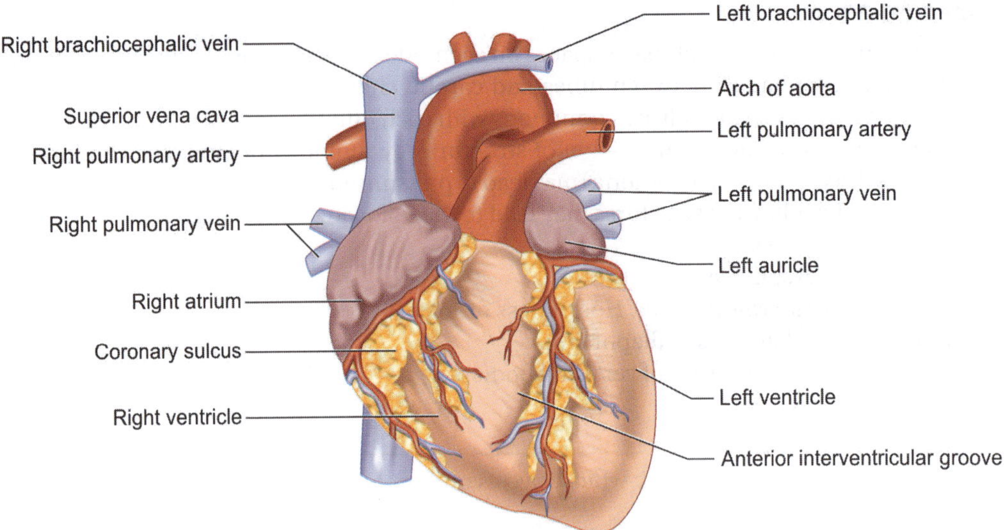

Fig. 6.1: Anterior view of the heart.

- The right 2/3 of the ventricular part is formed by right ventricle and the left 1/3 by the left ventricle. The anterior interventricular groove intervenes between them and lodges the anterior interventricular branch of the left coronary artery and the great cardiac vein.
- **Inferior or diaphragmatic surface:** The right 1/3 of this surface is formed by the right ventricle and the left 2/3 by the left ventricle and in between them is the posterior interventricular groove which lodges posterior interventricular branch of right coronary artery and middle cardiac vein.
- Between the base and inferior surface of the heart is the posterior part of the coronary sulcus in which (a) the terminal parts of the right and left coronary arteries meet in the middle, (b) the coronary sinus runs from left to right towards its termination into the right atrium, (c) the small cardiac vein is situated in the right edge.
- **Right margin** is formed by right atrium.
- Inferior margin is sharp and is formed mainly by the right ventricle. A very small part of this margin near the apex is formed by the left ventricle.
- **Left margin** is formed by left ventricle and a small part of left atrium in the upper part.
- **Superior margin** is formed by left atrium with right and left pulmonary arteries running on it. It is masked by the roots of the pulmonary trunk and the ascending aorta with the auricles overlapping them on both sides.

Chambers of the Heart

Right Atrium (Fig. 6.2)

External features

- From its upper and anterior aspect, a conical, ear-like muscular process, called right auricle projects forward and overlaps roots of pulmonary trunk and aorta on right side.
- The superior vena cava enters the chamber posterosuperiorly, the inferior vena cava enters posteroinferiorly.

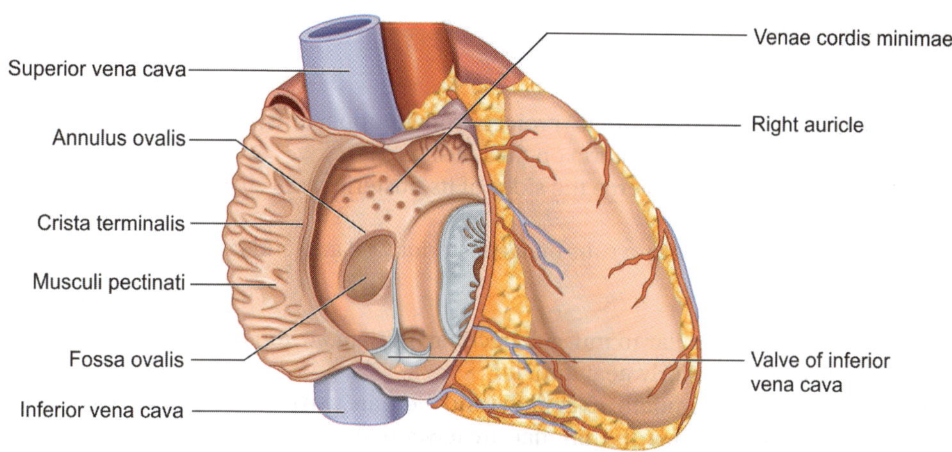

Fig. 6.2: Interior of the right atrium.

- Sulcus terminalis is a groove on surface of the right atrium extending between the right sides of superior and inferior vena cavae.
- It is separated by the right ventricle by the right atrioventricular groove which lodges the right coronary artery and small cardiac vein.

Internal features

Two portions: Anterior and posterior parts, separated by a vertical muscular ridge called crista terminalis which corresponds to sulcus terminalis on the surface.

Anterior rough part or atrium proper

- It has a rough ridged wall which is continuous with auricle.
- There are a number of transverse muscular ridges arising from crista terminalis and passing on the lateral and anterior walls. They resemble teeth of a comb and are called musculi pectinati.
- **Medial wall separates right atrium from left atrium and is called septal wall. It shows:** (i) An oval depression in the lower part called fossa ovalis which represents septum primum. (ii) Limbus fossa ovalis is the prominent margin of fossa ovalis which represents lower free edge of septum secundum. (iii) Occasionally slit like opening, foramen ovale is present which is normally occluded after birth.

Posterior smooth part or sinus venarum

Has a smooth inner lining receiving the following veins: Superior vena cava, inferior vena cava, coronary sinus, venae cordis minimae, anterior cardiac veins.

Tricuspid opening

- It connects right atrium with right ventricle.
- It is guarded by tricuspid valve with three cusps (anterior, inferior, medial or septal) which are directed towards ventricle.
- Each cusp gives attachment to chordae tendineae of ventricle.

Left Atrium

External features

- A small conical process (left auricle) projects from its upper and left corner and overlaps the roots of pulmonary trunk and aorta on the left side.
- The four pulmonary veins pierce the sides of its posterior wall (two on each side) to open into it.
- The oblique vein of left atrium runs on its posterior wall and ends in coronary sinus.

Internal features

- The muscular ridges similar to musculi pectinati of right atrium are fewer in this chamber and are seen more anteriorly near auricle.
- The posterior part has a smooth inner lining and there are two pairs of openings of pulmonary veins, openings of venae cordis minimae are fewer than in right atrium.

Bicuspid/Mitral opening

- It is the communicating orifice between left atrium and left ventricle.
- It is guarded by mitral valve with two cusps (anterior and posterior) which are directed towards ventricle.
- Each cusp gives attachment to chordae tendineae of ventricle.

Right Ventricle

External features

- At the upper left end of this chamber is a conical dilatation called infundibulum from which pulmonary trunk arises.
- The walls of ventricles are more muscular and thicker than those of atria.
- The right ventricular wall is thinner than the left ventricular wall as it has to pump the blood only to the lungs.
- Right ventricle is crescentic in cross-section since its posterior wall or interventricular septum bulges into it.

Internal features

- Inflowing and outflowing part separated by a muscular ridge called supraventricular crest.
- The inlet opening is tricuspid orifice or right atrioventricular orifice which is guarded by tricuspid valve which has three triangular cusps—anterior, medial or septal and inferior.
- **Inflowing part:** Its walls are rough due to presence of muscular ridges called trabeculae carneae.
- There are also three conical muscular projections called papillary muscles.
- The inflowing part receives blood from right atrium through tricuspid orifice.
- Fibrous strands called chordae tendineae connect papillary muscle with tricuspid valve.
- **The outflowing part or infundibulum:** It has a smooth inner wall and outlet opening of right ventricle is pulmonary orifice situated at the upper end of infundibulum.
- The opening is guarded by three semilunar valves, two anterior and one posterior.

Left Ventricle

External features

It forms the apex of the heart, which is directed downwards, forwards and to the left side.

Internal features

- Its walls are very thick as it has to pump blood through aorta to all parts of the body.
- The cavity is circular in cross section. It has inflowing and outflowing parts.
- **Inflowing part:** It has rough inner wall due to the presence of trabeculae carneae and two papillary muscles (anterior and posterior).
- **Mitral orifice:** It is the inlet opening in this part and ventricular surface of the cusps of its valve are connected by chordae tendineae to both papillary muscles.
- **Outflowing part:** It is the aortic vestibule, the portion below the outlet (aortic orifice) of left ventricle.
- It has a smooth inner lining and its walls are made of fibrous tissue only.
- The aortic orifice is guarded by three semilunar valves (two posterior and one anterior).
- **Interventricular septum:** It separates the two ventricles and is curved with the convexity bulging into right ventricle.
- Its margins correspond with anterior and posterior interventricular grooves on the surface of the heart.
- The major part of the septum is thick and muscular.
- A small, oval area in the upper part of the septum is thin and fibrous and is called membranous part of the septum.

Nerve Supply

Branches from superficial cardiac plexus and deep cardiac plexus.

Blood Supply

Arterial Supply (Fig. 6.3)

Right coronary artery

- Arises from anterior aortic sinus.
- It runs downwards and to the right side, in the anterior part of coronary sulcus.
- It curves around the right side of the heart and continues its course in the posterior part of the coronary sulcus.
- Finally ends by anastomosing with terminal end of left coronary artery.

Branches

- Right marginal artery runs along inferior margin of heart from right to left.
- Posterior interventricular branch runs forward in posterior interventricular groove on inferior surface of heart.

Areas supplied

- Right atrium
- A portion of left atrium
- Right ventricle except the area near the anterior interventricular groove.
- Small part of left ventricle near the posterior interventricular groove.
- Vasa vasorum to bases of pulmonary artery and aorta.
- Posterior part of interventricular septum and bundle of His.

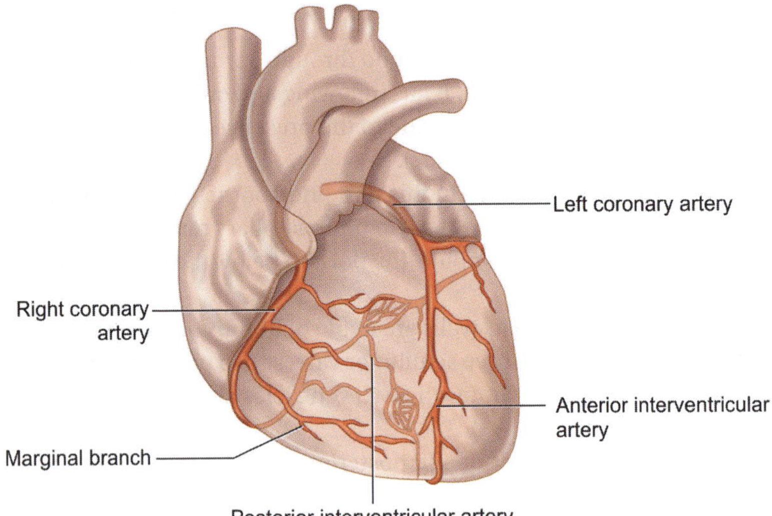

Fig. 6.3: Arterial supply of the heart.

Left coronary artery

- It is larger than right coronary artery.
- It arises from left posterior aortic sinus.
- It runs in a leftward direction in coronary sulcus, to end by anastomosing with terminal end of right coronary artery.

Branches

- A large descending or anterior interventricular branch descends in anterior interventricular groove of heart. It ends by anastomosing with terminal end of posterior interventricular branch of the right coronary artery near apex of the heart.
- A marginal branch which runs on the left ventricle.

Areas supplied

- Left atrium.
- Small part of right atrium.
- Left ventricle except near the posterior interventricular groove.
- Small part of right ventricle near anterior interventricular groove.
- Anterior part of interventricular septum.

Venous Drainage (Fig. 6.4)

Coronary Sinus

- It is the chief vein of the heart.
- It is the continuation of great cardiac vein which starts in the anterior interventricular groove and runs up in the groove to reach the coronary sulcus where it becomes coronary sinus.

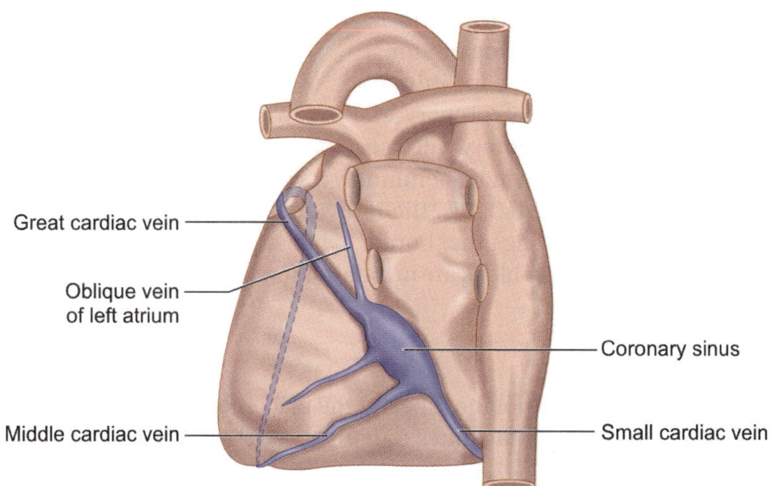

Fig. 6.4: Venous drainage of the heart.

- It turns towards the left in the anterior part of the coronary sulcus curving round the left side of the heart.
- It runs from left to right in the posterior part of the coronary sulcus.
- It gradually increases in size and finally ends by opening into right atrium.

Tributaries

- Great cardiac vein
- Oblique vein of left atrium
- Posterior vein of LV
- Middle cardiac vein
- Small cardiac veins.

Anterior cardiac veins: Drain directly into right atrium.

Venae cordis minimae: These are small minute veins which drain the musculature of the heart directly into all chambers of the heart mainly into atria.

Lymphatic Drainage

The lymph from the anterior lymph trunk drains into superior mediastinal nodes and the posterior lymph trunk to the right tracheobronchial nodes.

Applied Anatomy

- The first heart sound is produced by closure of the atrioventricular valves. The second heart sound is produced by closure of semilunar valves.
- **Narrowing of the valve orifice due to fusion of the valve cusps is called as stenosis. For example:** Mitral stenosis.
- Dilatation of the valve orifice or stiffening of the cusps causes imperfect closure of the valves leading to backflow of blood. This is called regurgitation, e.g., mitral and aortic regurgitation.
- **Tachycardia:** Increased heart rate.
- **Bradycardia:** Decreased heart rate.
- **Arrhythmia:** Irregular heart rate.

- **Pericarditis:** Inflammation of pericardium.
- **Myocarditis:** Inflammation of myocardium.
- **Endocarditis:** Inflammation of endocardium.
- Sudden obstruction of a branch of coronary artery by an embolus or a gradual obstruction due to a thrombus formation in the artery will cause sudden death and anterior interventricular branch of left coronary artery is more commonly involved.
- In incomplete or partial obstructions, the individual will suffer from severe pain in the precordial region radiating along ulnar border of left upper extremity (angina pectoris).
- The common sites for coronary block are in anterior interventricular branch, right coronary artery and circumflex branch.

Fetal Circulation (Fig. 6.5)

- Source of oxygenated blood is not the lung but the placenta.
- Oxygenated blood from placenta comes to fetus through umbilical vein, which joins left branch of portal vein.
- A small portion of this blood passes through the liver to IVC, but the greater part passes direct to IVC through ductus venosus.
- The oxygen-rich blood reaching right atrium through IVC is directed by the valve of IVC towards foramen ovale.
- Most of the blood passes through foramen ovale into left atrium.
- The rest of it gets mixed up with the blood returning to the right atrium through SVC and passes into the right ventricle.

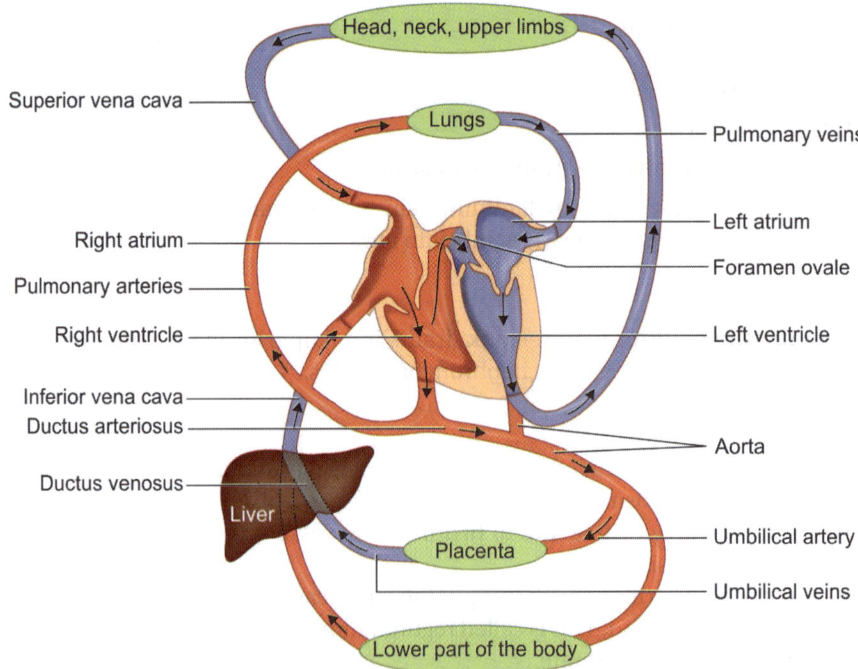

Fig. 6.5: Schematic diagram of fetal circulation.

- From right ventricle, blood (mostly deoxygenated) enters pulmonary trunk.
- Only a small portion of this blood reaches the lungs and passes through it to the left atrium. The greater part is short-circuited by ductus arteriosus into aorta.
- Hence the left atrium receives oxygenated blood from right atrium and a small amount of deoxygenated blood from lungs.
- This oxygen-rich blood passes into left ventricle and then into aorta.
- Some of this gets mixed up with poorly oxygenated blood from ductus arteriosus.
- Much of the blood from aorta is carried by umbilical arteries to placenta where it is again oxygenated and returned to the heart.

Changes Taking Place at Birth

- The following changes in the fetal blood vessels lead to the adult type of circulation.
- The distal part of the lumen of the umbilical arteries occludes which prevents loss of fetal blood into the placenta and is converted into fibrous tissue called medial umbilical ligaments.
- A few minutes after birth the lumen of the left umbilical vein and ductus venosus are also occluded which are replaced by fibrous tissue and forms ligament of teres of the liver and ligamentum venosum respectively.
- The lumen of the ductus arteriosus is closed and forms ligamentum arteriosum.
- Pulmonary vessels increase in size so that more blood reaches the left atrium increasing the pressure. Simultaneously the pressure in the right atrium decreases since the placental blood does not reach it. Because of the increased pressure in the left atrium than the right atrium, the foramen ovale closes.

ARTERIES OF THE BODY (FIG. 6.6)

Arteries of Thorax and Abdomen

Aorta

- It is one of the great vessels arising from left ventricle and distributes the oxygenated blood to all parts of the body.
- **It is divided into 3 parts:** Ascending aorta, arch of aorta, descending aorta (descending thoracic aorta and abdominal aorta).

Ascending Aorta

- It is 5 cm long and lies in middle mediastinum.
- **Extent:** It arises from left ventricle at the level of lower border of 3rd costal cartilage and ends in arch at the level of upper border of 2nd right costal cartilage and enclosed in pericardium.
- **Branches:** Right and left coronary arteries.

Arch of Aorta

- It connects ascending aorta with descending aorta and lies in superior mediastinum behind lower half of manubrium sterni.
- **Extent:** Starts behind right margin of sternum and ends on the left side at the level of the body of 4th thoracic vertebra.
- **Branches:** Brachiocephalic artery, left common carotid artery, left subclavian artery and occasionally thyroidea ima or vertebral arteries.

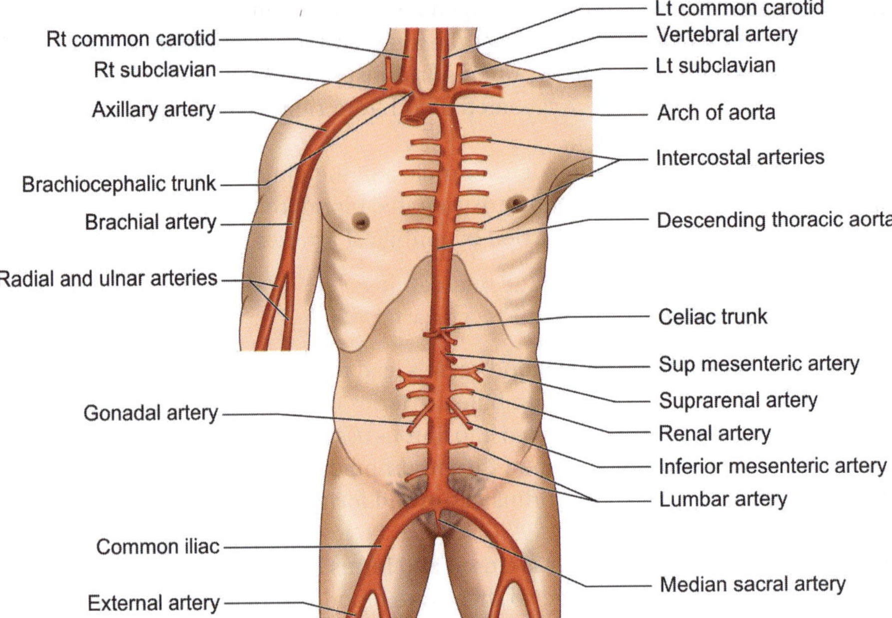

Fig. 6.6: Arteries of the body.

Descending Thoracic Aorta

- It continues from arch of aorta and lies in posterior mediastinum.
- **Extent:** Starts on the left side at the level of the lower border of the body of the 4th thoracic vertebra and ends at the level of lower border of 12th thoracic vertebra.
- **Branches:** Nine posterior intercostal arteries, subcostal artery, two left bronchial arteries, esophageal branches, pericardial branches, mediastinal branches, superior phrenic arteries.

Abdominal Aorta

- **Extent:** It begins as the continuation of descending thoracic aorta in the midline at the aortic opening of the diaphragm at the level of lower border of 12th thoracic vertebra and ends by dividing into two terminal branches, right and left common iliac arteries.
- **Branches:** Ventral branches: Celiac trunk, superior and inferior mesenteric artery; Dorsal branches: Lumbar arteries, median sacral artery; lateral branches (paired): Inferior phrenic, middle suprarenal, renal, gonadal (testicular or ovarian) arteries; terminal branches: Right and left common iliac arteries.

Celiac Trunk

- **Extent:** It is the artery of the foregut arising from the front of the abdominal aorta at the level of the disc between 12th thoracic vertebra and 1st lumbar vertebra.
- **Branches:** Left gastric, splenic (branches—pancreatic, left gastroepiploic, short gastric), hepatic (branches—cystic, right gastric, supraduodenal, gastroduodenal which again branches into right gastroepiploic and superior pancreaticoduodenal).

Superior Mesenteric

- **Extent:** It is the artery of the midgut arising from the front of the abdominal aorta at the level of 1st lumbar vertebra 1 cm below the celiac trunk.
- **Branches:** Inferior pancreaticoduodenal, jejunal, ileal, ileocolic, right colic, middle colic arteries.

Inferior Mesenteric

- **Extent:** It is artery of the hindgut arising from the front of the abdominal aorta at the level of 3rd lumbar vertebra, 3–4 cm above the bifurcation of aorta behind the duodenum.
- **Branches:** Left colic, sigmoid, superior rectal arteries.

Arteries of Head and Neck

Common Carotid Artery

- **Extent:** The origin of the right and left common carotid arteries differs. The right common carotid artery arises from brachiocephalic trunk and left from arch of aorta.
- **Branches:** Both the arteries end by dividing into external and internal carotid arteries at the level of upper border of thyroid cartilage or between 3rd and 4th cervical vertebrae.

External Carotid Artery

- **Extent:** One of the terminal branches of the common carotid artery arises at the level of the upper border of thyroid cartilage and ends by dividing into two terminal branches behind the neck of the mandible.
- **Branches:** Ascending pharyngeal, superior thyroid, lingual, facial, occipital, posterior auricular, maxillary and superficial temporal arteries.

Internal Carotid Artery

- **Extent:** One of the terminal branches of the common carotid artery arises at the level of the upper border of thyroid cartilage and ends inside the cranial cavity supplying the brain.
- **It is divided into four parts:** Cervical, petrous, cavernous and cerebral.
- **Branches:** Cervical part: No branches in the neck; petrous part: Caroticotympanic, pterygoid branches; cavernous part: Cavernous branches, superior and inferior hypophyseal branches; cerebral part: Ophthalmic, anterior cerebral, middle cerebral, posterior communicating, anterior choroidal.

Subclavian Artery

- **Extent:** On the left side, it directly arises from arch of aorta but on the right side, from brachiocephalic trunk. At the level of the outer border of the first rib, it continues as axillary artery in the axilla.
- The scalenus anterior muscle crosses in front of the artery and divides it into three parts. The 1st part is medial to the muscle, 2nd part is behind the muscle and 3rd part is lateral to the muscle.
- **Branches:** Vertebral, internal thoracic, thyrocervical, costocervical, dorsal scapular arteries.

Vertebral Artery

- **Extent:** It arises from the upper surface of first part of subclavian artery. It passes through the foramina transversaria of upper six cervical vertebrae and enter cranial cavity through foramen magnum. The two vertebral arteries unite to form basilar artery.

- **Branches:** Muscular, meningeal, medullary posterior spinal, anterior spinal, posterior inferior cerebellar arteries.

Blood Vessels of Brain

Two systems of arteries supply the brain—vertebral system and the carotid system.

Vertebral System

- A pair of vertebral arteries, which ascend upwards, and form the basilar artery.
- **Branches:** Muscular meningeal branches, medullary branches, anterior spinal, posterior spinal, posterior inferior cerebellar arteries.
- **Branches of basilar artery:** Pontine branches, anterior inferior cerebellar arteries, labyrinthine branches, superior cerebellar, posterior cerebellar arteries.

Carotid System

See under internal carotid artery.

Arterial Circle of Willis (Fig. 6.7)

This is an arterial circle situated at the base of the brain. It is formed as follows:

- Anteriorly—anterior communicating artery.
- Anterolaterally—anterior cerebral arteries.
- Laterally—posterior communicating arteries.
- Posteriorly—posterior cerebral arteries.

Arteries of Upper Limb

Axillary Artery

- **Extent:** It continues from subclavian artery at the level of the outer border of the first rib and ends at the level of lower border of teres major muscle. It continues as brachial artery.
- The pectoralis minor divides the artery into three parts, 1st part is medial to, 2nd part is behind and 3rd part is lateral to the muscle.

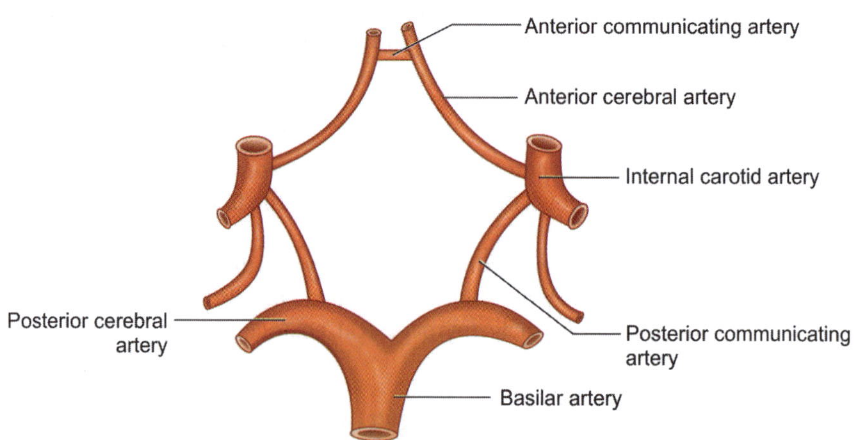

Fig. 6.7: Circle of Willis.

- **Branches:** 1st part: Superior thoracic artery; 2nd part: Lateral thoracic and acromiothoracic artery; 3rd part: Anterior and posterior circumflex humeral, subscapular artery.

Brachial Artery

- **Extent:** It is the continuation of the axillary artery at the level of the lower border of the teres major muscle and ends in front of the elbow at the level of neck of radius. It divides here into terminal branches—radial and ulnar arteries.
- **Branches:** Unnamed muscular branches, profunda brachii, superior ulnar collateral, inferior ulnar collateral, nutrient, radial and ulnar.

Radial Artery

- **Extent:** One of the terminal branch of the brachial artery given off in the cubital fossa and ends in the hand by anastomosing with deep branch of ulnar artery forming deep palmar arch.
- **Branches:** Radial recurrent artery, muscular branches, palmar carpal branch, superficial palmar branch, 1st dorsal metacarpal artery, princeps pollicis, radialis indices.

Ulnar Artery

- **Extent:** Larger terminal branch of the brachial artery given off in the cubital fossa and ends in the hand by dividing into superficial and deep branches.
- **Branches:** Anterior ulnar recurrent, posterior ulnar recurrent, common interosseous artery in turn dividing into anterior interosseous and posterior interosseous, muscular branches, palmar carpal, dorsal carpal and terminal superficial and deep branches.

Superficial Palmar Arch

- **Formation:** It is an arterial arch situated superficially in the palm deep to palmar aponeurosis. It is formed by superficial branch of ulnar artery joining any one of the branch of radial artery (superficial palmar branch or princeps pollicis or radialis indicis).
- **Branches:** Four digital arteries and cutaneous branches to palm.

Deep Palmar Arch

- **Formation:** It is formed by union of deep branch of ulnar artery with terminal part of radial artery. It is the second arch connecting radial and ulnar arteries in the hand deep to the long flexor tendons.
- **Branches:** Three palmar metacarpal arteries, three perforating arteries, recurrent branches.

Arteries of Lower Limb

Common Iliac Arteries

- **Extent:** The terminal branches of abdominal aorta begins in front of the 4th lumbar vertebra and ends in front of the sacroiliac joint at the level of lumbosacral intervertebral disc by dividing into terminal branches.
- **Branches:** Internal and external iliac arteries.

Internal Iliac Artery

- **Extent:** Smaller terminal branch of the common iliac artery, arises in front of the sacroiliac joint, at the level of the intervertebral disc between the 5th lumbar vertebra and sacrum and ends near the upper margin of the greater sciatic notch by dividing into anterior and posterior trunks.

- **Branches:** Anterior trunk: Superior vesical, obturator, middle rectal, inferior vesical, inferior gluteal, internal pudendal. In females the inferior vesical is replaced by vaginal and an extra branch—uterine artery is present; posterior trunk: Iliolumbar, lateral sacral, superior gluteal.

External Iliac Artery

- **Extent:** It is the larger branch which continues into the thigh as femoral artery. It starts in front of the sacroiliac joint and at the mid-inguinal point it becomes continuous with femoral artery.
- **Branches:** Inferior epigastric, deep circumflex iliac, twigs to ureter.

Femoral Artery

- **Extent:** The chief artery of the lower limb begins at the mid-inguinal point behind the inguinal ligament as the continuation of external iliac artery and ends by piercing the adductor magnus muscle at the junction of middle third and lower third of the thigh to become continuous with popliteal artery.
- **Branches:** Superficial arteries: Superficial external pudendal, superficial circumflex iliac and superficial epigastric; deep arteries: Profunda femoris, deep external pudendal artery, muscular branches.

Profunda Femoris Artery

- **Extent:** Largest branch of the femoral artery arises from the lateral side about 4 cm below the inguinal ligament and terminates as the 4th perforating branch by piercing the adductor magnus muscle to reach the posterior compartment of the leg.
- **Branches:** Medial circumflex femoral, lateral circumflex femoral, muscular, four perforating branches.

Popliteal Artery

- **Extent:** It starts as the continuation of the femoral artery at the junction of middle third and lower third of the thigh and ends at the lower border of popliteus muscle by dividing into anterior and posterior tibial arteries.
- **Branches:** Muscular branches, cutaneous branches, five genicular branches (medial and lateral superior genicular, medial and lateral inferior genicular, middle genicular), terminal anterior and posterior tibial arteries.

Anterior Tibial Artery

- **Extent:** The main artery of the anterior compartment of the leg begins as the smaller terminal branch of the popliteal artery at the lower border of the popliteus muscle in the posterior compartment of the leg. It enters the dorsum of foot as dorsalis pedis artery.
- **Branches:** Muscular, anterior and posterior tibial recurrent branches, anterior medial malleolar, anterior lateral malleolar branches.

Posterior Tibial Artery

- **Extent:** The main artery of the posterior and lateral compartment of the leg begins as the larger terminal branch of the popliteal artery at the lower border of the popliteus. It ends deep to flexor retinaculum, enters the sole of foot and divides into medial and lateral plantar arteries.

- **Branches:** Peroneal artery, muscular branches, nutrient artery, circumflex fibular, communicating branch to peroneal artery, malleolar branch, calcaneal branch, terminal medial and lateral plantar branches.

Plantar Arch

- **Formation:** It is formed by the lateral plantar artery and dorsalis pedis artery.
- **Branches:** Four plantar metatarsal arteries, three proximal perforating arteries.

Applied Anatomy

- Peripheral pulses are felt at radial, brachial, dorsalis pedis, popliteal, femoral and carotid arteries.
- Sudden occlusion of the popliteal artery may cause gangrene up to the knee, but usually prevented by the collateral circulation around the knee. This artery is more prone to aneurysm than many other arteries of the body.

VEINS OF THE BODY (FIG. 6.8)

Veins of Upper Limb

Dorsal Venous Arch

Lies on dorsum of hand and drains metacarpal veins, veins to five fingers and palm.

Basilic Vein

- Starts from medial end of dorsal venous arch of hand.
- Ascends on medial side of upper limb and continues as axillary vein.

Cephalic Vein

- Starts from lateral end of venous arch of hand.
- Ascends up on the lateral side of the upper limb and drains in the axillary vein.
- At the elbow the greater part of its blood is drained into the basilic vein through the median cubital vein and partly into the deep veins through a perforator.

Median Cubital Vein

- A large communicating vein that shunts blood from the cephalic to basilic vein.
- It begins from the cephalic vein 2.5 cm below the bend of the elbow and runs upwards and medially to end in the basilic vein 2.5 cm above the elbow.
- It is connected by a perforator with the deep veins; since it is fixed by this perforator, it is ideal to give intravenous injections just in front of the elbow.

Axillary Vein

- It is a continuation of the basilic vein.
- It lies medial to the axillary artery.
- At the outer border of the first rib, it continues as the subclavian vein.

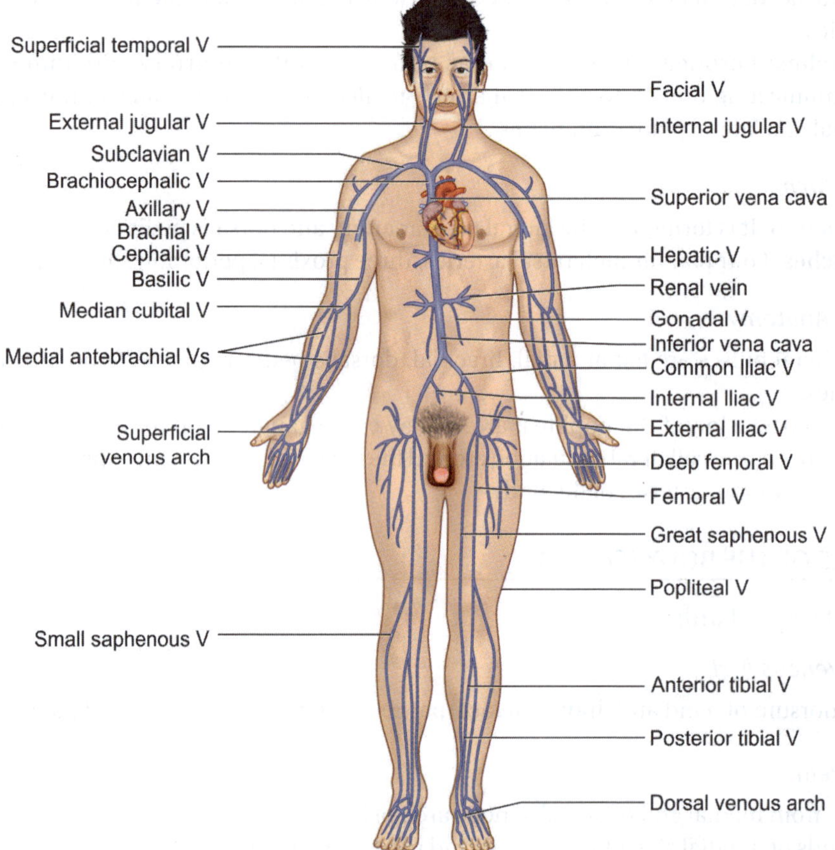

Fig. 6.8: Veins of the body.

- In addition to receiving tributaries corresponding to the branches of the axillary artery, it also receives the cephalic vein in its upper part.
- It is not covered by the axillary sheath so it is free to expand during increased venous return.

Veins of Thorax

Intercostal Veins

- There are two anterior intercostal veins in each of the upper nine intercostal spaces.
- They accompany the arteries.
- In the upper six spaces, they end in the internal thoracic vein and in the next three spaces; they end in the musculophrenic veins.
- There is one posterior intercostal vein in each space which accompanies the artery and lies superior to it.
- The tributaries correspond to the branches of arteries and include veins from the vertebral canal, vertebral venous plexus and muscles of skin and back.
- On the right side, the 1st posterior intercostal vein drains into the right brachiocephalic vein, 2nd and 3rd form the right superior intercostal vein that drains into the azygos vein, 5th to 12th vein drain into the azygos vein.

- On the left side, the 1st posterior intercostal vein drains into the left brachiocephalic vein, 2nd and 3rd form the left superior intercostal vein that drains into the left brachiocephalic vein. 5th to 8th vein drain into the accessory hemiazygos and 9th to 12th drain into the hemiazygos vein.

Azygos Vein

- Drains the thoracic wall and the lumbar regions.
- It is an important channel connecting the superior and inferior vena cavae.
- It is formed by the union of the lumbar azygos, right subcostal and the right ascending lumbar vein.
- It receives the right superior intercostal vein, 4th to 11th right posterior intercostal veins, hemiazygos vein at the level of T9, accessory hemiazygos vein at T8, the right bronchial vein and esophageal, mediastinal and pericardial veins.
- It enters the thoracic cavity by passing through the aortic opening of the diaphragm and end by draining into the superior vena cava.

Hemiazygos Vein

- It is the mirror image of the lower part of azygos vein.
- It originates either from the left renal vein or from the union of the left subcostal vein and the left ascending lumbar vein.
- It receives the left 9th to 12th intercostal veins and ends in the azygos vein at the level of T9.

Accessory Hemiazygos Vein

- It is the mirror image of the upper part of azygos vein.
- It originates at the medial end of the 4th or 5th intercostal space and receives the left 5th to 8th posterior intercostal veins and ends in the azygos vein at T8.
- It sometimes receives the left bronchial veins.

Superior Vena Cava

- It is a large venous channel that collects blood from the upper part of the body and drains it into the right atrium.
- It is formed by the union of the right and left brachiocephalic veins behind the lower border of the first right costal cartilage.
- It receives the azygos veins and some small mediastinal and pericardial veins.

Veins of Lower Limb

Dorsal Venous Arch

It lies on the dorsum of foot and receives four dorsal metatarsal veins each of which is formed by the union of two dorsal digital veins.

Great Saphenous Vein

- It is the largest and the longest superficial vein of the lower limb.
- It begins from the medial side of the dorsal venous arch of the foot, ascends up and ends in the femoral vein at the saphenous opening in the upper part of the thigh.

- Before it ends in the femoral vein it receives the superficial epigastric, superficial circumflex iliac and superficial external pudendal veins.
- It contains about 10–20 valves which prevent the back flow of blood.
- If valves are defective, vein becomes dilated and tortuous and are called varicose veins.
- It is also connected to the deep veins through the perforator veins. They permit flow of blood only to the deep veins from the superficial veins.

Small Saphenous Vein

- Formed from lateral side of the dorsal venous arch and ends in the popliteal vein.
- It drains the lateral border of the foot, the heel and the back of leg.

Popliteal Vein

- It is formed by the union of veins accompanying the anterior and posterior tibial arteries at the lower border of popliteus muscle.
- It continues as the femoral vein and receives the small saphenous vein and the veins corresponding to the branches of popliteal artery.

Femoral Vein

- It begins as a continuation of the popliteal vein at the lower end of adductor canal and ends as the external iliac vein.
- Receives great saphenous vein, veins accompanying branches of femoral artery, i.e., profunda, external pudendal and muscular, lateral and medial circumflex femoral.

Veins of Abdomen and Pelvis

Superior Mesenteric Vein

- It drains blood from small intestine, appendix, cecum, ascending colon and transverse colon.
- It begins in right iliac fossa by union of tributaries from ileocecal region.
- It terminates behind the neck of pancreas, by joining splenic vein to form portal vein.
- Its tributaries are veins corresponding to branches of superior mesenteric artery, right gastroepiploic vein and occasionally, inferior mesenteric vein.

Inferior Mesenteric Vein

- It drains blood from rectum, sigmoid colon and descending colon.
- It begins as superior rectal vein from upper part of internal rectal venous plexus.
- It opens into splenic vein.
- Its tributaries correspond to branches of inferior mesenteric artery.

Portal Vein (Fig. 6.9)

- It collects blood from abdominal part of alimentary tract, gall bladder, pancreas, spleen and conveys it to liver.
- In the liver, portal vein breaks up into sinusoids which are drained by hepatic veins to inferior vena cava.
- **Formation:** By union of superior mesenteric and splenic veins behind the neck of pancreas at the level of L2 vertebra.

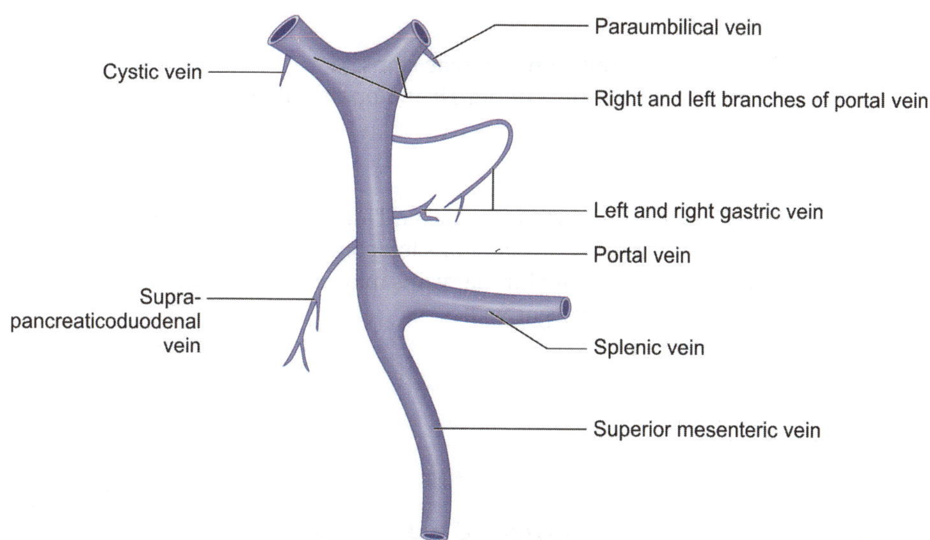

Fig. 6.9: Tributaries of portal vein.

- The vein ends at the right side of porta hepatis by dividing into right and left branches which enter the liver.
- **Tributaries:** Splenic, superior mesenteric, left gastric, right gastric, superior pancreaticoduodenal, cystic, paraumbilical veins.

Portosystemic/Portocaval anastomosis

These communications form important routes of collateral circulation in portal obstruction. The following are the important sites of portosystemic anastomosis.

- **Umbilicus:** Left branch of portal vein with veins of anterior abdominal wall (systemic) with paraumbilical veins (portal). In portal obstruction, veins around the umbilicus enlarge forming caput medusae.
- **Lower end of esophagus:** Esophageal tributaries of accessory hemiazygos vein (systemic) with esophageal tributaries of left gastric vein (portal).
- **Anal canal:** Middle and inferior rectal veins (systemic) with superior rectal vein (portal).
- **Bare area of liver:** Phrenic and intercostal veins (systemic) with hepatic venules (portal).
- **Posterior abdominal wall:** Retroperitoneal veins of abdominal wall and of renal capsule (systemic) with veins of retroperitoneal organs, like duodenum, ascending colon and descending colon (portal).
- **Liver:** Rarely, ductus venosus remains patent and connects inferior vena cava with left branch of portal vein.

Applied anatomy

- **Portal pressure:** Normal pressure in portal vein is 5–15 mm Hg.
- **Portal hypertension:** Pressure above 40 mm Hg, caused by cirrhosis of liver, thrombosis of portal vein.

Inferior Vena Cava

Formation: By union of right and left common iliac veins.
It pierces the diaphragm at the level of vertebra T8 and opens into lower and posterior part of right atrium.

Tributaries

- Common iliac veins (formed by union of external and internal iliac veins). Each vein receives an iliolumbar vein. The median sacral vein joins left common iliac vein.
- 3rd and 4th lumbar veins. 1st and 2nd lumbar veins may end in 3rd lumbar vein, ascending lumbar vein, azygos vein or hemiazygos vein.
- Right testicular or ovarian vein.
- Renal vein.
- Right suprarenal vein.
- Hepatic veins.

Applied anatomy

- Tumors of head of pancreas can press on IVC and cause obstruction.
- Obstruction due to thrombosis causes edema of lower extremities and back without ascites.

Common Iliac Veins

- They are formed by the union of external and internal iliac veins at the level of pelvic brim.
- They both unite to form the inferior vena cava.
- The internal iliac vein drains the pelvic organs, the perineum, greater part of gluteal region and the iliac fossa.
- The external iliac vein is a continuation of the femoral vein and drains the lower limb.

Veins of Head and Neck

Dural Venous Sinuses (Fig. 6.10)

- They are the venous spaces present between two layers of dura mater—endosteal and meningeal layers.
- The dural venous sinuses are classified as paired and unpaired venous sinuses.
- **Unpaired sinuses** are superior sagittal sinus, inferior sagittal sinus, straight sinus, occipital sinus, anterior and posterior intercavernous sinuses.
- **Paired sinuses** are cavernous sinuses, superior and inferior petrosal sinuses, transverse sinuses, sigmoid sinuses.
- **Superior sagittal sinus** lies in the upper convex part of the falx cerebri. It ends near the internal occipital protuberance posteriorly and drains into the right transverse sinus.
- **Inferior sagittal sinus** lies in the posterior part of the free margin of the falx cerebri. It ends by joining the great cerebral vein to form the straight sinus.
- **Straight sinus** lies in the junction of the falx cerebri with the tentorium cerebelli. It ends by continuing as the transverse sinus on the left side.
- **Transverse sinuses** are large sinuses situated on the posterior attached margins of the tentorium cerebelli. The right is a continuation of the superior sagittal sinus and the left one of the straight sinus.

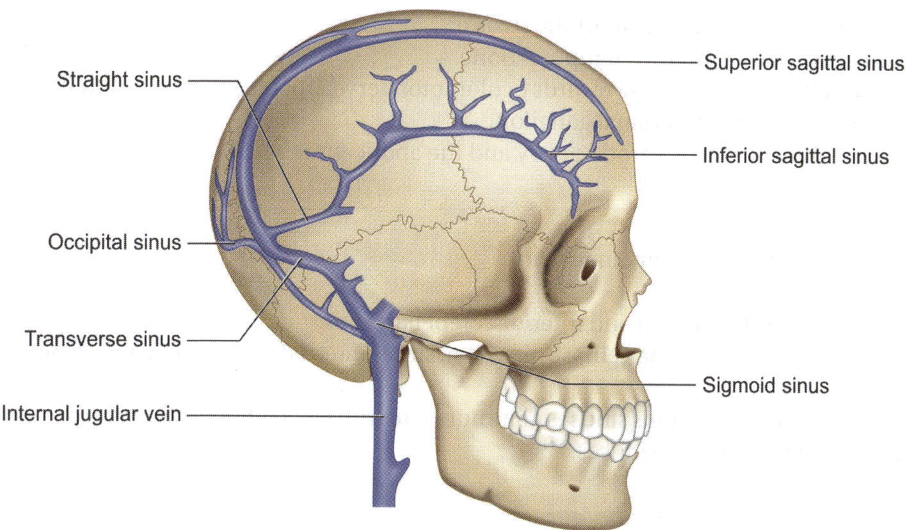

Fig. 6.10: Dural venous sinuses.

- **Sigmoid sinuses** are direct continuation of straight sinus on either side. Each sinus lies in the parietal bone and then becomes the superior bulb of the jugular vein.

Cavernous Sinus (Fig. 6.11)

Situation

Each cavernous sinus (right and left) is situated on either side of the body of sphenoid bone in the middle cranial fossa.

Relations

- **Floor:** Endosteal dura mater.
- **Roof, medial wall and lateral walls:** Meningeal layer of dura mater.

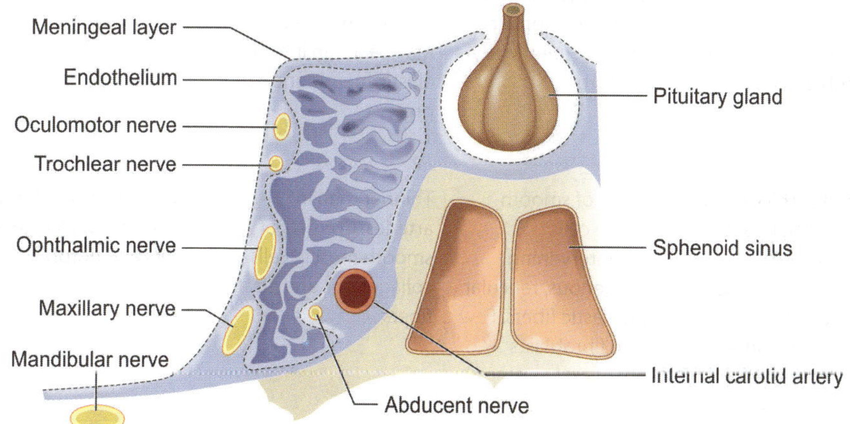

Fig. 6.11: Cavernous sinus.

- **Anterior:** Extends to superior orbital fissure.
- **Posteriorly:** Apex of petrous temporal bone.
- **Lateral wall:** From above downwards oculomotor nerve, trochlear nerve, ophthalmic nerve, maxillary nerve and trigeminal ganglion.
- **Through sinus:** Internal carotid artery and the abducent nerve.

Tributaries

- Superior and inferior ophthalmic veins.
- Central vein of retina.
- Superficial middle cerebral and inferior cerebellar veins.
- **It drains into the following veins:** Transverse sinus, internal jugular vein, pterygoid venous plexus, and facial vein.
- The right and left cavernous sinuses communicate with each other through the anterior and posterior intercavernous sinuses.

Histological Structure of Blood Vessels

- The entire blood vascular system is lined by single layer of flattened epithelium called as endothelium.
- **In all the vessels usually three layers are present. From within outwards:** Tunica intima (single layer of endothelial cells), tunica media (fibromuscular coat) and tunica adventitia (connective tissue with largely longitudinal arrangement).

The differences between arteries and veins are listed in Table 6.2.

Table 6.2: Differences between arteries and veins.

Large artery (Figs. 6.12A and B)	*Medium sized artery (Figs. 6.13A and B)*	*Medium sized vein (Fig. 6.14)*	*Large vein (Figs. 6.15A and B)*
Tunica intima: Thick, lining endothelium with basal lamina, subendothelial layer with CT having collagenous and elastic fibers and smooth muscle cells. Fibroblasts absent. Internal elastic lamina not distinct	Endothelial cells with basal lamina. Subendothelial CT sparse. Internal elastic membrane appears as well defined wavy structure	Endothelial cells with basal lamina. Small amount of subendothelial CT with smooth muscle cells. May be a thin internal elastic membrane present	Endothelial layer with basal lamina, small amount of subendothelial CT with smooth muscle cells
Tunica media: Thickest of three layers. Abundant elastic fibers with intervening smooth muscle cells, collagenous fibers and ground substance. Elastic fibers in the form of membranes	Mainly of smooth muscle cells with intervening collagenous, reticular and elastic fibers. Few or no fibroblasts	Thinner than in arteries. Consists of smooth muscle cells, collagenous and elastic fibers	Thin consisting of smooth muscle cells, collagenous fibers and fibroblasts

Contd...

Contd…

Large artery (Figs. 6.12A and B)	***Medium sized artery (Figs. 6.13A and B)***	***Medium sized vein (Fig. 6.14)***	***Large vein (Figs. 6.15A and B)***
Tunica adventitia: Less than half the thickness of tunica media. Mainly of collagenous fibers with loose network of elastic fibers. Fibroblasts and macrophages are present. Vasa vasorum seen	As thick as tunica media. Mainly collagenous fibers, concentrating adjacent to tunica media to form prominent external elastic lamina	Usually thicker than tunica media. Consists of bundles of smooth muscle cells and collagenous and elastic fibers	Thick consisting of longitudinally running smooth muscle cells, some fibroblasts, collagenous fibers and some elastic fibers. Vasa vasorum extends up to the tunica media
Lumen: Round, intact	Round, intact	Collapsed, irregular, larger lumen than artery	Collapsed, irregular, larger lumen than artery
For example: Aorta, pulmonary trunk	Radial, ulnar, tibial	Saphenous veins	Superior vena cava, inferior vena cava

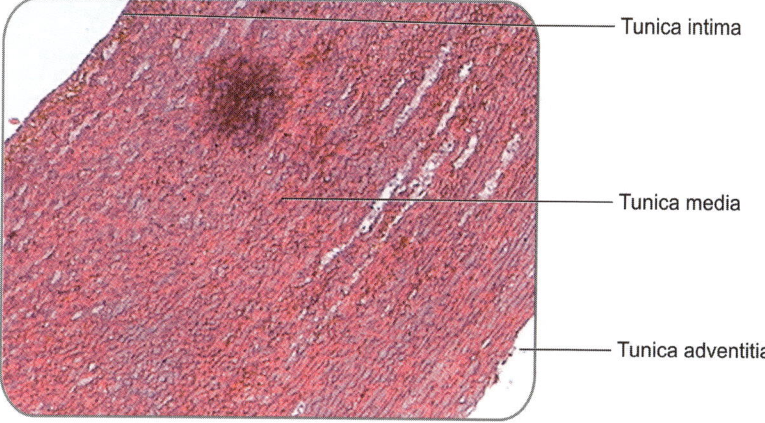

Fig. 6.12A: Photomicrograph of histology of elastic artery.

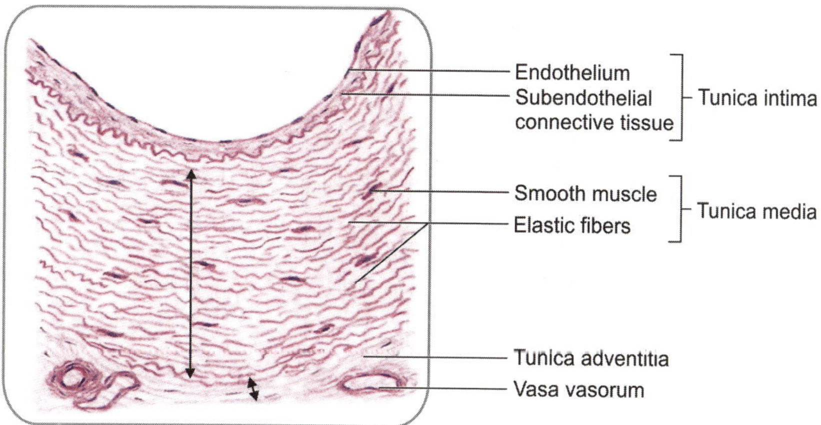

Fig. 6.12B: Diagrammatic representation of histology of elastic artery.

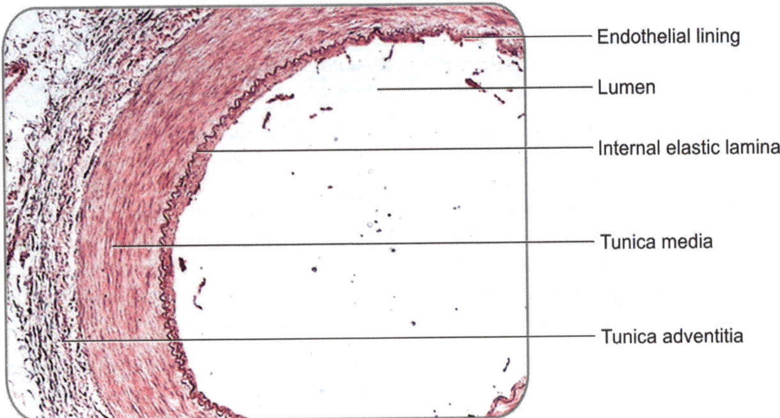

Fig. 6.13A: Photomicrograph of histology of medium sized artery.

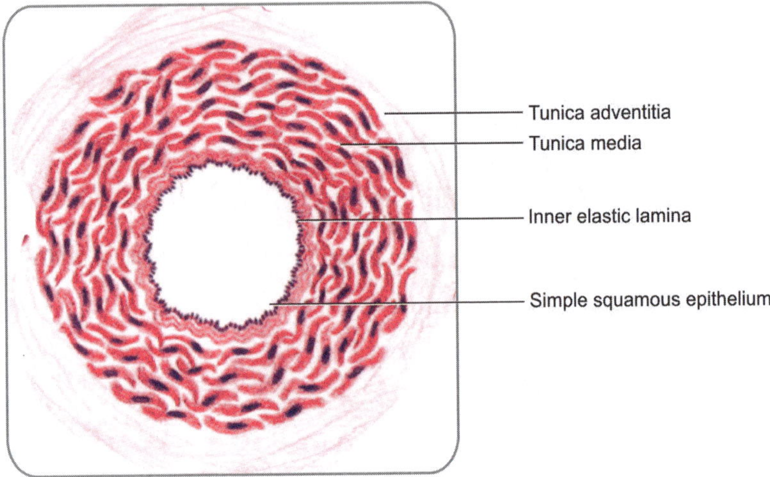

Fig. 6.13B: Diagrammatic representation of histology of medium sized artery.

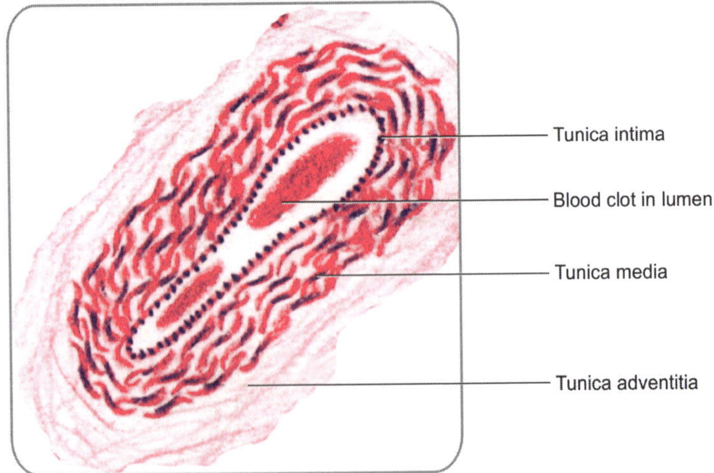

Fig. 6.14: Medium sized vein.

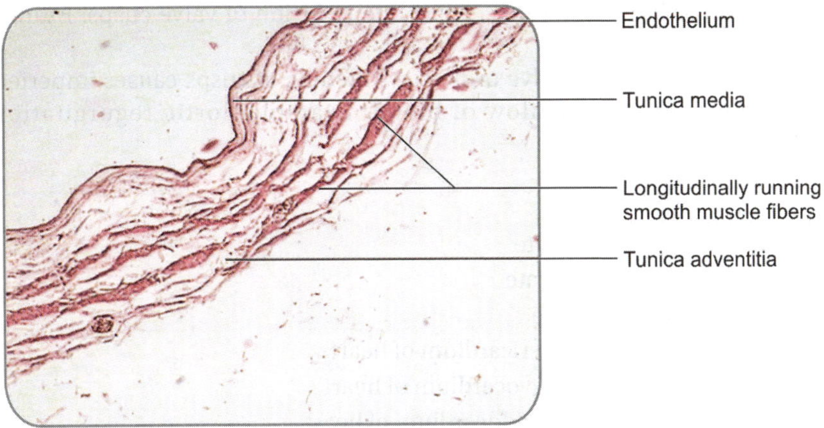

Fig. 6.15A: Photomicrograph of histology of large vein.

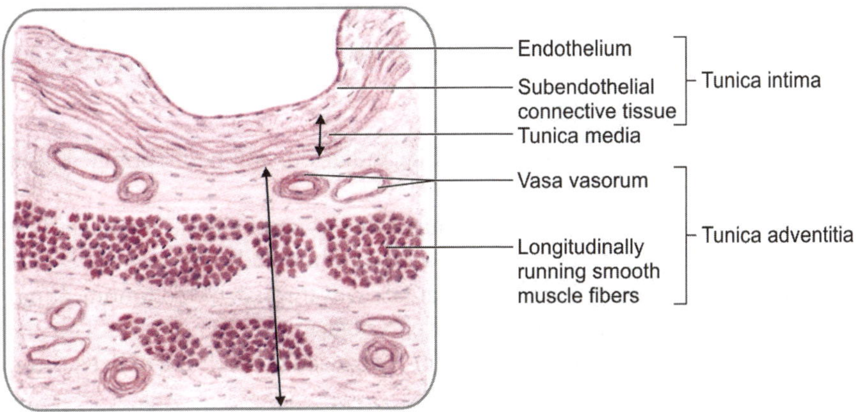

Fig. 6.15B: Diagrammatic representation of histology of large vein.

APPLIED ANATOMY

Mediastinum

- Infection in mediastinum may spread from one to another since the spaces between the organs are continuous with each other.
- **Mediastinal syndrome:** Tumor may lead to compression of adjacent structures. Pressure on the structures lead to following symptoms:
  - Trachea-dyspnea
  - Esophagus-dysphagia
  - Left recurrent laryngeal nerve-hoarseness of voice
  - Phrenic nerve-paralysis of diaphragm
  - Vertebral column-erosion of vertebral bodies

- Stenosis-narrowing of the valve orifice due to fusion of valve cusps. Example-mitral stenosis
- Regurgitation-dilation of valve orifice or stiffening of cusps causes imperfect closure of valves leading to backflow of blood. Example-aortic regurgitation, mitral regurgitation.

Heart

- **Tachycardia:** Increased heart rate
- **Bradycardia:** Decreased heart rate
- **Arrhythmia:** Irregular heart rate
- **Pericarditis:** Inflammation of pericardium of heart
- **Myocarditis:** Inflammation of myocardium of heart
- **Endocarditis:** Inflammation of endocardium of heart
- **Angina pectoris:** Partial obstructions in the coronary artery will lead to reduced blood supply to the heart and in turn severe pain in the chest radiating along ulnar border of left upper extremity.
- **Sudden cardiac arrest:** Complete obstruction of a branch of coronary artery by embolus or thrombus formation leads to sudden cardiac arrest.

Vessels

- Peripheral pulse can be felt at carotid, brachial, radial, dorsalis pedis, popliteal, and femoral arteries.
- Sudden occlusion of the popliteal artery may cause gangrene up to the knee. The artery is more prone to aneurysm than many other arteries of the body.
- Infection in the face can be transmitted to cranial cavity through the communicating channels between cavernous sinus and the external veins of face.
- **Portal hypertension:** Pressure above 40 mm Hg caused by cirrhosis of liver, thrombosis of portal vein.
- Tumors of head of pancreas can compress inferior vena cava and cause obstruction.

SUMMARY

- **Mediastinum:** Superior, middle, anterior and posterior mediastina
- **Pericardium:** Parietal, visceral layers and pericardial cavity
- **Heart:**
  - Apex, base/posterior surface, anterior/sternocostal surface, inferior/diaphragmatic surface, right margin, inferior margin, left margin, superior margin.
  - Four chambers right and left atria, right and left ventricles.
  - *Interior of right atrium:* Musculi pectinati, fossa ovalis, limbus fossa ovalis, openings of superior vena cava, inferior vena cava, coronary sinus, tricuspid opening, triangle of Koch.
  - *Blood supply:* Arteries right and left coronary arteries, vein coronary sinus.

Fetal Circulation

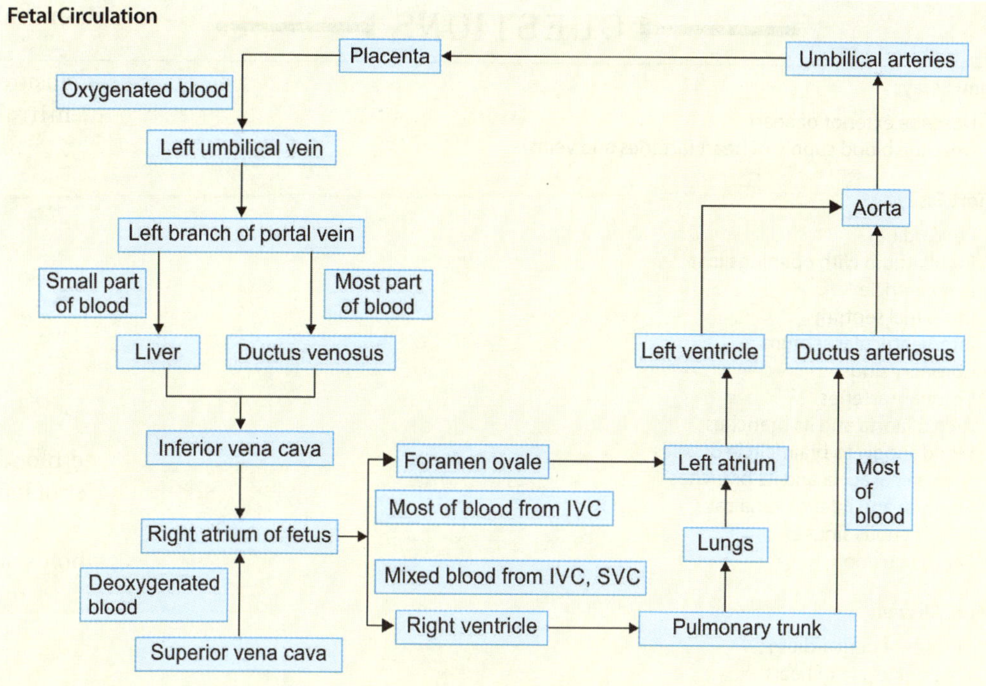

Arteries and Veins of the Body

Region	*Major arteries*	*Major veins*
Head and neck	Common carotid, external carotid, internal carotid, subclavian, vertebral	Facial, internal jugular, external jugular
Brain	Vertebral, circle of Willis, anterior cerebral, middle cerebral, posterior cerebral	Dural venous sinuses, cavernous sinus
Upper limb	Axillary, brachial, radial, ulnar, superficial palmar arch, deep palmar arch	Dorsal venous arch, basllic, cephalic, median cubital, axillary
Thorax	Ascending aorta, arch of aorta, descending thoracic aorta	Intercostal, azygos, hemiazygos, accessory hemiazygos, superior vena cava
Lower limb	Common iliac, internal iliac, external iliac, femoral, profunda femoris, popliteal, anterior tibial, posterior tibial, plantar arch	Dorsal venous arch, great saphenous, small saphenous, popliteal, femoral
Abdomen and pelvis	Abdominal aorta, celiac trunk, superior mesenteric, inferior mesenteric, internal iliac	Superior mesenteric, inferior mesenteric, portal, inferior vena cava, common iliac

QUESTIONS

Long Essays

- Describe exterior of heart.
- Describe blood supply of heart (arteries and veins).

Short Essays

- Pericardium
- Right atrium with openings in it
- Left ventricle
- Interatrial septum
- Interventricular septum
- Coronary sinus
- Coronary arteries
- Arch of aorta and its branches
- Blood supply to brain/circle of Willis
- Abdominal aorta and its branches
- Superior and inferior vena cava
- Dural venous sinuses
- Fetal circulation.

Short Answers

- Sinuses of pericardium
- Foramen ovale of heart
- Name the valves of the heart
- Branches of external carotid artery
- Branches of subclavian artery
- Branches of axillary artery
- Superficial palmar arch
- Branches of femoral artery
- Popliteal artery
- Dorsalis pedis artery
- Median cubital vein
- Cephalic and basilic vein
- Peripheral pulses
- Portal vein
- Great saphenous vein

CHAPTER 7

Respiratory System

LEARNING OBJECTIVES

The student should be able to:

- Name the parts of respiratory system, describe in detail about nasal cavity (septum and lateral wall), olfactory pathway, paranasal air sinuses, larynx, trachea, lungs—differences between left and right lungs, bronchopulmonary segments.
- Describe pleura and its layers.
- Give the names of paranasal air sinuses.

INTRODUCTION

Parts of respiratory system are nose, paranasal air sinuses, nasopharynx, larynx, trachea, bronchi and lungs.

NASAL CAVITY

- It is pyramidal in shape and is divided into two halves by a septum.
- The two halves open on the face through anterior nasal apertures and posteriorly into nasopharynx, through posterior nasal apertures.
- Each half has a roof, floor, lateral wall and medial wall (septum).

Septum (Fig. 7.1)

- It has a posterior bony part formed by perpendicular plate of ethmoid bone and vomer and an anterior cartilaginous part.
- Roof is formed by cribriform plate of ethmoid which transmits olfactory nerve filaments to anterior cranial fossa.
- Floor is formed by maxilla and palatine bone.
- 90% of nasal bleeding (epistaxis) occurs from anteroinferior part of nasal septum.

Blood Supply

Arterial supply: The nasal septum is supplied by the following arteries:

- Anterosuperiorly by the anterior ethmoidal artery—branch of ophthalmic artery.
- Posteroinferiorly by the saphenopalatine and greater palatine branches of the maxillary artery.

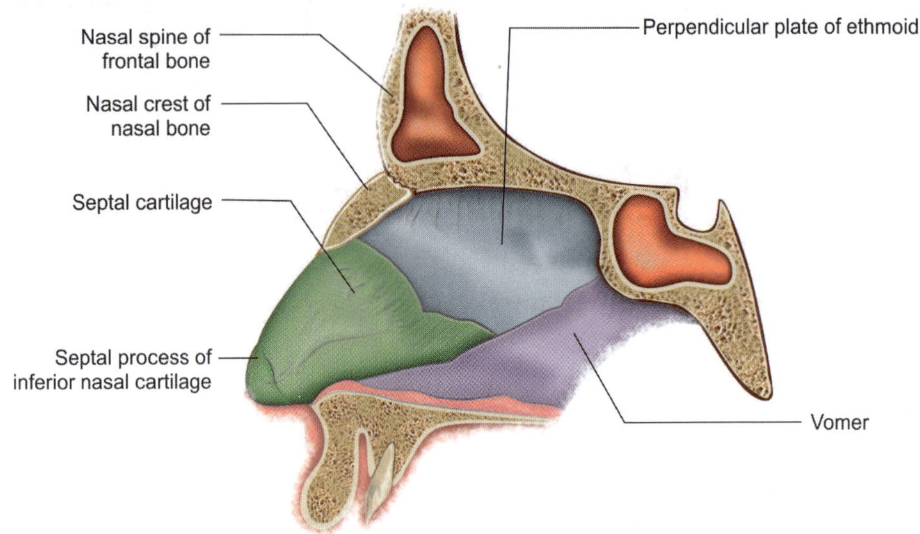

Fig. 7.1: Formation of nasal septum.

- Mobile part of the septum by the superior labial branch of facial artery.
- Anteroinferior part is a highly vascular area, where septal branch of the facial, sphenopalatine and terminal branches of greater palatine arteries anastomose. This area is known as Little's area or Kiesselbach's area where epistaxis due to a small ulcer can lead to profuse arterial hemorrhage.

Venous drainage

The veins drain into the superior ophthalmic, pterygoid venous plexus and the facial vein.

Lateral Wall of the Nose (Fig. 7.2)

- The following bones contribute to form the lateral wall of the nasal cavity. They are nasal, frontal process of maxilla, lacrimal, middle and superior nasal conchae of the labyrinth of ethmoid, inferior concha, perpendicular plate of the palatine and the medial pterygoid plate of the sphenoid.
- The bony wall is covered by mucous membrane and projects medially as curved plates of three nasal conchae, superior, middle and inferior concha. The superior and the middle are parts of the ethmoid labyrinth. The inferior concha is a separate bone.
- There are 3 meatuses (spaces) between these conchae; they are the superior, middle and the inferior meatuses. The space under cover of the superior concha is known as superior meatus into which posterior ethmoidal sinus open.
- Above and behind the superior concha lies a depression, the supreme meatus the sphenoethmoidal recess, this receives the opening of the sphenoidal sinus.
- The space under cover of the middle concha forms the middle meatus, which receives the openings of the following paranasal sinuses—maxillary, frontal, anterior and middle ethmoidal air sinuses.

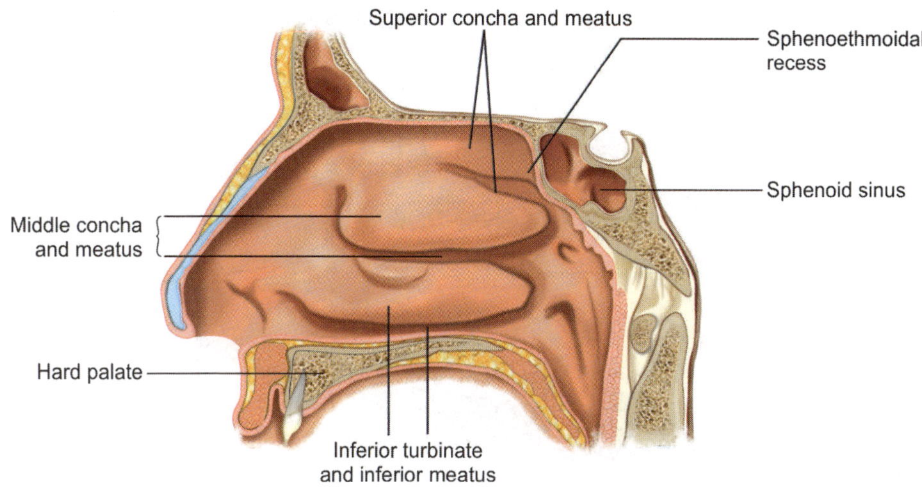

Fig. 7.2: Lateral wall of nose.

- The inferior meatus is the space under cover of the inferior concha which receives the opening of the nasolacrimal duct.

Blood Supply

Arterial supply

The lateral wall of the nose is supplied by branches of ophthalmic, maxillary and facial arteries.

Venous drainage

Veins drain into facial, retropharyngeal and pterygoid venous plexus.

PARANASAL AIR SINUSES (FIG. 7.3)

- They are air-filled spaces lined by mucous membrane present around and communicate with the nasal cavity.
- These are pairs of maxillary, ethmoidal, frontal, sphenoidal sinuses.

Maxillary Air Sinuses

- They are the largest of the air sinuses, situated in the body of the maxilla on other side.
- Each sinus resembles a pyramid with an apex directed laterally and base medially.
- It opens into the hiatus semilunaris in the middle meatus of the nose. The opening is at a higher level than the floor of the sinus. Hence fluids tend to collect in the sinus and can be drained into the nasal cavity by tilting the head to one side (postural drainage) or by surgical puncture.
- **Blood supply:** Branches of maxillary artery, infraorbital artery.
- **Nerve supply:** Branches of maxillary nerve, infraorbital nerve.

Frontal Sinus

- Lies in the frontal bone deep to the superciliary arch.

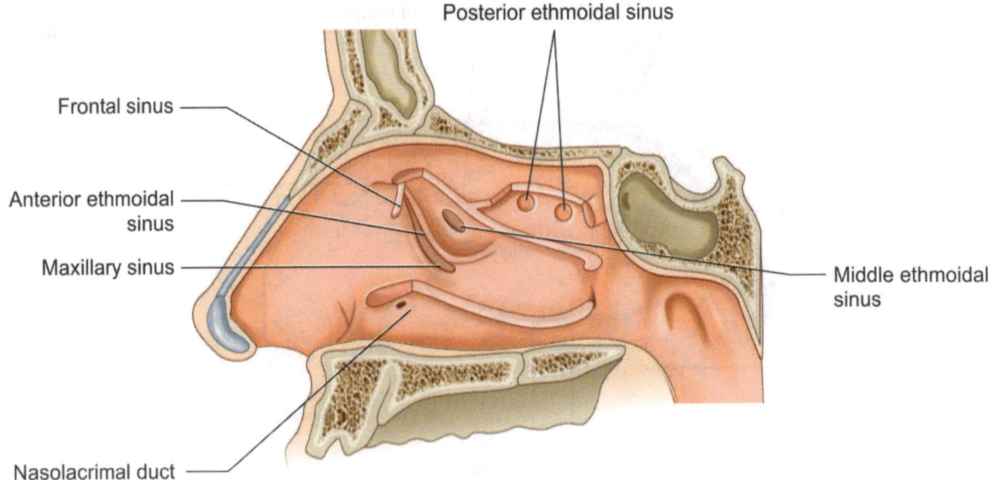

Fig. 7.3: Openings of the paranasal air sinuses.

- It opens into the middle meatus of the nose at the anterior end of the hiatus semilunaris through the infundibulum.
- It is absent at birth and well developed by 7–8 years of life. It is supplied by the supraorbital artery and vein and the supraorbital nerve.

Sphenoidal Sinuses

- Lie within the body of the sphenoidal bone and are usually separated by a septum.
- Each sinus opens into the sphenoethmoidal recess on the supreme meatus of the nasal cavity.
- They are supplied by the posterior ethmoidal arteries and nerves.

Ethmoidal Sinuses

- They are numerous intercommunicating spaces that lie in the ethmoid bone.
- They are divided into the anterior, middle and the posterior groups.
- The anterior ethmoidal sinus opens into the hiatus semilunaris and is supplied by the anterior ethmoidal nerves and vessels.
- The middle ethmoidal sinus opens into the middle meatus of the nose and is supplied by the posterior ethmoidal nerve and vessels.
- The posterior ethmoidal sinus opens into the superior meatus and is supplied by the posterior ethmoidal nerve and vessels.

Nasopharynx is dealt with in the Chapter: Gastrointestinal Tract.

LARYNX

- Larynx is the voice box and also serves as an air passage.
- **Extent:** From root of tongue to the commencement of trachea, i.e. opposite to 3rd to 6th cervical vertebra in adults.
- **Cartilages:** Unpaired: Thyroid, cricoid and epiglottis; Paired: Arytenoids, corniculate and cuneiform.
- **Muscles:** Cricothyroid, posterior and lateral cricoarytenoid, transverse oblique arytenoideus, aryepiglotticus, thyroarytenoideus, vocalis, and thyroepiglotticus.

- **Two pairs of folds project into the cavity from the lateral walls:** The upper vestibular and the lower vocal folds/vocal cords.
- **Blood supply:** Superior laryngeal branch of superior thyroid artery, inferior laryngeal branch of inferior thyroid artery.
- **Lymphatic drainage:** Above the level of vocal folds, to upper deep cervical, below to prelaryngeal and pretracheal nodes.
- **Nerve supply:** Motor: All muscles except cricothyroid by recurrent laryngeal, cricothyroid by external laryngeal nerve; Sensory: Mucosa above vocal folds by internal laryngeal, below the vocal folds by recurrent laryngeal nerve.

TRACHEA

- It is the windpipe which serves to conduct air to both lungs for respiration.
- It continues from larynx at the level of C6 and ends by dividing into right and left principal bronchi at the lower border of T6 in the living.
- **Blood supply:** Inferior thyroid arteries and veins.
- **Lymphatics:** Paratracheal and pretracheal nodes.
- **Nerve supply:** Parasympathetic from vagus and recurrent laryngeal nerve, sympathetic from middle and lower cervical sympathetic trunk.
- **Microscopic structure (Figs. 7.4A and B):** Mucous membrane: (1) epithelial layer lined by pseudostratified ciliated columnar epithelium with numerous goblet cells, (2) lamina propria rich in longitudinal elastin fibers, (3) submucous coat with loose irregular connective tissue containing blood vessels, nerves and seromucous glands; fibrocartilaginous layer: Anterior 2/3rds of trachea has C-shaped hyaline cartilages (16–20) and posteriorly the gap is filled by fibromuscular layer which contains smooth muscle fibers called trachealis. It allows expansion of esophagus during passage of food.

Pleura

- Each lung is present in the pleural cavity covered by pleura, a fibroserous membrane.
- Pleura is a completely closed serous sac which is invaginated from medial side by developing lung and so is converted into a double layered sac, an outer parietal and an inner visceral layer.

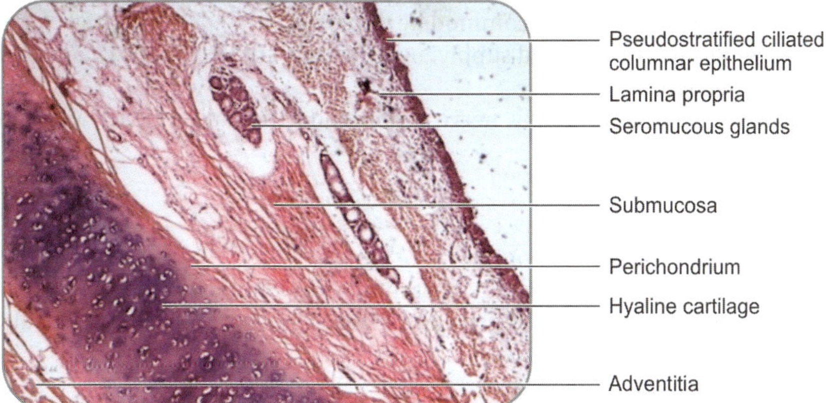

Fig. 7.4A: Photomicrograph of histology of trachea.

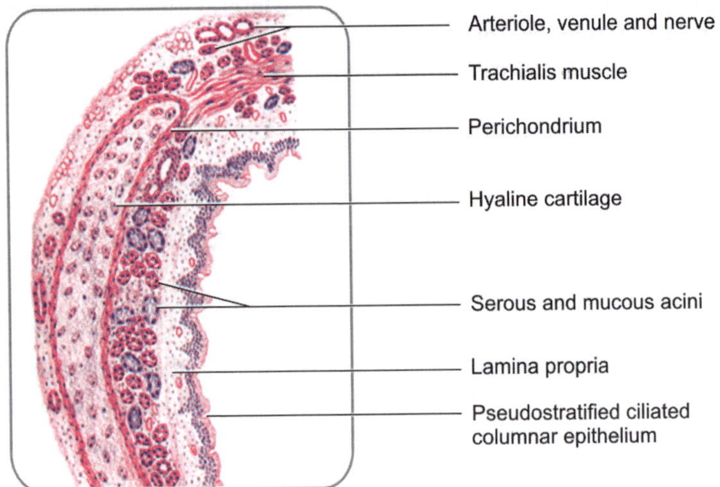

Fig. 7.4B: Diagrammatic representation of histology of trachea.

- Outer parietal layer lines the inner walls of the cavity in which the lung lies. It is divided into diaphragmatic pleura, costal pleura, mediastinal pleura and cervical pleura depending on the region which it lines.
- Inner pulmonary or visceral pleura is very closely adherent to the surface of the lung, dips into its fissures and is responsible for the shiny appearance of the surface of the lung.
- Inner and outer layers are in contact with each other and potential space between them is called pleural cavity, which is filled with a thin film of lymph-like fluid. This fluid serves to lubricate adjoining surfaces of the pleural membrane and prevents friction during movements of the lung.
- Parietal and visceral layers are continuous with each other along the sheath which covers the root of lung and also along the layers of pulmonary ligament.
- Pulmonary ligament is a triangular fold stretching below the root of lung as far down as diaphragm between the lung and mediastinum.
- Pulmonary ligament serves to accommodate the engorged veins during high venous return.
- Parietal layer has the same blood supply, nerve supply and lymphatic drainage as the wall to which it is related.
- Visceral layer has its blood supply, nerve supply and lymphatic drainage as the lung which it covers.

LUNGS (FIG. 7.5)

- Lungs are paired organs of respiration.
- **Situation:** One on each side of the mediastinum within thoracic cavity.
- **Shape:** Resembles a half cone having an apex; a base; 2 surfaces: Medial and lateral; 3 borders: Anterior, inferior and posterior.
- **Size:** Right lung is broader than left.
- **Right lung has 3 lobes:** Upper, middle and lower; 2 fissures: Oblique and horizontal.
- **Left lung has 2 lobes:** Upper and lower; one oblique fissure.

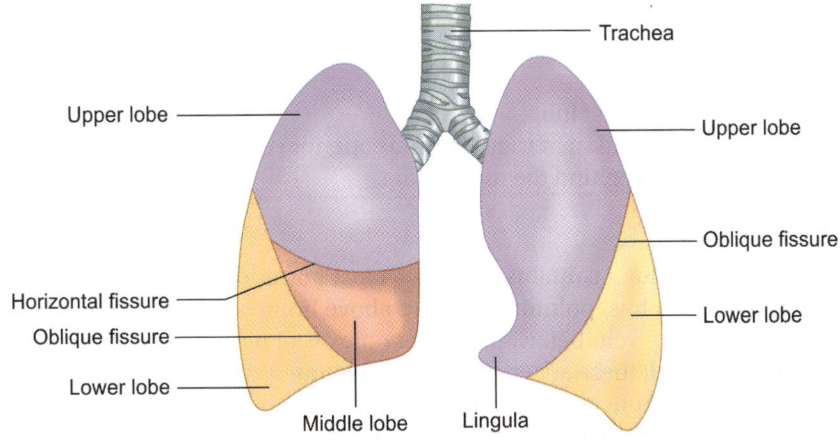

Fig. 7.5: Lobes of right and left lung.

- Apex of lung projects into the root of neck above the level of 1st rib.
- Base is concave and is related to the convex dome of diaphragm (diaphragmatic surface).
- Lateral or costal surface is convex and is related to ribs.
- Medial surface is divided into vertebral surface (related to thoracic vertebrae) and mediastinal surface which has different relations in left and right side.

Right Lung (Fig. 7.6)

- Cut end of root of right lung presents eparterial and hyparterial bronchi most posteriorly, bronchial arteries on the posterior wall of the bronchi, pulmonary artery in front and between the two bronchi, upper pulmonary vein in front, lower pulmonary vein below, pulmonary plexus of nerves around the root, hilar lymph nodes. All these are enclosed by a layer of pleura.
- Cardiac impression in front and below the root.
- Right phrenic nerve and pericardiophrenic vessels.

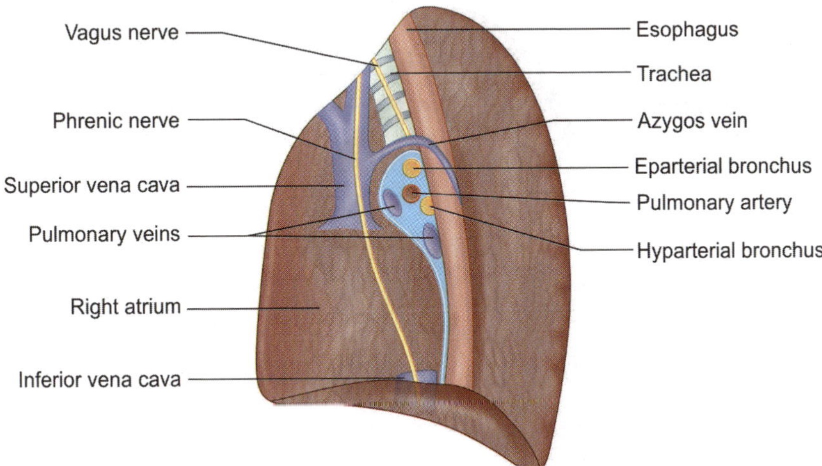

Fig. 7.6: Relations of right lung.

- Superior vena cava and lower part of right brachiocephalic vein.
- Ascending aorta and remains of thymus in front of the above.
- Inferior vena cava.
- Azygos arch above the root of lung.
- Right surface of trachea and right vagus behind superior vena cava.
- Right edge of esophagus behind the root of lung.

Left Lung (Fig. 7.7)

- Cut end of root of left lung contains bronchus most posteriorly, bronchial arteries on the posterior wall of bronchus, pulmonary artery above bronchus, upper pulmonary vein in front, lower pulmonary vein below, pulmonary plexus of nerves around the structures in the root, hilar nodes. All these are ensheathed by pleura.
- Cardiac impression in front and below the root.
- Left phrenic nerve and pericardiophrenic vessels.
- Arch of aorta makes an impression above the root and descending aorta behind the root.
- Left subclavian artery and left common carotid artery.
- Left vagus between the two arterial grooves.
- Left edge of esophagus and thoracic duct behind groove for left subclavian artery and just behind lower end of pulmonary ligament.
- Left brachiocephalic vein in front of groove for subclavian artery.

Bronchopulmonary Segments (Fig. 7.8 and Table 7.1)

- Each bronchus, on entering the hilum divides into primary, secondary and tertiary/segmental bronchi.
- Each segmental bronchus and accompanying division of pulmonary artery supply a definite part of the lung called as bronchopulmonary segment.
- The radicals of pulmonary veins are not segmental, but are intersegmental in position and function.

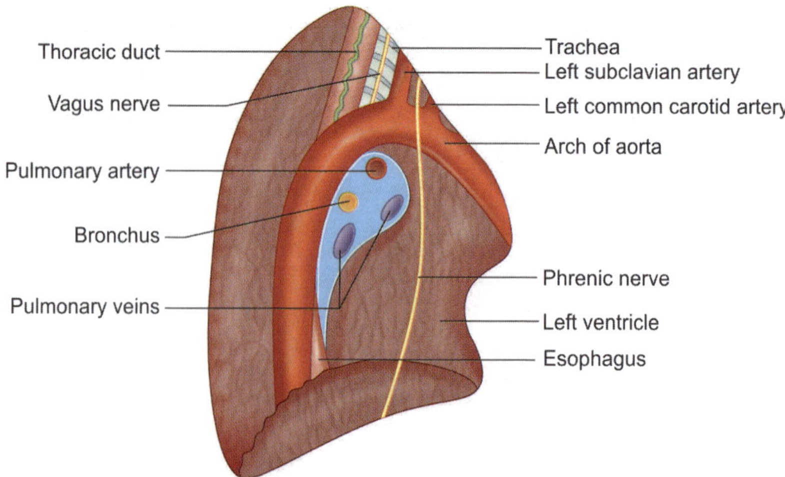

Fig. 7.7: Relations of left lung.

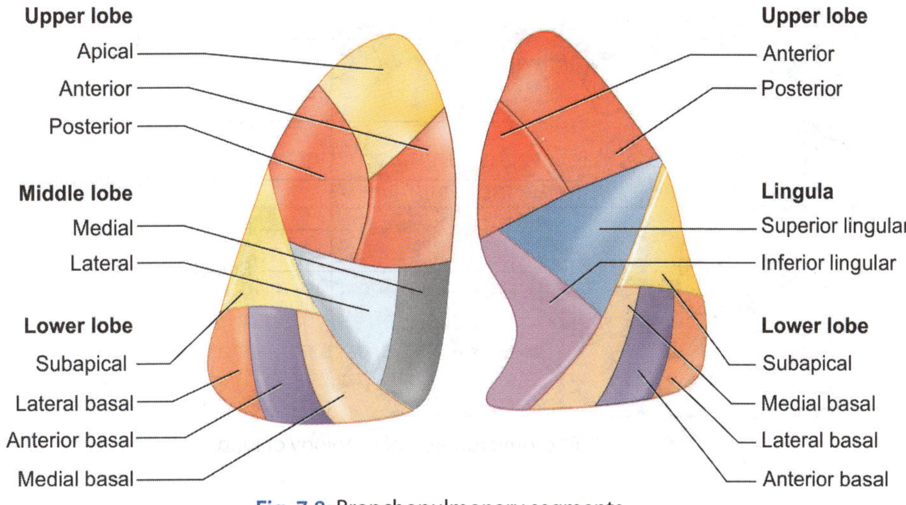

Fig. 7.8: Bronchopulmonary segments.

Table 7.1: Bronchopulmonary segments.

Lobe	*Name of bronchopulmonary segments*	
	Right lung	*Left lung*
Upper	• Apical • Anterior • Posterior	• Apicoposterior • Anterior • Posterior
Middle	• Medial • Lateral	• Superior lingular • Inferior lingular
Lower	• Subapical • Anterior basal • Posterior basal • Medial basal • Lateral basal	• Subapical • Anterior basal • Posterior basal • Medial basal • Lateral basal

Blood Supply

Pulmonary artery and veins, bronchial artery.

BRONCHIAL TREE

Trachea → right and left principal (primary) bronchi → intrapulmonary (secondary) bronchi → segmental (tertiary) bronchi → bronchiole → terminal bronchiole → respiratory bronchiole → alveolar duct → atria → air saccules. The alveolar duct, atria, air saccules are studded with alveoli.

Structure (Figs. 7.9A and B)

- Each lung is covered by serous coat which consists of mesothelium and lamina propria. The connective tissue extends into the lungs and separates into lobules.
- Each lobule is a small polyhedral mass of lung tissue with a bronchiole surrounded by alveoli, terminal ramification of pulmonary arteriole and venule, lymphatics and nerves.
- The alveoli are thin walled pouches. The wall of each alveolus is composed of a thin epithelial lining supported by a basement membrane.

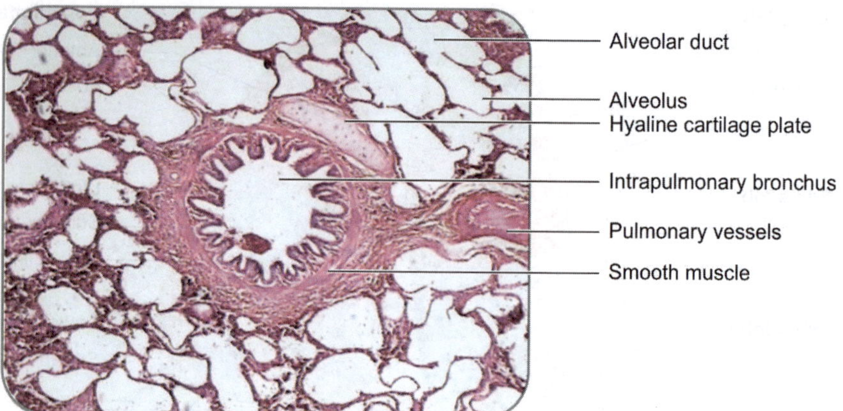

Fig. 7.9A: Photomicrograph of histology of lung.

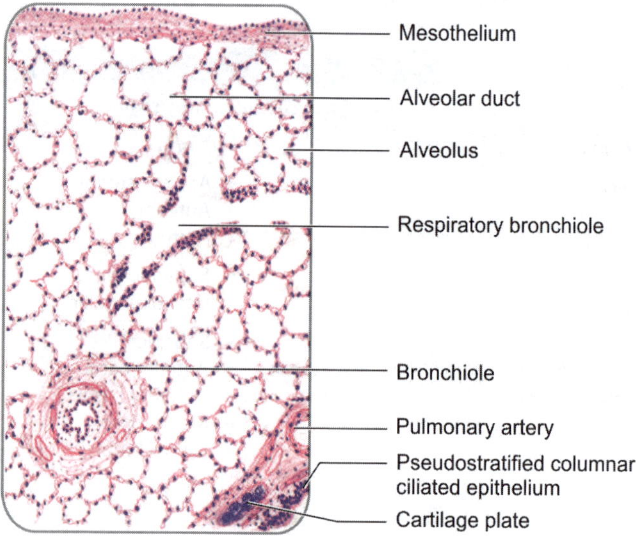

Fig. 7.9B: Diagrammatic representation of histology of lung.

- The walls of adjacent alveoli are separated from each other by a thin irregular lamina of connective tissue and its contained blood vessels forming an interalveolar septum.
- The connective tissue of the interalveolar septa is composed of fibroblasts, mesenchymal cells, macrophages and a loose matrix containing blood capillaries and lymphatics; widely dispersed elastin fibers, numerous fine reticulin fibers and nongranular leukocytes.
- The epithelium includes cells supported by basement membrane, squamous cells (type 1 pneumocytes), secretory cells (type 2 pneumocytes) and alveolar phagocytes.
- The secretory cells secrete fluid which spreads over the squamous cells and acts as surfactant by reducing surface tension. This prevents the collapse of alveoli during expiration.
- **Blood-air barrier:** Flattened epithelium of alveoli; basement membrane of alveoli; basement of underlying capillary; cells lining the capillary.

DIAPHRAGM (FIG. 7.10)

It is a dome-shaped musculoaponeurotic partition which intervenes between the thorax and the abdomen. The thoracic surface is convex on the right and left sides, and is depressed in the middle; the summits of the convexities are known as cupolae. The right cupola is slightly higher than the left one due to presence of the liver.

The peripheral part of the diaphragm is muscular (striated) and the central part is tendinous which is occupied by the central tendon.

Origin: It arises from the oblique circumference of the inner surface of the thoracic outlet and the origins are arranged in three groups—sternal, costal and vertebral (lumbar).

Sternal: By two fleshy slips from the back of the xiphoid process.

Costal: From the inner surface of the lower six ribs and their costal cartilages interdigitating with the transversus abdominis.

Vertebral: On either side, it arises from two crurae; a right crus that takes origin from the front of bodies of first three lumbar vertebrae, a left crus that takes origin from the front of bodies of first two lumbar vertebrae; a pair of medial arcuate ligaments; and a pair of lateral arcuate ligaments.

Insertion: All fibers are inserted into the central tendon. It is shaped like 3 leaflets presenting median, right and left leaflets. At the junction of the median and right leaflets it presents the vena caval opening, and to the left of that opening it presents a central point of decussation from which four diagonal bands radiate.

Openings of Diaphragm

Major openings and structures passing through:

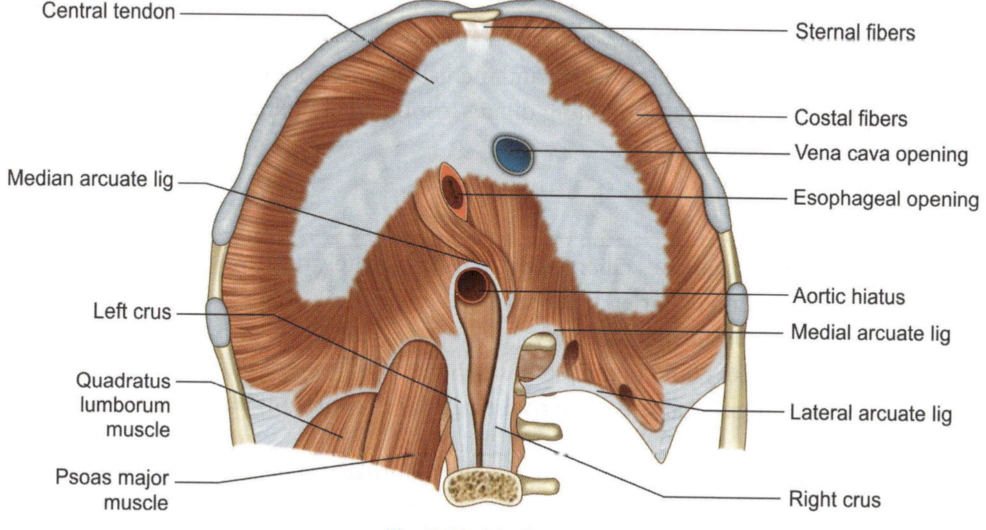

Fig. 7.10: Diaphragm.

Vena Caval Opening

- IVC
- A few branches of right phrenic nerve
- A few lymph vessels from liver

Esophageal Opening

- Esophagus
- Anterior and posterior vagal trunks
- Esophageal branches of the left gastric artery and the corresponding tributaries of the left gastric vein
- Lymphatics from liver
- Phrenoesophageal ligament

Aortic Opening

- Abdominal aorta
- Thoracic duct
- Azygos vein

Nerve Supply

Motor: Phrenic nerve (C3,4,5), sensory: Phrenic nerves, lower 6 or 7 intercostal nerves, sympathetic: Celiac plexus via inferior phrenic plexus.

Blood supply: Musculophrenic and pericardiophrenic arteries (branches of internal thoracic artery), lower 5 or 6 posterior intercostal arteries, superior phrenic artery (last branch of descending thoracic aorta), inferior phrenic artery (first branch of abdominal aorta). Veins correspond with the arteries and drain into systemic veins.

Actions

- It is the principal muscle of inspiration.
- It is a compressor of abdominal viscera and increases intra-abdominal pressure.
- During inspiration vena caval opening dilates, esophageal opening constricts and aortic opening undergoes no change.

APPLIED ANATOMY

- **Sinusitis:** Smoking diminishes ciliary activity and ultimately destroys cilia.
- **Pleuritis:** Inflammation of parietal pleura.
- **Pneumothorax:** Air in the pleural cavity.
- **Pleural effusion:** Excess fluid in the pleural cavity.
- **Foramen of Morgagni:** Failure of sternal origin of diaphragm; abdominal viscera may herniate to thorax.
- **Bochdalek's triangle:** Triangular gap formed by failure of origin of diaphragm from lateral arcuate ligament; abdominal viscera may herniate to thorax.

SUMMARY

Paranasal air sinuses:

- Maxillary, frontal, sphenoidal and ethmoidal.

Trachea:

- Extends from larynx to principal bronchi.
- Wall has 4 layers from inside out-mucous membrane with epithelium (pseudostratified ciliated columnar) and lamina propria (connective tissue), submucosa (connective tissue, blood vessels, nerves, seromucous glands), fibromusculocartilaginous layer (fibrous tissue, C-shaped hyaline cartilage, trachealis smooth muscle) and adventitia (connective tissue).

Lungs: Differences between right and left lung

Features	*Right lung*	*Left lung*
Size	Broad, short	Narrow, long
Lobes	3 (upper, middle, lower)	2 (upper, lower)
Fissures	2 (oblique, horizontal)	1 (oblique)
Anterior border	Straight	Presents cardiac notch, lingula
Hilar structures	• 2 bronchi (eparterial, hyparterial) • Pulmonary artery • Superior and inferior pulmonary vein • Pulmonary plexus of nerves • Lymph nodes	• 1 bronchus • Pulmonary artery • Superior and inferior pulmonary vein • Pulmonary plexus of nerves • Lymph nodes
Visceral impressions	Cardiac, right phrenic nerve, superior vena cava, right brachiocephalic vein, ascending aorta, inferior vena cava, azygos vein, trachea, esophagus	Cardiac, left phrenic nerve, arch of aorta, descending aorta, left subclavian artery, left common carotid artery, left vagus, esophagus, left brachiocephalic vein

Diaphragm:

- Origin: Posterior surface of xiphoid process, inner surface of lower 6 ribs, bodies of upper 3 lumbar vertebrae on right and upper 2 on left side
- Insertion: Central tendon
- Nerve supply: Phrenic nerve
- Action: Principal muscle of inspiration, increases intra-abdominal pressure; major openings: Vena caval, esophageal, aortic

QUESTIONS

Long Essay

- Name the parts of respiratory system. Describe lungs in detail.

Short Essays

- Paranasal air sinuses
- Nasal septum
- Lateral wall of nasal cavity
- Trachea—gross and histology
- Differences between right and left lungs
- Bronchopulmonary segments
- Pleura

CHAPTER

Digestive System

LEARNING OBJECTIVES

The student should be able to:

- Describe the peritoneum and its reflections.
- Name the parts of digestive system, describe salivary glands, tonsil, tongue, palate, pharynx, stomach, intestines (duodenum, jejunum, ileum, cecum, appendix, colon), liver, gallbladder, pancreas, spleen—gross and histology.

INTRODUCTION

- The gastrointestinal tract (GIT) is concerned with mastication, deglutition, digestion and absorption of food and elimination of waste products from the body.
- It extends from mouth to anus where in both regions it becomes continuous with epidermis of skin.
- Parts of GIT are mouth, pharynx, esophagus, stomach, small intestine, large intestine and associated glands. The associated glands are salivary glands (parotid, submandibular, sublingual), liver, gallbladder and pancreas.

PERITONEUM

- A large serous membrane (made up of mesothelial cells) lining abdominal cavity.
- It is in the form of a closed sac, which is invaginated by many viscera.
- Visceral peritoneum (lines the external part of the organ).
- Parietal peritoneum (lines the body wall).
- Peritoneal cavity contains serous fluid (reduces friction and enables digestive organs to have freedom of movement).
- It has been named differently with different organs.
- **Peritoneal folds:** Greater and lesser omentum (lining stomach), the mesentery (lining jejunum and ileum), mesoappendix (lining appendix), transverse and sigmoid mesocolon (lining transverse and sigmoid colon).
- **Peritoneal cavity:** The cavity is divided into two main parts. The larger part is called greater sac and the smaller part which is situated behind the stomach and lesser omentum is called lesser sac. Greater and lesser sacs communicated by epiploic foramen (of Winslow), subphrenic spaces, hepatorenal pouch (of Morisson), rectouterine pouch (of Douglas).

- There are certain organs that are covered by peritoneum only on the anterior surface. These are called retroperitoneal organs: Pancreas, duodenum and parts of large intestine, kidneys and suprarenal glands.

MOUTH

- Mouth is divided into vestibule, the outer smaller portion present between lips, cheeks externally and gums, teeth internally and mouth proper, the inner larger portion present between the teeth, gums and alveolar arches anterolaterally; hard palate above and dorsum of tongue below.
- Mouth consists of lips, cheeks, teeth, hard palate, soft palate and tongue.
- Teeth are a part of masticatory apparatus which are fixed to jaws. It is replaced only once between 6 and 12 years. The first set is known as milk or deciduous teeth (20 in number) and the second set as permanent teeth (32 in number: 8 incisors, 4 canines, 8 premolars, 12 molars).
- Hard palate is a partition between the oral cavity below and nasal cavity above. It is formed by palatine process of maxilla and horizontal process of palatine bone. The posterior margin is continuous with soft palate.

Teeth (Fig. 8.1)

- **Three parts:** Crown that projects upwards from gum, root that is embedded in the gum and neck that is between the crown and root. Each crown has a central pulp cavity that has the nerves and blood supply to the tooth. This is covered by dentin and then the enamel that is the hardest part of the tooth. The root is covered by a similar structure called cementum. The tooth is covered by a periodontal membrane that attaches it to the gum.
- **Eruption of deciduous teeth is as follows:**
  - Lower jaw teeth erupt earlier than upper jaw.
  - *Central incisor:* 7 months
  - *Lateral incisor:* 8–9 months
  - *1st molar:* 1 year

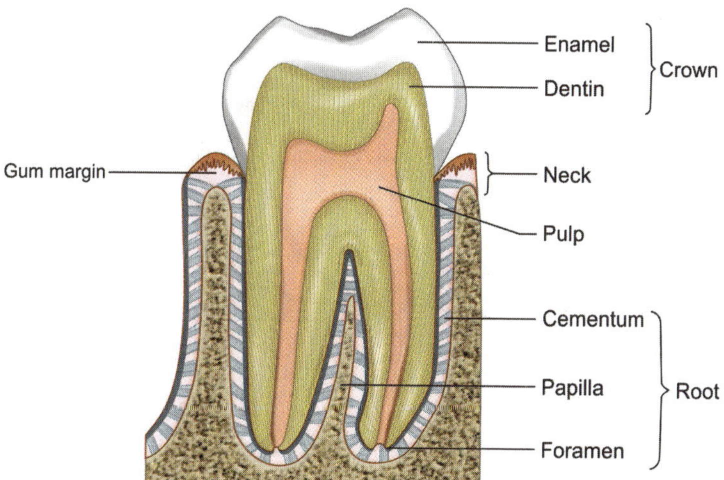

Fig. 8.1: Parts of tooth.

- *Canine:* 18 months
- *2nd molar:* 2 years.

- **Eruption of permanent teeth is as follows:**
  - *1st molar:* 6 years
  - *Medial incisor:* 7 years
  - *Lateral incisor:* 8 years
  - *1st premolar:* 9 years
  - *2nd premolar:* 10 years
  - *Canine:* 11 years
  - *2nd molar:* 12 years
  - *3rd molar:* 17–25 years (or later).

Soft Palate (Fig. 8.2)

- It is a movable muscular fold, suspended from the posterior border of the hard palate. It separates nasopharynx from oropharynx.
- The muscles forming soft palate are tensor palati, levator palati, musculus uvulae, palatoglossus and palatopharyngeus.
- **Blood supply:** Greater palatine branch of maxillary, palatine branch of ascending pharyngeal, ascending palatine of facial, tonsillar branch of lingual arteries. Veins drain into pterygoid plexus and pharyngeal plexus of veins.
- **Lymphatics:** Upper deep cervical, retropharyngeal nodes.
- **Nerve supply:** The muscles are supplied by cranial part of accessory nerve except tensor palati supplied by mandibular nerve. General sensory from greater, lesser, middle palatine, nasopalatine, tonsillar branch of glossopharyngeal. Secretomotor fibers come from facial nerve through branches of pterygopalatine ganglion. Taste fibers from lesser palatine nerves.

Tongue (Fig. 8.3)

- Tongue is a muscular organ situated in the floor of the mouth.
- Functions—taste, speech, mastication and deglutition.

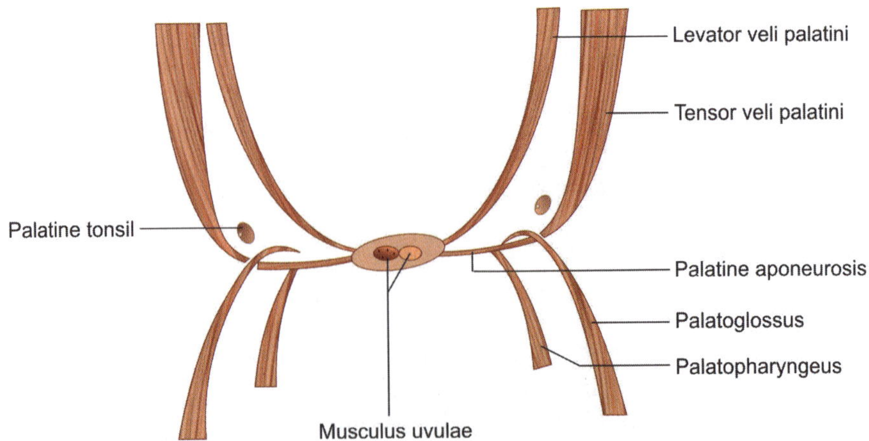

Fig. 8.2: Muscles of soft palate.

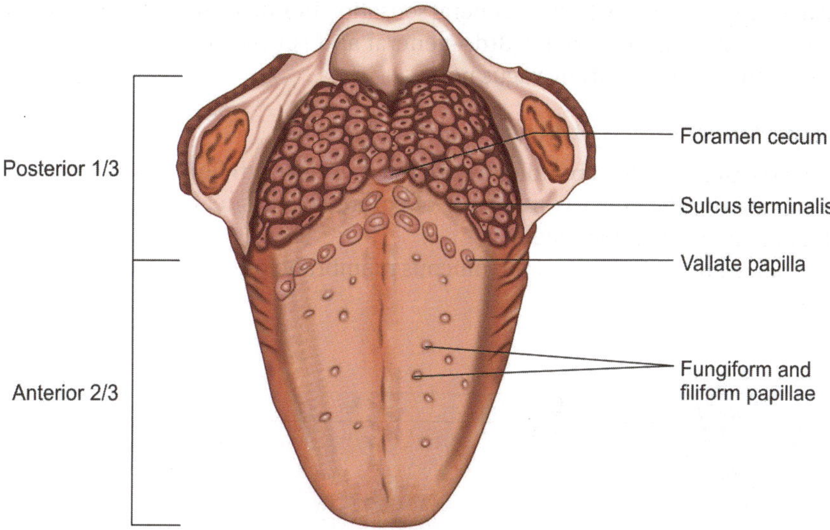

Fig. 8.3: Tongue.

- **External features:** The tongue has a root, a tip, two surfaces—ventral and dorsal and two lateral borders.
- By its root, the tongue is attached to the hyoid bone. The tip is free.
- Dorsal surface is covered with mucous membrane. A "V"-shaped groove (called the sulcus terminalis) divides this surface into anterior 2/3rds and posterior 1/3rd. The apex of the "V" shows a blind opening, the foramen cecum.
- The mucous membrane is rough on the anterior 2/3rds showing papillae. The mucous membrane on the posterior 1/3rd is smooth and papillae are absent.
- Collection of lymphatic tissue under the mucous membrane is called lingual tonsils.
- Ventral surface is covered with smooth mucous membrane. No papillae seen here.

Muscles

- Intrinsic muscles—Superior longitudinal, inferior longitudinal, transverse and vertical.
- Extrinsic muscles—Genioglossus, hyoglossus, styloglossus, palatoglossus.

Blood Supply

- Lingual artery (a branch of the external carotid artery).
- Venae comitantes (accompanying lingual artery and hypoglossal nerve) and deep lingual vein unite to form the lingual vein which terminates in common facial vein or internal jugular vein.

Lymphatic Drainage

Submental nodes, submandibular nodes, jugulo-omohyoid nodes.

Nerve Supply

- **Motor supply:** All muscles by hypoglossal nerve, except palatoglossus by pharyngeal plexus.

- **Sensory supply:** Anterior 2/3rd—general sensation by lingual nerve; special sensation (taste) by chorda tympani; posterior 1/3rd—general and special sensation by glossopharyngeal nerve; posterior-most part by vagus nerve.

Microscopic Structure (Figs. 8.4A and B and 8.5A and B)

- Tongue is chiefly made of bundles of striated muscles with fibroelastic tissue.
- Mucous membrane consists of a layer of connective tissue, lined by stratified squamous epithelium along with papillae.
- The papillae are projections of the mucous membrane present in the anterior 2/3rds of the tongue.

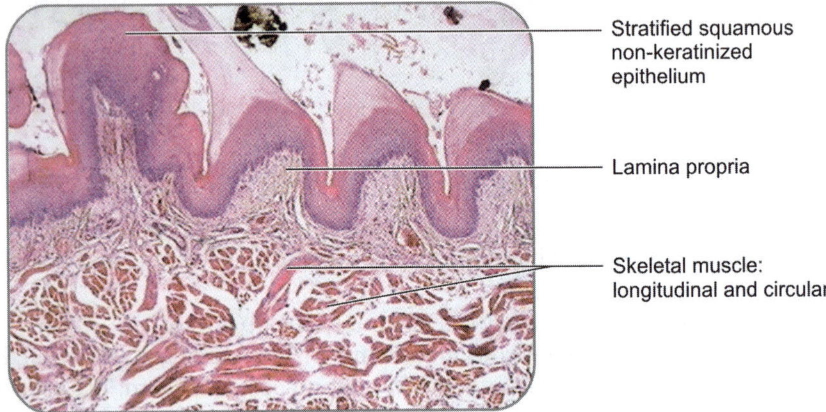

Fig. 8.4A: Photomicrograph of histology of filiform and fungiform papillae.

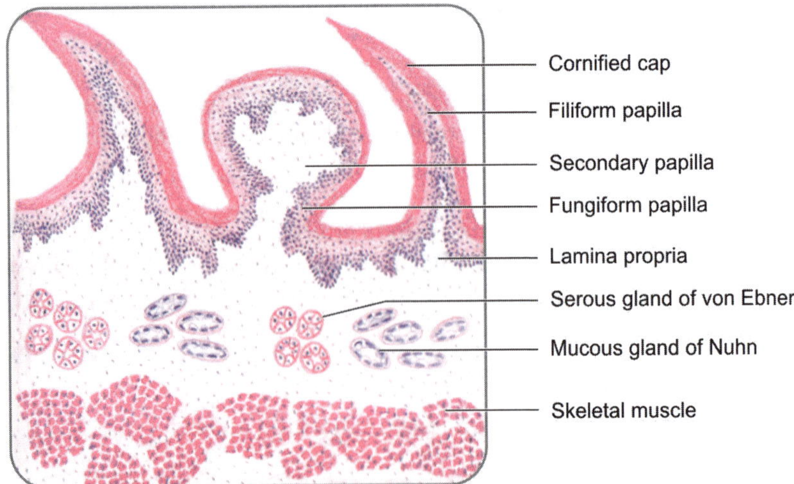

Fig. 8.4B: Diagrammatic representation of histology of filiform and fungiform papillae.

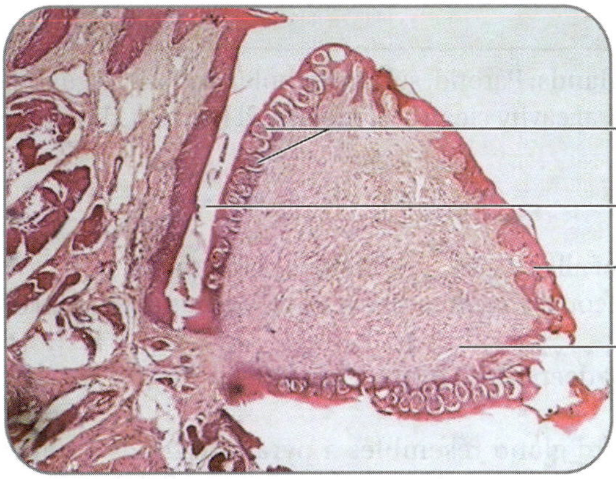

Taste buds
Deep furrow
Non-keratinized stratified squamous epithelium
Lamina propria

Fig. 8.5A: Photomicrograph of histology of circumvallate papilla.

Stratified squamous epithelium
Secondary papilla
Circular furrow
Taste buds
Skeletal muscle
Excretory ducts
von Ebner's gland

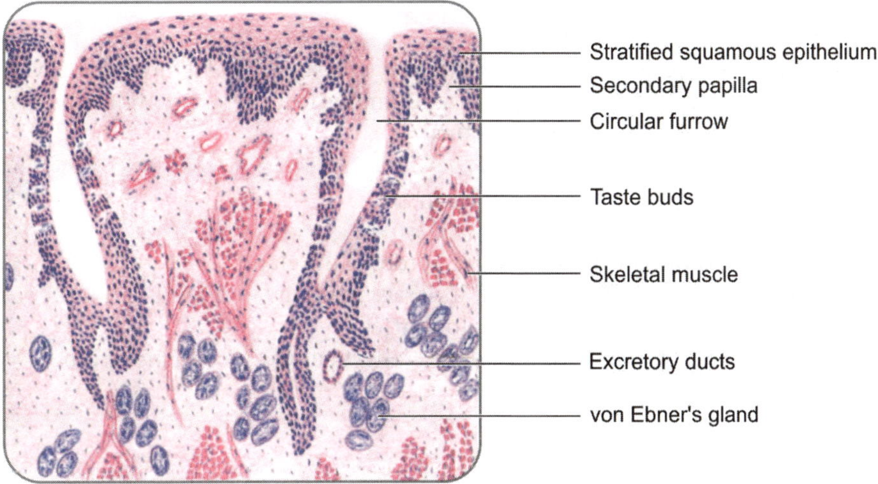

Fig. 8.5B: Diagrammatic representation of histology of circumvallate papilla.

- *Vallate papillae:* Large, 8–12 in number, seen with naked eyes, situated in a row in front of the sulcus terminalis **(Figs. 8.5A and B)**.
- *Fungiform papillae—numerous, present near the tip of the tongue. They have a bright red color* ***(Figs. 8.4A and B)***.
- *Filiform papillae:* Conical projections, with pointed tips, in the presulcal area, smallest of all the papillae **(Figs. 8.4A and B)**.

- Taste buds are numerous in fungiform, vallate papilla, posterior 1/3rd of tongue, soft palate, epiglottis and pharynx.

Applied Anatomy

- Injury to the hypoglossal nerve causes paralysis of the muscles.
- Carcinoma of tongue is common.

SALIVARY GLANDS

There are three pairs of salivary glands: Parotid, submandibular and sublingual glands. These produce saliva, which keeps the oral cavity clean and moist and helps in chewing, swallowing and phonation.

Parotid Gland (Fig. 8.6)

- The parotid gland, the largest of all the salivary glands, is of a serous type.
- **Situation:** Below the external acoustic meatus, between the ramus of the mandible and the sternocleidomastoid muscle.
- **Capsule:** The investing layer of deep fascia forms a capsule for the gland. It splits into two layers and encloses the gland.
- **External features:** The parotid gland resembles a pyramid. It has an apex, directed downwards. The gland has 4 surfaces—superior (base), superficial, anteromedial and posteromedial and 3 borders—anterior, posterior and medial.

Structures within the Parotid Gland

- **Arteries:** External carotid artery, maxillary artery and superficial temporal artery.
- **Veins:** Maxillary and superficial temporal veins uniting to form retromandibular vein, which divides into anterior and posterior divisions.
- **Nerves:** Facial nerve and its branches.

Parotid Duct

- It emerges from the middle of the anterior border of the gland.
- At the anterior border of the masseter, it passes medially and pierces buccal pad of fat, buccopharyngeal fascia and the buccinator muscle.
- Opens into vestibule of mouth, opposite the crown of upper second molar tooth.

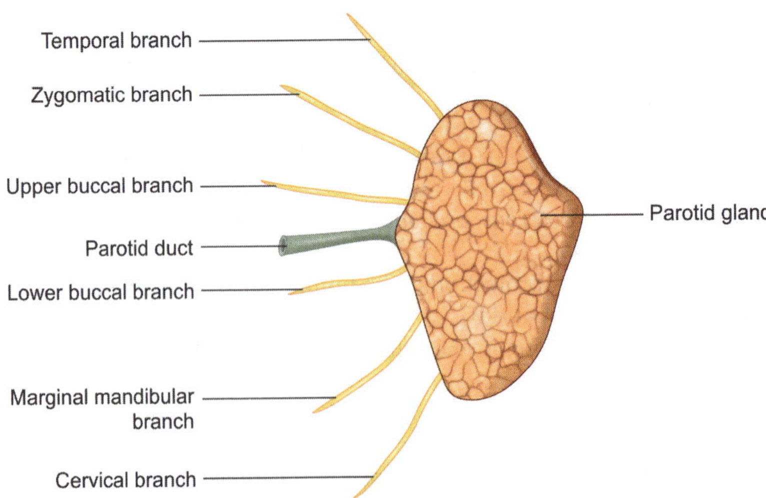

Fig. 8.6: Structures emerging from the parotid gland.

Blood Supply

- Branches of external carotid artery
- Veins drain into the external jugular vein through retromandibular vein.

Nerve Supply

- **Parasympathetic:** Secretomotor fibers by glossopharyngeal nerve through the otic ganglion and auriculotemporal nerve.
- **Sympathetic:** Vasomotor fibers arising from superior cervical ganglion forming plexus around external carotid artery.
- **Sensory:** Auriculotemporal nerve.

Lymphatic Drainage

- Superficial part to parotid lymph nodes and deep part to retropharyngeal lymph nodes.

Applied Anatomy

- **Mumps:** Infectious disease caused by specific virus.
- During surgical removal of the gland, facial nerve should be preserved.

Submandibular Gland

- It is a mixed type of salivary gland.
- **Situation:** In the anterior part of digastric triangle.
- It is J-shaped and has superficial and deep parts which communicate around posterior border of mylohyoid muscle.
- **Superficial part:** Has inferior, lateral and medial surfaces, enclosed between the two layers of the deep cervical fascia.
- Deep part is small in size

Submandibular Duct

It is thin walled and about 5 cm long. It opens on the floor of the mouth.

Blood Supply

- Facial and lingual arteries
- The veins drain into the facial or lingual veins.

Nerve Supply

- **Parasympathetic:** Secretomotor fibers from the facial nerve through chorda tympani, submandibular ganglion and its branches.
- **Sympathetic:** Vasomotor fibers from superior cervical ganglion forming plexus around the facial artery.
- **Sensory:** Lingual nerve.

Lymphatic Drainage

Submandibular lymph nodes.

Sublingual Gland

- It is a mucous type of salivary gland.

- **Situation:** In the floor of the mouth between the mucous membrane and mylohyoid muscle.
- Fifteen to twenty small ducts open at the summit of sublingual fold in the mouth cavity directly or to submandibular duct.
- Blood supply, nerve supply and lymphatic drainage are similar to that of submandibular gland.

PHARYNX (FIG. 8.7)

Pharynx is a wide muscular tube situated behind the nose, the mouth and the larynx. It is 12 cm in length and its cavity is divided into three parts.

Parts of Pharynx

- Nasal part is called the nasopharynx and lies behind the nose and above the soft palate.
- The oral part is called the oropharynx and lies behind the oral cavity. It communicates above with the nasopharynx through the nasopharyngeal isthmus. Below it opens into the laryngopharynx at the level of upper border of epiglottis.
- The laryngeal part is called the laryngopharynx and extends from the upper border of epiglottis to the lower border of cricoid cartilage.

Muscles of the Pharynx

- The main muscles of the pharynx are superior constrictor, middle constrictor and inferior constrictor. They are all inserted into a median raphe in the posterior wall of pharynx.
- The three longitudinal muscles are stylopharyngeus (coming from the styloid process), palatopharyngeus (coming from the palate) and salpingopharyngeus (coming from the auditory tube).

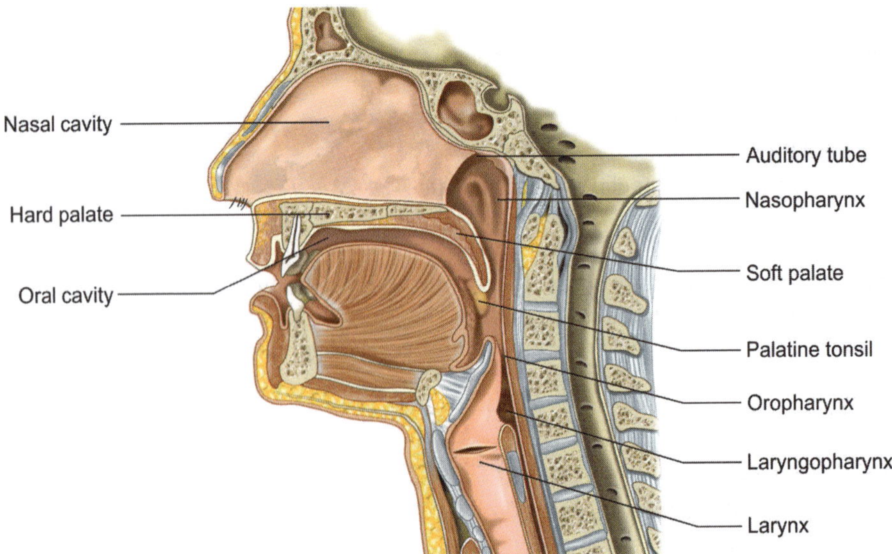

Fig. 8.7: Parts of pharynx.

Nerve Supply

- All the muscles of pharynx are supplied by the pharyngeal plexus of nerves except the stylopharyngeus which is supplied by the glossopharyngeal nerve.
- Sensory supply is by the glossopharyngeal nerve.

Blood Supply

- Pharynx is supplied by branches of external carotid artery, and maxillary artery.
- The veins drain into the facial veins and the internal jugular veins.

ESOPHAGUS

- A narrow muscular tube, forming the food passage between pharynx and stomach.
- It is about 25 cm long.
- Begins in the neck at lower border of cricoid cartilage. It is a continuation of the lower end of the pharynx.
- It passes down in front of the vertebral column, pierces the diaphragm at T10.
- It ends by opening into the cardiac end of the stomach.

Constrictions

Four constrictions:

1. At its beginning (6 inches from the incisor teeth).
2. Where it is crossed by the aortic arch (9 inches from the incisor teeth).
3. Where it is crossed by the left bronchus (11 inches from the incisor teeth).
4. Where it pierces the diaphragm (15 inches from the incisor teeth).

Blood Supply

- **Cervical part:** Inferior thyroid arteries.
- **Thoracic part:** Esophageal branches of aorta.
- **Abdominal part:** Branches of left gastric artery.
- Veins drain into brachiocephalic, azygos, left gastric veins.

Lymphatic Drainage

Deep cervical, posterior mediastinal and left gastric nodes.

Nerve Supply

- **Parasympathetic nerves:** Recurrent laryngeal nerves, esophageal plexus.
- **Sympathetic nerves:** Middle cervical ganglion, thoracic ganglia (upper 4).

Microscopic Structure (Figs. 8.8A and B)

- **Mucosa:** It is lined by stratified squamous epithelium. Beneath it is lamina propria and muscularis mucosae.
- **Submucosa:** Made of loose connective tissue and mucous glands.
- **Muscularis externa:** Containing smooth muscles—inner circular and outer longitudinal layers.
- **Adventitia:** Connective tissue and mesothelial cells.

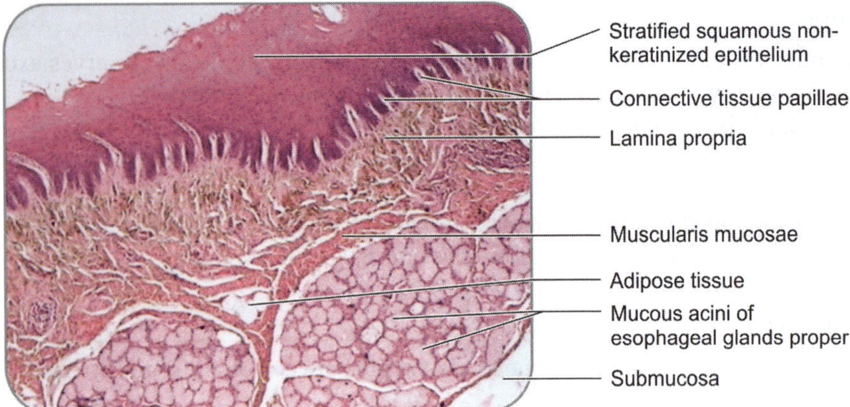

Fig. 8.8A: Photomicrograph of histology of esophagus.

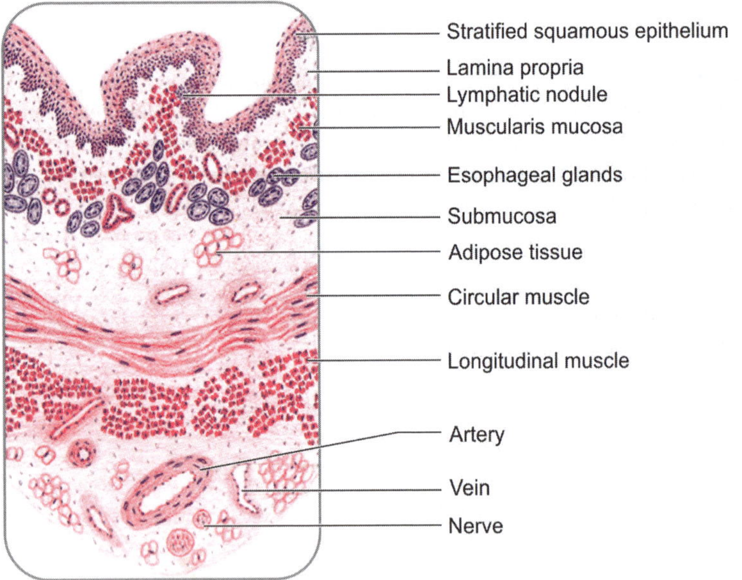

Fig. 8.8B: Diagrammatic representation of histology of esophagus.

Applied Anatomy

- In portal hypertension, the veins at the lower end of the esophagus dilate—esophageal varices. Rupture of these varices causes vomiting of blood (hematemesis).
- The normal constrictions should be noted during esophagoscopy.
- Compression of the esophagus in cases of mediastinal syndrome causes dysphagia (difficulty in swallowing).

STOMACH

- A muscular bag, connected above with lower end of esophagus and below with duodenum.
- The most dilated part of GIT.
- Acts as a reservoir of food and helps in digestion of proteins and fat.
- **Situation:** It occupies the upper and left part of the abdomen, occupying epigastric, umbilical and left hypochondriac regions.
- **Shape and size:** An empty stomach is J-shaped. It is about 10 cm long.

External Features (Fig. 8.9)

- The stomach has two orifices, two curvatures and two surfaces.
- Cardiac orifice is continuous with lower end of esophagus.
- Pyloric orifice opens into the duodenum. It bears a pyloric sphincter.
- Lesser curvature is concave, forms the right border of the stomach, and gives attachment to the lesser omentum.
- Greater curvature is convex, forms left border of stomach, provides attachment to greater omentum. At its upper end, it presents a cardiac notch which separates it from esophagus.
- **Two parts:** Cardiac and pyloric.
  1. Larger cardiac part is further subdivided into the fundus and the body.
  2. Smaller pyloric part is subdivided into pyloric antrum and pyloric canal.

Relations

Peritoneal Relations

- Lesser omentum is attached to lesser curvature and greater omentum is attached to greater curvature.

Visceral Relations

- **Anterior surface:** Liver, diaphragm, anterior abdominal wall.
- **Posterior surface (forming stomach bed):** Diaphragm, left kidney, left suprarenal, pancreas, transverse mesocolon, splenic flexure of the colon, splenic artery.

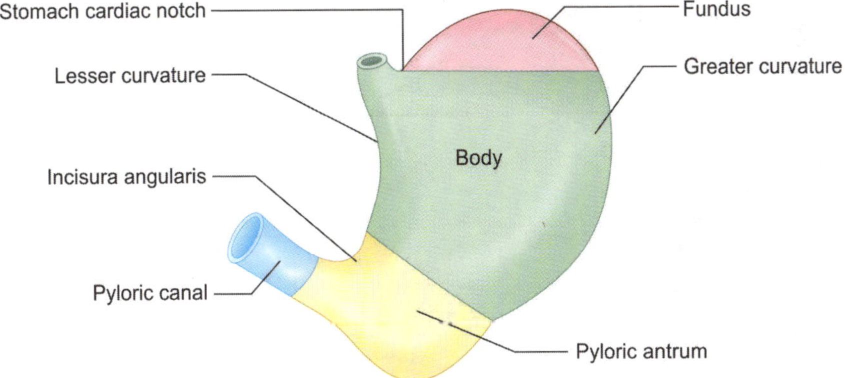

Fig. 8.9: Parts of stomach.

Blood Supply

- Left and right gastric, left and right gastroepiploic and short gastric arteries.
- Veins drain into superior mesenteric, portal and splenic veins.

Lymphatic Drainage

Stomach is divided into four lymphatic territories.

1. **Fundus:** Pancreaticosplenic nodes.
2. **Lesser curvature:** Left gastric nodes.
3. **Greater curvature:** Right gastroepiploic, splenic and hepatic nodes.
4. **Pylorus:** Pyloric, hepatic and left gastric nodes.

Nerve Supply

- **Sympathetic nerves:** T6–T10 segments via splanchnic nerves (vasomotor), motor to the pyloric sphincter (but inhibitory to the rest of the musculature).
- **Parasympathetic nerves:** Derived through the vagus.

Microscopic Structure

Fundus and Body of Stomach (Figs. 8.10A and B)

- **Mucosa:** Lined by simple columnar epithelium forming small depressions at luminal surface called gastric pits. Beneath it is the connective tissue, lamina propria, which contains the gastric glands opening at the bottom of the gastric pits. Deep to the lamina propria, is a layer of smooth muscles called muscularis mucosa. The mucous membrane is thrown into folds called rugae when the stomach contracts and gets obliterated when it distends. The gastric pits are shallow in fundus and body. Three types of glands are seen. Longer glands with zymogenic (chief) cells that are basophilic and secrete pepsin, parietal (oxyntic) cells that are eosinophilic and secrete hydrochloric acid and mucous neck cells which are light staining and secrete mucus.
- **Submucosa:** Made up of loose connective tissue.

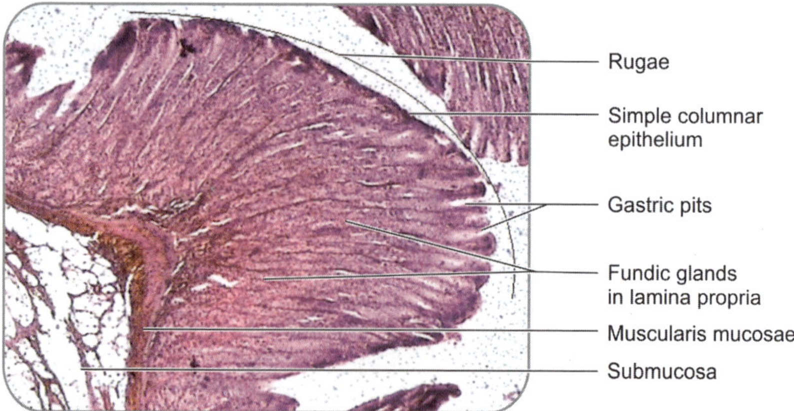

Fig. 8.10A: Photomicrograph of histology of stomach fundus.

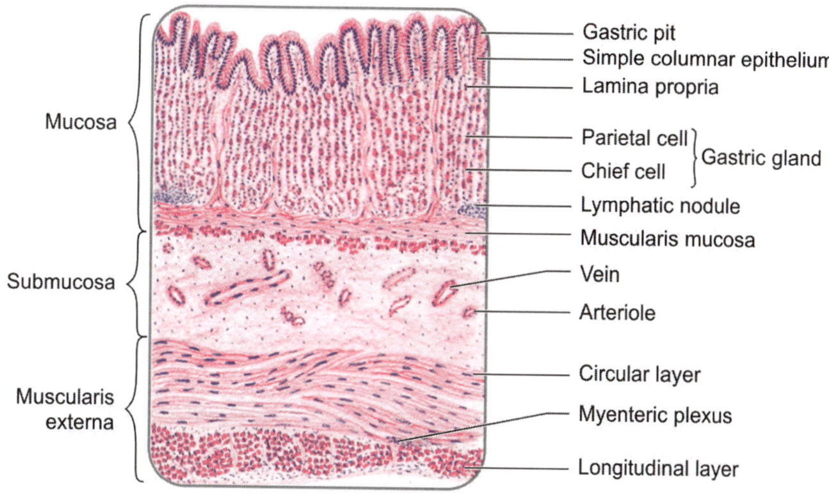

Fig. 8.10B: Diagrammatic representation of histology of stomach fundus.

- **Muscularis externa:** Outer longitudinal, middle circular and inner oblique smooth muscle fibers.
- **Serosa:** Made of a single layer of flattened mesothelium.

Pylorus of Stomach (Figs. 8.11A and B)

- **Mucosa:** Lined by simple columnar epithelium forming small depressions at luminal surface called gastric pits. Beneath it is the connective tissue, lamina propria, which contains the gastric glands opening at the bottom of the gastric pits. Deep to the lamina propria, is a layer of smooth muscles called muscularis mucosa. The mucous membrane is thrown into folds called rugae when the stomach contracts and gets obliterated when it distends. The pits are longer and deeper in pylorus. The glands are mucus secreting with long, coiled ducts.
- **Submucosa:** Made up of loose connective tissue.

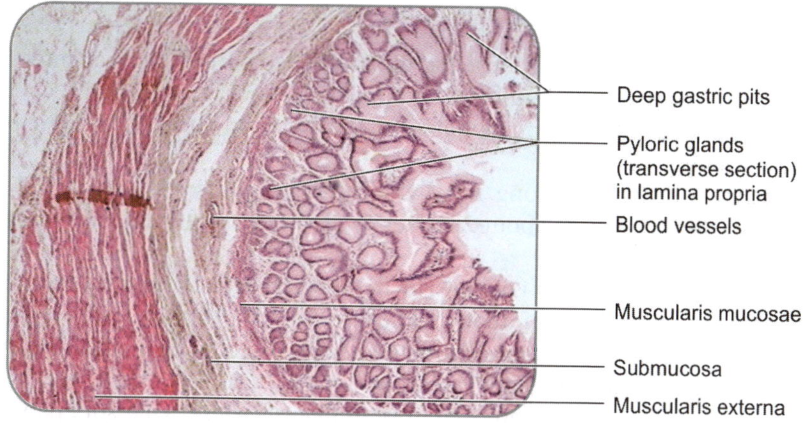

Fig. 8.11A: Photomicrograph of histology of stomach pylorus.

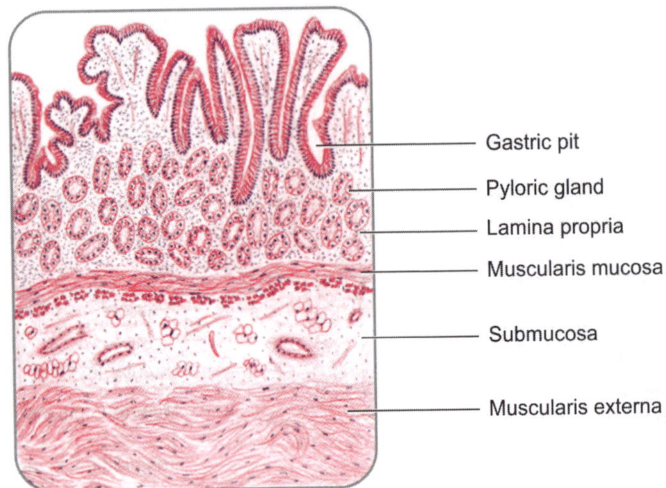

Fig. 8.11B: Diagrammatic representation of histology of stomach pylorus.

- **Muscularis externa:** Outer longitudinal, middle circular and inner oblique smooth muscle fibers.
- **Serosa:** Made of a single layer of flattened mesothelium.

Functions of the Stomach

- Reservoir of food
- Softens and mixes the food with the gastric juice.
- Gastric glands produce gastric juice, HCl.

SMALL INTESTINE

- **Extent:** From the pylorus to the ileocecal junction.
- It is about 6 m long.
- **Divided into three parts:** Duodenum, jejunum and the ileum.

Duodenum (Fig. 8.12)

- The duodenum is the shortest, widest and the most fixed part of the small intestine.
- **Situation:** In the posterior abdominal wall, opposite vertebrae L1, L2 and L3.
- **Extent:** From pylorus to duodenojejunal flexure. It is curved round the head of pancreas in the form of a letter, "C".
- Duodenum is about 10 inches long. It is divided into four parts:
  1. **First (superior) part:** It is about 2 inches long. It begins at pylorus of the stomach to superior duodenal flexure.
  2. **Second (descending) part:** It is about 3 inches long. It begins at superior duodenal flexure, passes down to reach inferior duodenal flexure.
     Interior of 2nd part shows major duodenal papilla: An elevation present 8–10 cm away from pylorus. Bile and pancreatic ducts open at this region.
     Minor duodenal papilla is seen 6–8 cm from pylorus. Here, accessory pancreatic duct opens.

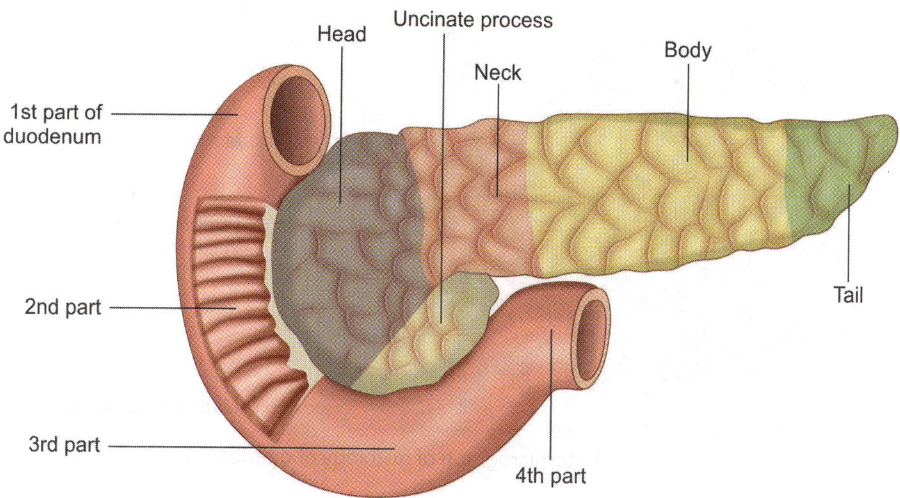

Fig. 8.12: Duodenum and pancreas.

3. **Third (horizontal) part:** It is about 4 inches long, begins at inferior duodenal flexure, and passes horizontally.
4. **Fourth (ascending) part:** It is 1 inch long, ends at the duodenojejunal flexure.

Blood Supply

- Superior pancreaticoduodenal artery supplies parts of duodenum up to major duodenal papilla; rest by inferior pancreaticoduodenal artery.
- Veins drain into splenic, superior mesenteric and portal veins.

Lymphatic Drainage

Pancreaticoduodenal nodes.

Nerve Supply

Sympathetic nerves: T9, T10; Parasympathetic nerves: Vagus.

Microscopic Structure (Figs. 8.13A and B)

- **Mucosa:** It is lined by simple columnar epithelium. Beneath it is lamina propria with loose connective tissue, blood vessels, lymphatics, nerves, intestinal glands (crypts of Lieberkuhn) with Paneth cells (secreting enzymes), argentaffin cells (secreting serotonin) surrounding lamina propria is muscularis mucosae.
- **Submucosa:** It is made of dense connective tissue, blood vessels, nerves, and mucus -ecreting glands (duodenal glands of Brunner).
- **Muscularis externa:** It contains smooth muscles—inner circular and outer longitudinal layers.
- **Adventitia or serosa:** Posterior part covered by adventitia (connective tissue), anterior part by serosa (connective tissue and mesothelium).

Applied Anatomy

- In skiagrams taken after a barium meal, the first part of the duodenum is seen as a triangular shadow called duodenal cap.
- The first part of duodenum is the commonest site for peptic ulcers.

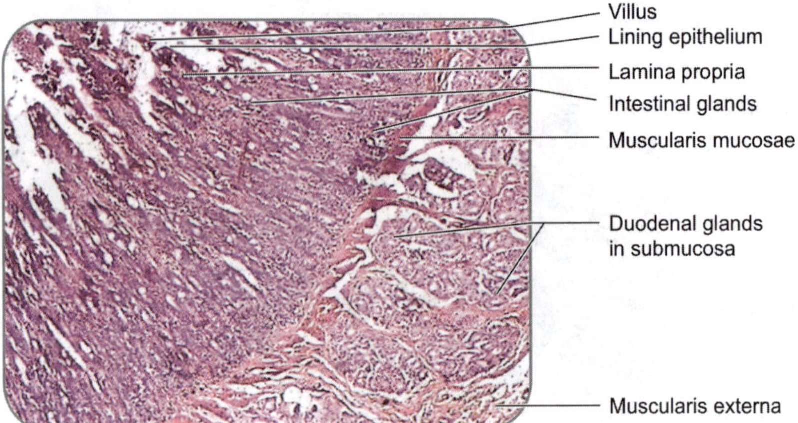

Fig. 8.13A: Photomicrograph of histology of duodenum.

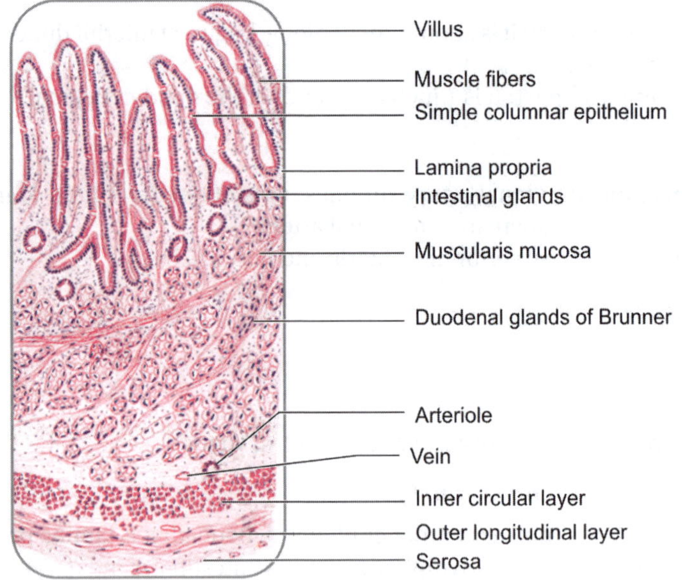

Fig. 8.13B: Diagrammatic representation of histology of duodenum.

Jejunum and Ileum

- Jejunum forms upper 2/5ths of the small intestine and ileum forms the lower 3/5ths of the small intestine.
- Both are suspended from a fold of mesentery from posterior abdominal wall and are therefore mobile.
- Jejunum begins at duodenojejunal flexure and ileum terminates at ileocecal junction. The differences between duodenum, jejunum and ileum are listed in **Table 8.1**.

Table 8.1: Differences between duodenum, jejunum and ileum.

Features	*Duodenum*	*Jejunum*	*Ileum*
Location	C-shaped 1st part of intestine	Upper and left part of intestine	Lower and right parts of intestine
Walls		Thicker and more vascular	Thinner and less vascular
Lumen		Wider and empty	Narrow and full
Mesentery	Retroperitoneal, fixed except at two ends	Has windows, less fat, 1–2 arterial arcades and longer and fewer vasa recta	No windows, more fat, 3–6 arterial arcades and shorter and more vasa recta
Villi	Leaf shaped, numerous	Tall, tongue shaped, numerous	Short, finger shaped, few
Peyer's patches	Absent	Absent	Present
Plicae circularis	Absent in 1st part	Larger and more closely set	Smaller and sparse
Epithelium	Simple columnar with few goblet cells	Same with little more of goblet cells	Same with more number of goblet cells
Lamina propria	Crypts with more argentaffin cells, loose lymphatic tissue	Crypts with less argentaffin cells, diffuse lymphatic nodules	Crypts with less argentaffin cells, lymphatic nodules aggregated to form Peyer's patches
Muscularis mucosa	Continuous	Interrupted	Interrupted
Submucosa	Presence of Brunner's glands along with CT, blood vessels and nerves	CT with blood vessels and nerves	Presence of Peyer's patches along with CT, blood vessels and nerves

Function

Absorption of nutrients from food.

Blood Supply

- Superior mesenteric artery
- Drained by the superior mesenteric veins.

Lymphatic Drainage

- Lymph passes from lacteals present in intestines to those in mesentery.
- They finally drain into lymph nodes present in front of the aorta at origin of superior mesenteric artery.

Nerve Supply

- **Sympathetic:** T9–T10 segments.
- **Parasympathetic:** Vagus nerve.

Meckel's Diverticulum

- This is the persistent part of vitellointestinal duct.
- Seen in embryos; it normally disappears during the 6th week of intrauterine life.
- It is present in 2% of the subjects, is about 2 cm long and is situated 2 feet proximal to the ileocecal valve attached to the antimesenteric border of ileum.
- It may cause obstruction in the small intestine and its inflammation might simulate appendicitis.

Microscopic Structure (Figs. 8.14A and B and 8.15A and B)

The small intestine is made up of four layers:

- **Mucosa:** Is the innermost layer. It is lined by simple columnar epithelium with microvilli. The mucosa is thrown into finger-like folds called the villi which are long and leaf-like in jejunum

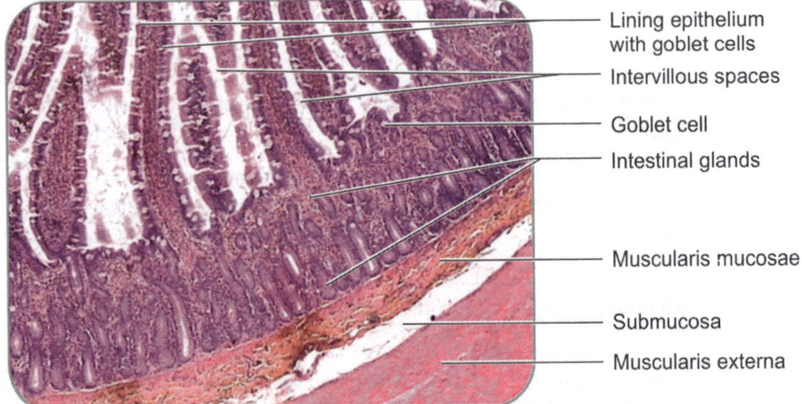

Fig. 8.14A: Photomicrograph of histology of jejunum.

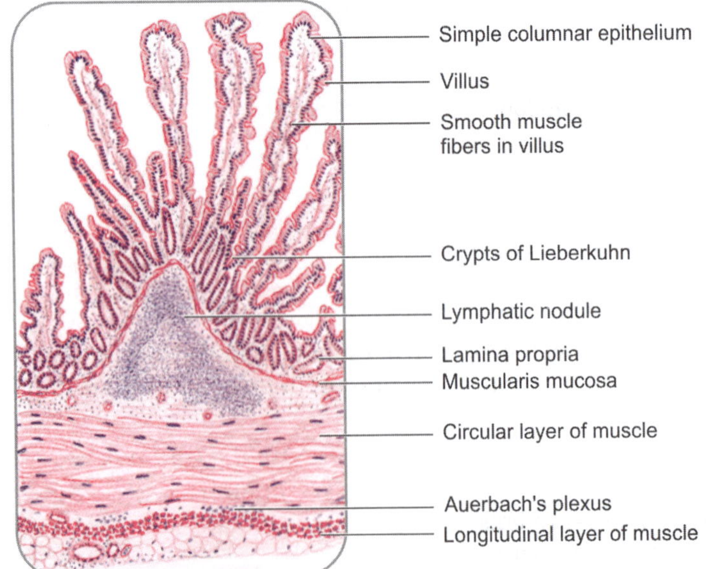

Fig. 8.14B: Diagrammatic representation of histology of jejunum.

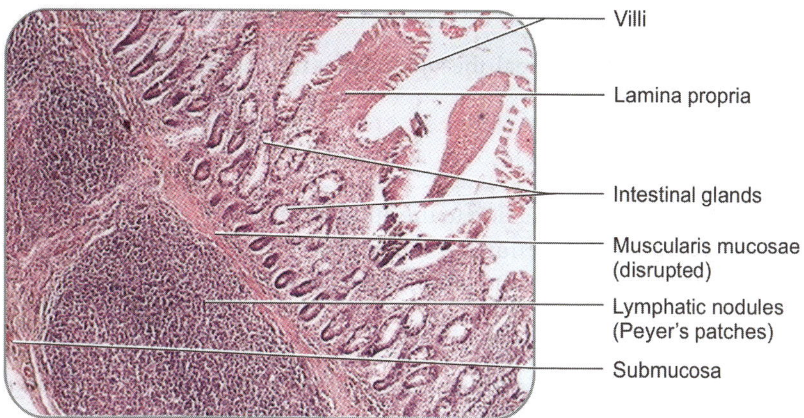

Fig. 8.15A: Photomicrograph of histology of ileum.

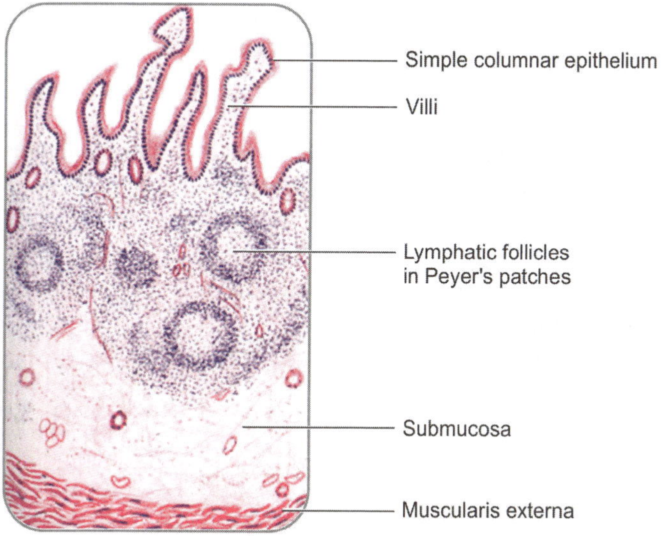

Fig. 8.15B: Diagrammatic representation of histology of ileum.

and short finger-like in ileum; mucosa dips inside the lamina propria to form crypts. Lamina propria is made up of connective tissue that has nerve fibers and blood vessels. The mucosa ends at the muscularis mucosa which is a layer of smooth muscle.

- **Submucosa:** Lies beneath the mucosa and is made up of connective tissue, blood vessels and nerve fibers. The mucosa and submucosa are folded to form the plicae circularis. Submucosal plexus of nerves are seen.
- In the jejunum the submucosa shows no special features but in the ileum aggregations of lymphatic tissue in the form of lymphatic follicles called Peyer's patches are seen.
- **Muscularis externa:** This is made up of smooth muscle arranged in two layers, inner circular and outer longitudinal. Between the two is present the myenteric plexus of nerves.
- **Serosa:** Outermost layer made up of connective tissue and mesothelium.

Applied Anatomy

In skiagrams taken after a barium meal, the jejunum has no features but the ileum looks feathery in appearance.

LARGE INTESTINE (FIG. 8.16)

- It extends from the ileocecal junction to the anus. It is about 1.5 m long.
- **Parts:** Cecum, ascending colon, transverse colon, descending colon, sigmoid colon, rectum and anal canal. Between cecum and terminal part of ileum is the appendix.

Features

- The longitudinal muscle coat is thrown into 3 ribbon-like bands called Taenia coli that encircle the large intestine. They are absent in rectum and anal canal.
- Taeniae are shorter than circular muscle coat and hence large intestine shows folds called sacculations or haustrations.
- The peritoneum shows small bags of fat called appendices epiploicae scattered over the whole of large intestine except rectum, appendix and cecum.

Function

- Absorption of water and storage of matter reaching it from the small intestine.
- Bacteria present in the large intestine help to synthesize Vitamin B.

Blood Supply

- Till the right 2/3rds of transverse colon, branches of superior mesenteric artery, thereafter by branches of inferior mesenteric artery.
- Drained by veins of the same name.

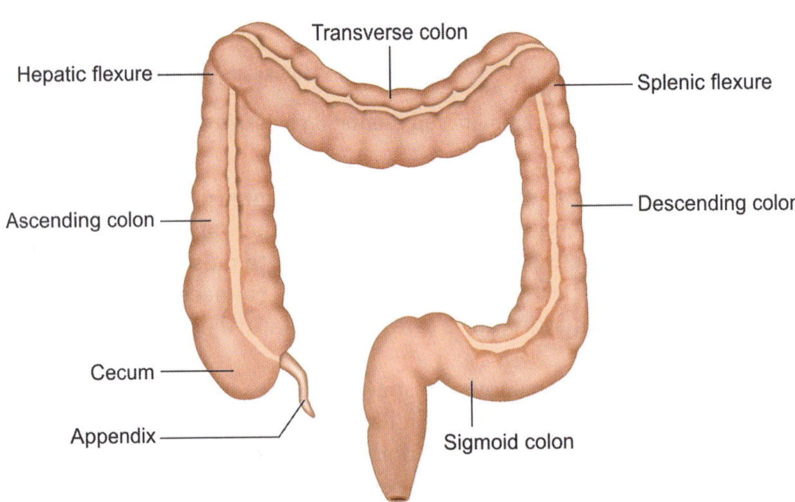

Fig. 8.16: Parts of large intestine.

Nerve Supply

- **Sympathetic supply:** Till the right 2/3rds of the transverse colon, the sympathetic supply is from the celiac and superior mesenteric ganglia (T11–L1). Thereafter, it is supplied by the lumbar sympathetic chain (L1–L2).
- **Parasympathetic supply:** Till the right 2/3rds of the transverse colon, the supply is from the vagus nerve and thereafter from pelvic splanchnic nerves.

Lymphatic Drainage

Epicolic and paracolic lymph nodes.

Microscopic Structure (Figs. 8.17A and B)

- **Mucosa:** Is the inner most layer. It is lined by simple columnar epithelium with microvilli and goblet cells. The epithelium dips inside the lamina propria to form crypts of Lieberkuhn. No villi are seen but there is abundance of goblet cells such that every 3rd cell is a goblet cell. Below the lining epithelium lies lamina propria made up of loose connective tissue with intestinal glands, nerve fibers and blood vessels. The mucosa ends at the muscularis mucosa which is a layer of smooth muscle, inner circularly arranged and outer longitudinally arranged.
- **Submucosa:** This lies beneath the mucosa and is made up of connective tissue, blood vessels and nerve fibers. Submucosal plexus of nerves is seen.
- **Muscularis externa:** This is made up of smooth muscle arranged in two layers, inner circular and outer longitudinal. The outer longitudinal layer is thickened into three ribbon-like bands called taenia coli. Between the two is present the myenteric plexus of nerves.
- **Adventitia or serosa:** Posterior part of ascending colon, descending colon, rectum covered by adventitia (connective tissue), anterior parts by serosa (connective tissue and mesothelium).

Applied Anatomy

In skiagrams taken after a barium meal, the large intestine shows characteristic haustrations.

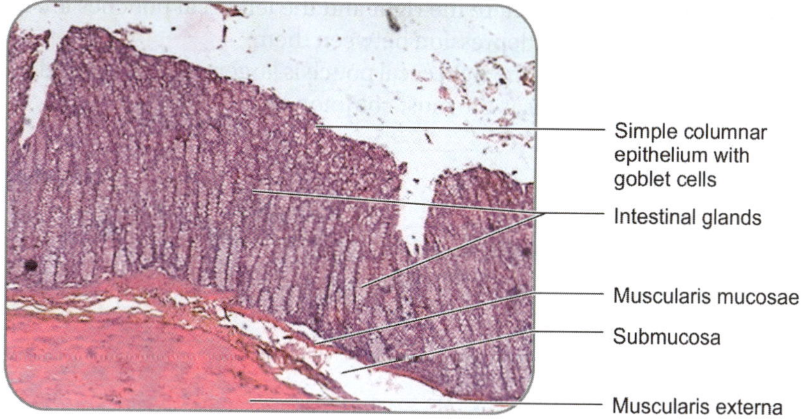

Fig. 8.17A: Photomicrograph of histology of large intestine.

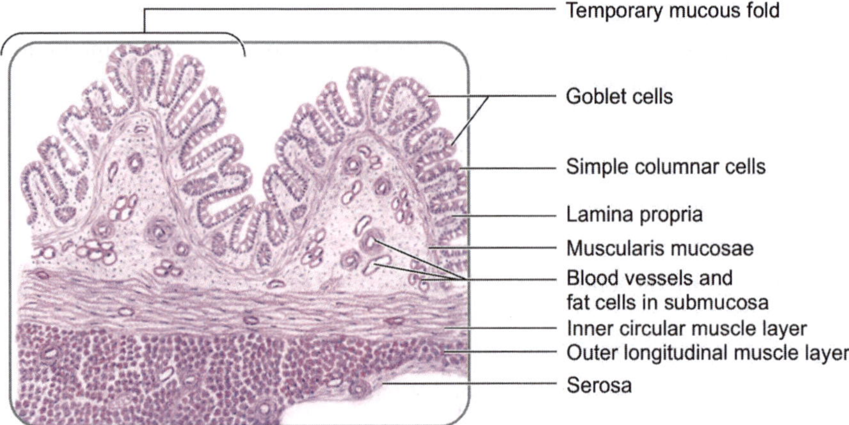

Fig. 8.17B: Diagrammatic representation of histology of large intestine.

CECUM

- It is a blind pouch formed at the beginning of large intestine.
- Situated in right iliac fossa.
- Continuous superiorly with ascending colon, it communicates medially with the ileum at the ileocecal junction and posteriorly with the appendix.

Relations

- **Anterior:** Coils of small intestine and the anterior abdominal wall.
- **Posterior:** Psoas major and iliacus muscles, genitofemoral, femoral and lateral cutaneous nerves of the thigh, testicular or ovarian vessels and appendix.

Types (Fig. 8.18)

- **Conical type:** Where the appendix arises from the apex (midpoint) of cecum.
- **Funicular intermediate type:** Where the right and the left cecal pouches are of equal size and the appendix arises from a depression between them.
- **Normal ampullary type:** Where the right cecal pouch is larger than the left and the appendix arises from the medial side. This is the most common type.

Blood Supply

- Cecal branches of ileocolic artery.
- Drained by the superior mesenteric veins.

Nerve Supply

- **Sympathetic:** T11–L1 segments.
- Parasympathetic is from the vagus nerve.

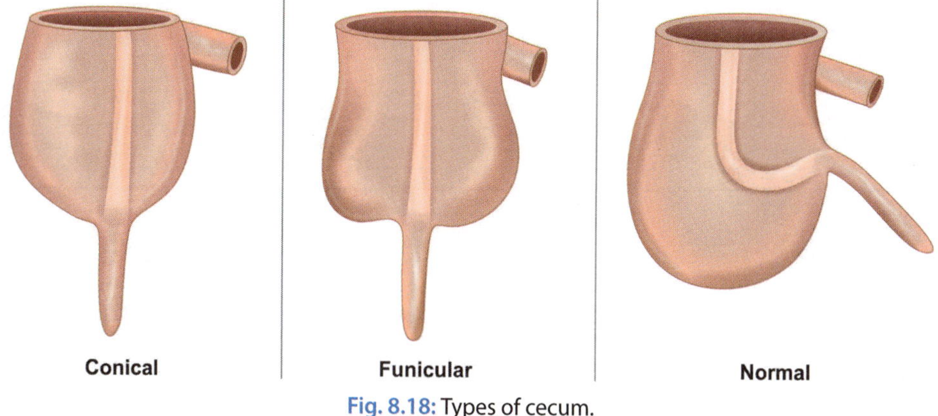

Fig. 8.18: Types of cecum.

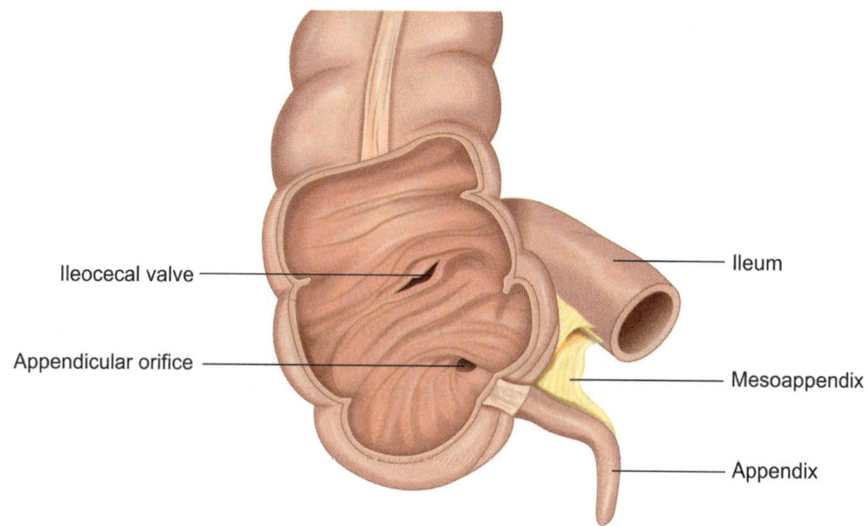

Fig. 8.19: Ileocecal valve.

Ileocecal Valve (Fig. 8.19)

- Lower end of the ileum opens into cecum and is guarded by a valve called ileocecal valve.
- The valve is closed by sympathetic nerves and by distension of cecum.
- It prevents the passage of food from cecum to the ileum. It also regulates the speed of ileal contents so that they do not pass too quickly into the cecum from the ileum.

VERMIFORM APPENDIX (FIG. 8.20)

- It is a worm-like diverticulum that arises from posteromedial wall of cecum.
- It is about 9 cm in length.
- Lies in right iliac fossa. The base of the appendix is fixed but the tip can point in any direction—pass upwards and to right—paracolic or 11 O'clock position; lie behind

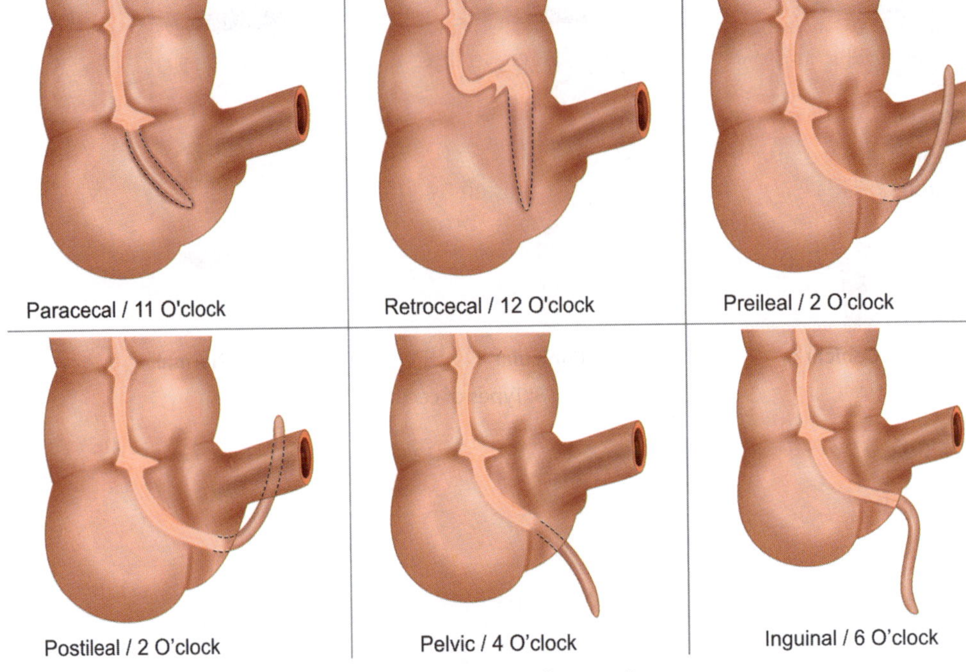

Fig. 8.20: Positions of appendix.

cecum or colon—retrocecal or 12 O'clock position—commonest; pass upwards and to left towards spleen—splenic or 2 O'clock position; pass horizontally and to left towards sacral promontory—promontoric or 3 O'clock; descend into pelvis - pelvic or 4 O'clock position—second most common; lie below cecum towards inguinal ligament—midinguinal or 6 O'clock position.

Blood Supply

- Appendicular artery
- Drained by appendicular, ileocolic and superior mesenteric veins.

Lymphatic Drainage

Ileocolic lymph nodes

Nerve Supply

- **Sympathetic:** T9–T10 segments.
- **Parasympathetic:** Vagus nerve.

Applied Anatomy

- Inflammation of the appendix is called appendicitis.
- Pain felt first at umbilicus (as both are supplied by T10 segment—referred pain).

- McBurney's point is the site of maximum tenderness in appendicitis. The point lies at the junction of the lateral 1/3rd and medial 2/3rds of the line joining umbilicus to right anterior superior iliac spine. It corresponds roughly to the base of the appendix.

Microscopic Structure (Figs. 8.21A and B)

The appendix is made up of four layers:

- **Mucosa:** This is the innermost layer. It is lined by simple columnar epithelium with goblet cells. The epithelium dips inside the lamina propria to form crypts of Lieberkuhn. No villi are seen but there is abundance of goblet cells such that every 3rd cell is a goblet cell. Below the lining epithelium lies the lamina propria made up of connective tissue that has nerve fibers and blood vessels. It also has abundant lymphatic follicles. The mucosa ends at the muscularis mucosa which is a layer of smooth muscle.

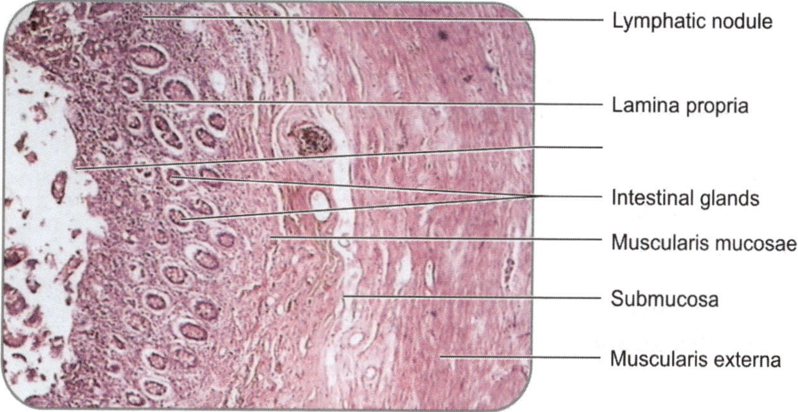

Fig. 8.21A: Photomicrograph of histology of vermiform appendix.

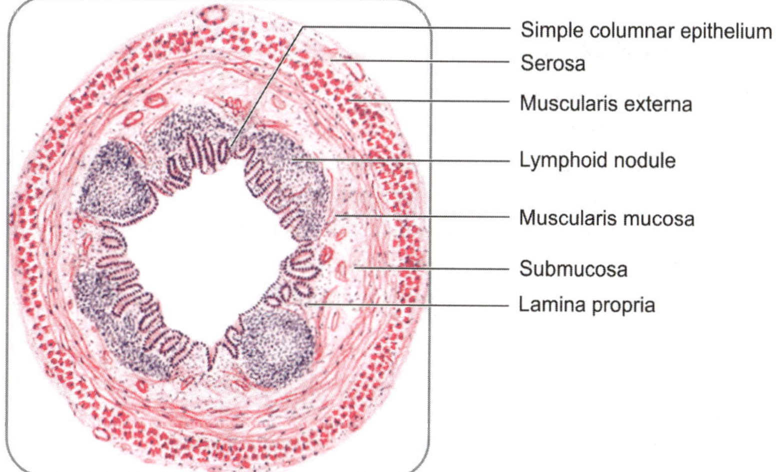

Fig. 8.21B: Diagrammatic representation of histology of vermiform appendix.

- **Submucosa:** This lies beneath the mucosa and is made up of connective tissue, blood vessels and nerve fibers.
- **Muscularis externa:** This is made up of smooth muscle arranged in two layers, inner circular and outer longitudinal.
- **Serosa:** Outer most layer made up of connective tissue and mesothelium.

RECTUM

- Begins at S3 as a continuation of sigmoid colon and ends at the anorectal junction as anal canal.
- 12 cm long, lower part shows a dilatation called the rectal ampulla.
- Shows two anteroposterior curves and three lateral curves.
- Related to urinary bladder in males and uterus in females by folds of peritoneum called the rectovesical pouch and the rectouterine pouch respectively.

Blood Supply

- Supplied by the superior and middle rectal arteries and median sacral artery.
- Drained by the superior and middle rectal veins.

Lymphatic Drainage

Internal iliac lymph nodes.

Nerve Supply

- **Sympathetic:** L1 and L2.
- **Parasympathetic:** S2, 3, 4.

Applied Anatomy

- **Prolapse of rectum:** Rectum protrudes out of the anal canal.
- **Perrectal examination:** Done in males to check for abnormalities in the accessory genital organs.

ANAL CANAL (FIG. 8.22)

- Terminal portion of large intestine
- 3.8 cms long, divided into three parts
  1. *Upper part:* 15 mm long, lined with mucous membrane thrown into folds called anal columns. Lower ends of valves form pectinate line.
  2. *Middle part:* 15 mm long, no valves, dense venous plexus, ends at white line of Hilton.
  3. *Lower part:* 8 mm long, true skin, shows glands and hair.
- Shows the external and internal sphincters for control of passage of feces.

Blood Supply

- Superior and inferior rectal arteries.
- Drained by internal and external rectal venous plexuses of veins.

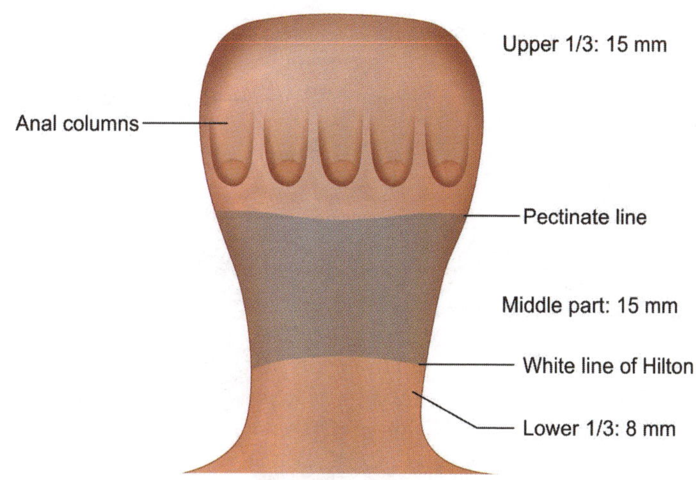

Fig. 8.22: Divisions of the anal canal.

Lymphatic Drainage

Internal iliac and superficial inguinal lymph nodes.

Nerve Supply

- **Sympathetic:** L1 and L2.
- **Parasympathetic:** S2, 3, 4.

Applied Anatomy

- Bleeding from veins causes a condition called hemorrhoids/piles.
- Discontinuity in anal valves called anal fistula.

The differences between large and small intestines are shown in **Table 8.2.**

ACCESSORY DIGESTIVE ORGANS

Spleen (Fig. 8.23)

- Spleen is a wedge-shaped organ lying mainly in the left hypochondrium.

Table 8.2: Differences between small and large intestines.

Feature	*Small intestine*	*Large intestine*
Villi	Present	Absent
Appendices epiploicae	Absent	Present
Taenia coli	Absent	Present
Sacculations	Absent	Present
Callber	Smaller	Larger
Peyer's patches	Present	Absent
Fixity	Most of it is free	Most of it is fixed

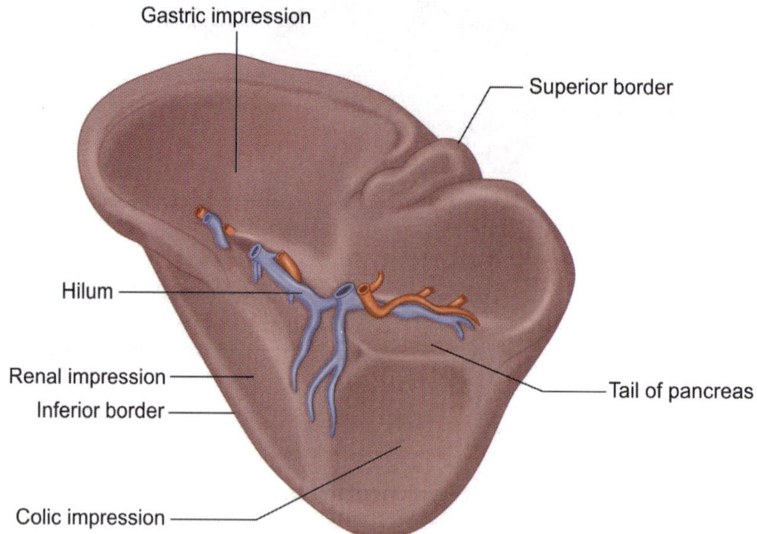

Fig. 8.23: Visceral surface of spleen.

- It is soft, highly vascular and dark purple in color. It is a lymphatic organ connected to the blood vascular system.
- **Function:** To act as a filter for blood and plays an important role in the immune responses of the body.
- **Position:** It lies obliquely along the long axis of the 10th rib. Thus, it is directed downwards, forwards and laterally, making an angle of 45° with the horizontal plane.
- The spleen has two ends, three borders and two surfaces.
- Anterior end is rounded and placed in the midaxillary line.
- Posterior end is rounded and rests on the upper pole of left kidney.
- Superior surface is notched near anterior end.
- Inferior border is rounded.
- Diaphragmatic surface is related to diaphragm which separates the spleen from the pleura, the lung and the 9th, 10th and 11th ribs.
- Visceral surface shows gastric (fundus of stomach), renal (left kidney), colic (splenic flexure of colon) and pancreatic (tail of pancreas) impressions.
- Intermediate border is the hilum of the spleen. It is the place where the splenic vessels and nerves enter the spleen and the splenic veins leave the spleen. It also provides attachment to the gastrosplenic and lienorenal ligaments.
- The spleen is covered on all sides by the visceral layer of the peritoneum.
- Two ligaments attach the hilum of spleen to stomach and kidney. It is attached to greater curvature of stomach by gastrosplenic ligament. It is attached to anterior surface of left kidney by lienorenal ligament.

Blood Supply

- Splenic artery
- Drained by splenic veins.

Lymphatic Drainage

Pancreaticosplenic lymph nodes.

Nerve Supply

Coeliac plexus.

Functions

- **Phagocytosis:** Phagocytes present in spleen remove cell debris and old RBC, thus filtering the blood.
- **Hemopoiesis:** Spleen manufactures blood cells in fetal life. In adult life, it produces lymphocytes.
- **Storage of RBCs:** RBCs can be stored in spleen and released when required. This function is more developed in animals.

Applied Anatomy

- In normal course, spleen is not palpable. It becomes palpable when it becomes two times its size and can be palpated under the left costal margin during inspiration.
- Enlargement of the spleen is called splenomegaly. It occurs in diseases like fever (typhoid and malaria), leukemias and carcinoma.
- Surgical removal of spleen is called splenectomy.
- **Splenic puncture:** A needle can be passed into the spleen through the 8th or 9th intercostal space in the midaxillary line. Dyes injected through the needle can help in the visualization of splenic veins.

Liver (Fig. 8.24)

- The liver is a large, solid gland situated to the right side of the abdominal cavity.
- It is reddish brown in color, soft in consistency.
- Liver is the largest gland in the body.
- It secretes bile and helps in metabolism.

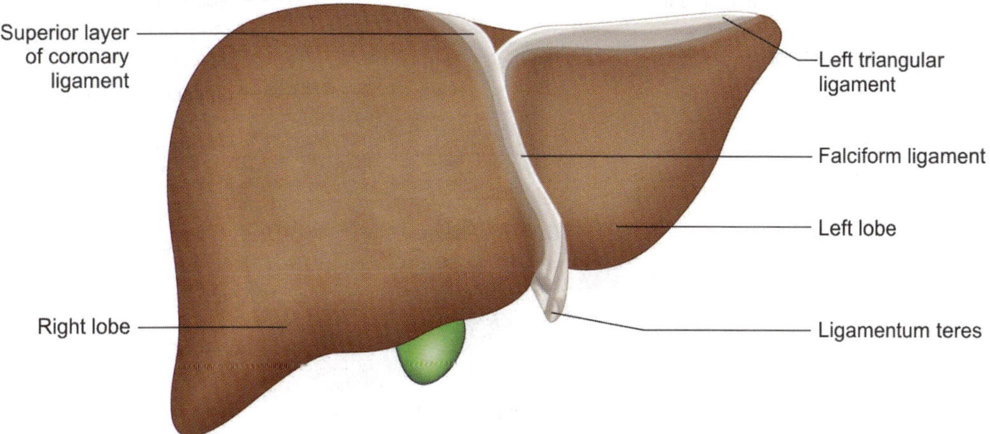

Fig. 8.24: Anterior view of liver.

- **External feature:** Is wedge shaped.
- **It has five surfaces:** Anterior, posterior, superior, inferior and right.
- It is divided into right and left lobes (by attachment of falciform ligament), caudate and quadrate lobes.
- Right lobe is larger than the left lobe, forms 5/6ths of the liver.
- Caudate lobe is situated on the posterior surface. It is bounded on the right by groove for inferior vena cava, left by fissure for ligamentum venosum and inferiorly by porta hepatis.
- Quadrate lobe is situated on inferior surface. It is bounded anteriorly by inferior border of the liver, posteriorly by porta hepatis, to the right by fossa for gallbladder, to the left by fissure for ligamentum teres.
- Porta hepatis is a deep, transverse fissure about 2 inches long, situated on the inferior surface of the right lobe of the liver. It lies between caudate lobe above and quadrate lobe below. Portal vein, hepatic artery, and hepatic plexus of nerves enter and right and left hepatic ducts exit at the porta hepatis.

Relations (Fig. 8.25)

Peritoneal relations

- Most of the liver is covered by peritoneum, except 'bare area' on posterior surface of right lobe, groove for inferior vena cava, fossa for gallbladder, porta hepatis.
- A number of peritoneal folds are attached to the liver.
- **Falciform ligament:** Connecting liver to anterior abdominal wall.
- **Left triangular ligament:** Connecting superior surface of left lobe to diaphragm.
- **Right triangular ligament:** Connecting right lobe to diaphragm.
- **Coronary ligament:** Superior and inferior layers, which enclose bare area of the liver.
- Lesser omentum

Visceral relations

- **Anterior surface:** Xiphoid process, anterior abdominal wall, diaphragm.
- **Posterior surface:** Vertebral column, diaphragm, inferior vena cava, esophagus.

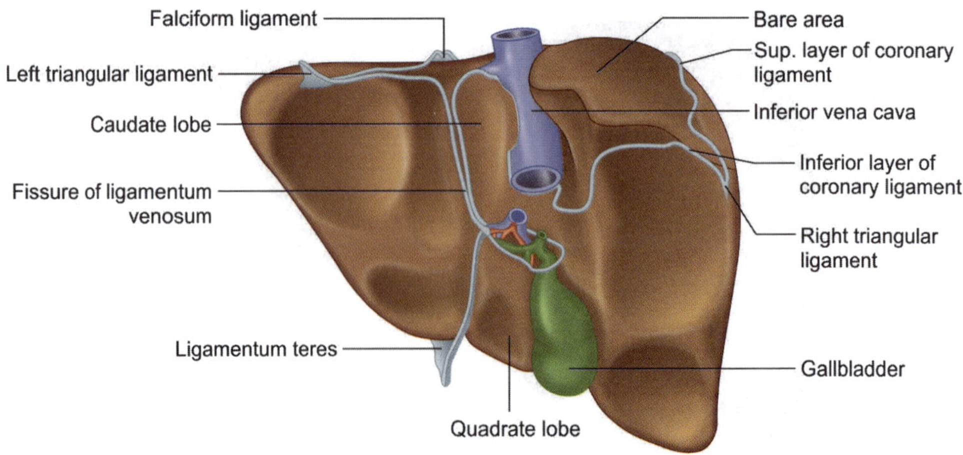

Fig. 8.25: Visceral relations of liver.

- **Superior surface:** Cardiac impression, diaphragm.
- **Inferior surface:** Gastric impression, fissure for ligamentum teres, fossa for gallbladder, colic impression, renal impression, duodenal impression.
- **Right surface:** Diaphragm (right kidney with right supracanal gland).

Blood Supply

- Hepatic artery and portal vein.
- **Veins:** Hepatic sinusoids → interlobar veins → sublobar veins → hepatic veins → inferior vena cava.

Lymphatic Drainage

Hepatic, paracardial, celiac nodes.

Nerve Supply

Hepatic plexus formed by sympathetic fibers from celiac plexus and parasympathetic fibers from both vagi via anterior gastric nerve.

Functions

- Metabolism of carbohydrates, fats and proteins.
- Synthesis of bile and prothrombin.
- Excretion of drugs, toxins, poisons, cholesterol, bile pigments and metals.
- Protection by destruction, phagocytosis, antibody formation.
- **Storage:** Glycogen, iron, fat, Vitamins A and D, blood.

Microscopic Structure (Figs. 8.26A and B)

- Liver is surrounded by a fibrous capsule.
- The parenchyma of liver is made up of liver cells (hepatocytes) which are polyhedral in shape, with a spherical nucleus.
- Inside the liver, cells are arranged in laminae, which branch and anastomose together.
- Spaces between hepatic laminae lodge hepatic sinusoids, which are lined by a layer of endothelium. Some of the lining cells have phagocytic property and are called Kupffer's cells.

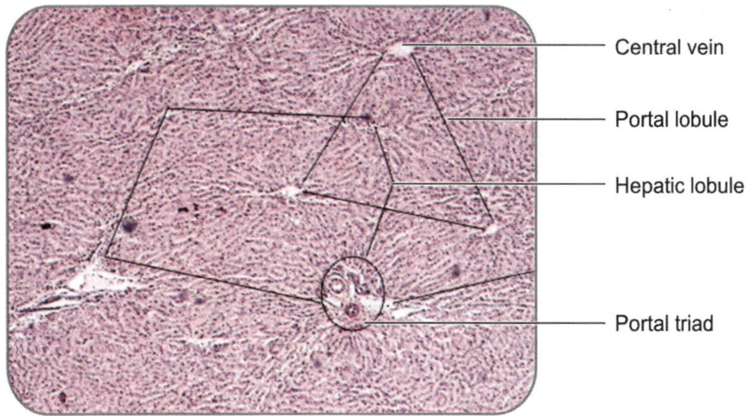

Fig. 8.26A: Photomicrograph of histology of liver.

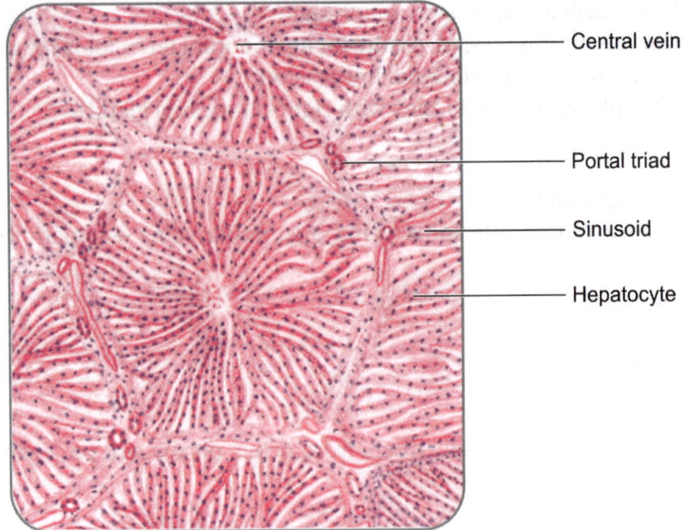

Fig. 8.26B: Diagrammatic representation of histology of liver.

- Hepatocytes are arranged in a number of polyhedral "hepatic lobules", with a central vein in the center and portal triads at the periphery. The liver cells are seen extending between the central veins and the portal triad.
- Each portal triad contains a branch of portal vein, a branch of hepatic artery, and interlobular bile ductule, enclosed in a thin connective tissue sheath.

Applied Anatomy

- **Hepatitis:** Inflammation of liver.
- **Cirrhosis:** Under certain conditions liver tissue undergoes fibrosis and shrinks.

Extrahepatic Biliary Apparatus (Fig. 8.27)

- The biliary apparatus collects bile from liver, stores it in gallbladder and transmits it to the second part of the duodenum.
- The apparatus consists of right and left hepatic ducts, common hepatic duct, gallbladder, cystic duct and bile duct.
- Right and left hepatic ducts emerge at porta hepatis from the two lobes of liver.
- Common hepatic duct is formed by right and left hepatic ducts at porta hepatis.
- It is joined by the cystic duct to form the bile duct.

Gallbladder

- Pear-shaped reservoir of bile.
- Situated in the fossa on inferior surface of right lobe of liver.
- Divided into fundus, body and neck.
- Fundus projects beyond the inferior border of the liver. Body lies in the fossa for gallbladder on the liver. The upper end of the body is continuous with the neck. The neck curves and continues as the cystic duct.

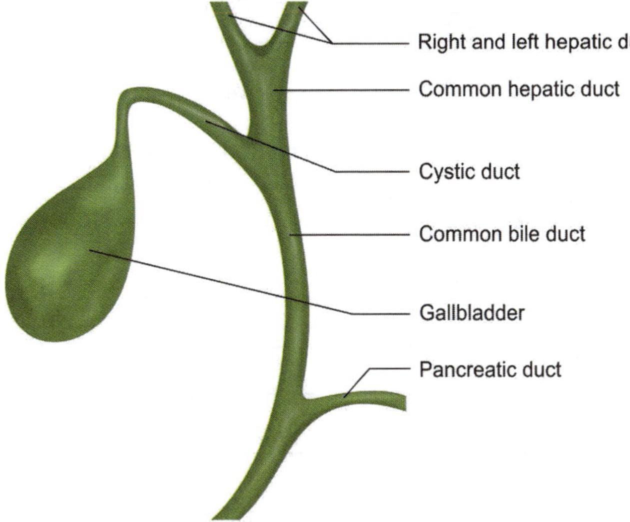

Fig. 8.27: Extrahepatic biliary apparatus.

Cystic Duct

- It is about 3–4 cm long.
- Begins at the neck of gallbladder and ends by joining common hepatic duct to form bile duct.

Microscopic Structure (Figs. 8.28A and B)

- Mucous membrane thrown into folds; lined by simple columnar epithelium with microvilli—brush border.
- Fibromuscular coat made of fibrous tissue with smooth muscles.
- Serous coat made of mesothelial cells.

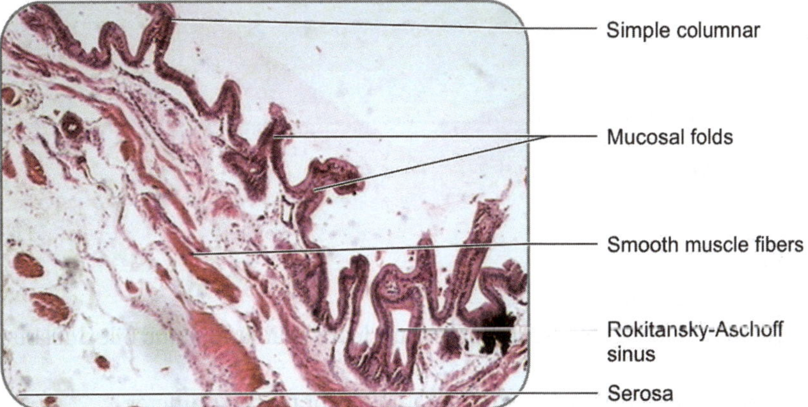

Fig. 8.28A: Photomicrograph of histology of gallbladder.

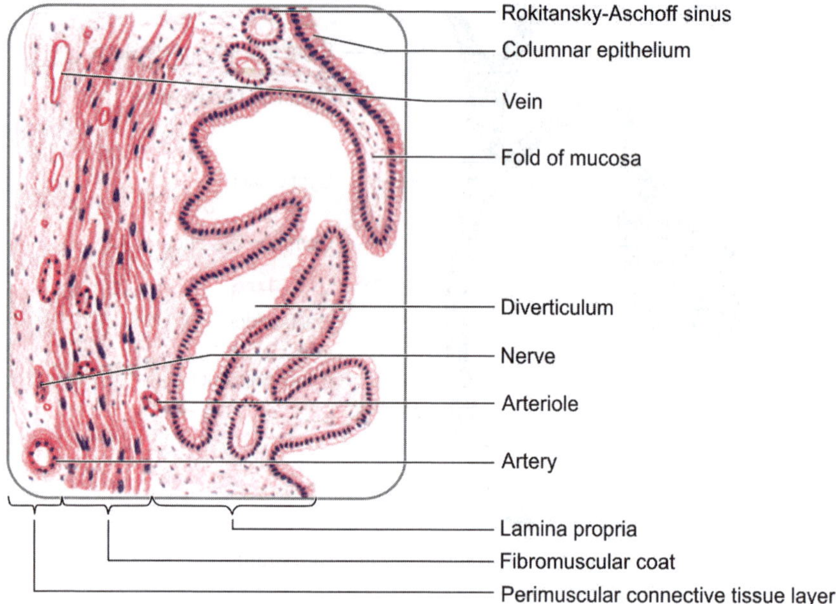

Fig. 8.28B: Diagrammatic representation of histology of gallbladder.

Functions

- Storage of bile and release into the duodenum when required.
- Absorption of water and concentration of bile.

Applied Anatomy

- Gallbladder function can be investigated by cholecystography.
- **Inflammation of gallbladder:** Cholecystitis.
- When the gallbladder is inflamed, the concentration function becomes abnormal and bile salts alone are absorbed, leaving behind cholesterol. This leads to precipitation of cholesterol and formation of gall stones.
- Removal of the gallbladder is called cholecystectomy.

Blood Supply

- Cystic artery.
- Veins drain into the portal vein.

Lymphatic Drainage

Cystic node.

Nerve Supply

- Cystic plexus of nerves.
- The parasympathetic nerves are motor to muscles of gallbladder and bile duct but inhibitory to sphincters.
- Sympathetic nerves T7–T8 are vasomotor and motor to the sphincter.
- Pain from gallbladder is felt in the inferior angle of scapula.

Pancreas (see Fig. 8.12)

- Pancreas is a soft lobulated elongated organ, partly exocrine and partly endocrine.
- The exocrine part secrets pancreatic juice and endocrine part secretes hormones.
- **Situation:** The pancreas lies on the posterior abdominal wall, at the level of L1 and L2 vertebrae. It is 15–20 cm long, about 3 cm broad and 2 cm thick.
- **Parts:** The pancreas is divided into a head, neck, body and tail.
- The head is enlarged and lies within the curve of the duodenum. The tail reaches the hilum of the spleen.

Head

The head has 3 borders (superior, inferior and right lateral), 2 surfaces (anterior and posterior) and one process, the uncinate process.

Relations

- **Superior border:** First part of duodenum; inferior border: Third part of the duodenum and the pancreatic duodenal artery.
- **Right border:** Second part of duodenum, terminal part of the bile duct.
- **Anterior surface:** Gastroduodenal artery, transverse colon and jejunum.
- **Posterior surface:** Inferior vena cava, terminal parts of the renal veins, right crus of the diaphragm, bile duct.
- **Uncinate process:** Anteriorly—superior mesenteric vessels, posteriorly—aorta.

Neck

- The neck is a constricted part, between the head and the body.
- **It has two surfaces:** Anterior and posterior.
- **Relations:** Anterior surface: Pylorus; posterior surface: Termination of the superior mesenteric vein and the beginning of the portal vein.

Body

The body is elongated. It extends from the neck to the tail. It is triangular in cross-section and has 3 borders—anterior, superior and inferior; and 3 surfaces—anterior, posterior and inferior.

Relations

- **Anterior border:** Root of transverse mesocolon.
- **Superior border:** Celiac trunk, hepatic artery and splenic artery.
- **Inferior border:** Superior mesenteric vessels.
- **Anterior surface:** Peritoneum, lesser sac, stomach.
- **Posterior surface:** Superior mesenteric artery, left crus of the diaphragm, left suprarenal gland, left kidney, left renal vessels, splenic vein.
- **Inferior surface:** Peritoneum, duodenojejunal flexure, coils of jejunum, left colic flexure.

Tail

The tail lies in the lienorenal ligament with the splenic vessels. It comes in contact with the gastric surface of the spleen.

Ducts

- The exocrine part of pancreas is drained by two ducts.
- **Main pancreatic duct (duct of Wirsung):** Lies near the posterior surface of the pancreas. It begins at the tail of pancreas and runs on the body, towards the head. The pancreatic duct, along with bile duct forms hepatopancreatic ampulla, which opens on the summit of the major duodenal papilla.
- **Accessory pancreatic duct:** Begins in the lower part of the head, crosses in front of main pancreatic duct, and opens into duodenum more proximally, at minor duodenal papilla.

Blood Supply

- Pancreatic branches of splenic, superior and inferior pancreaticoduodenal arteries.
- Venous blood is drained by splenic vein.

Lymphatic Drainage

Drain into pancreaticosplenic, celiac, superior mesenteric nodes.

Nerve Supply

- **Sympathetic:** Splanchnic nerves are vasomotor.
- **Parasympathetic:** Vagi control pancreatic secretion.

Microscopic Structure (Figs. 8.29A and B)

- **Exocrine part:** Pancreas shows a number of lobules, made up of serous acini. In the lumen of the acini centroacinar cells are present.
- Sections of intralobular and interlobular ducts can be seen. The ducts are lined by cuboidal cells.
- **Endocrine part:** Contains microscopic elements called pancreatic islets (of Langerhans). These are small isolated masses of cells, present throughout the pancreas.
- The islets have beta cells which produce insulin and alpha cells which produce glucagon.

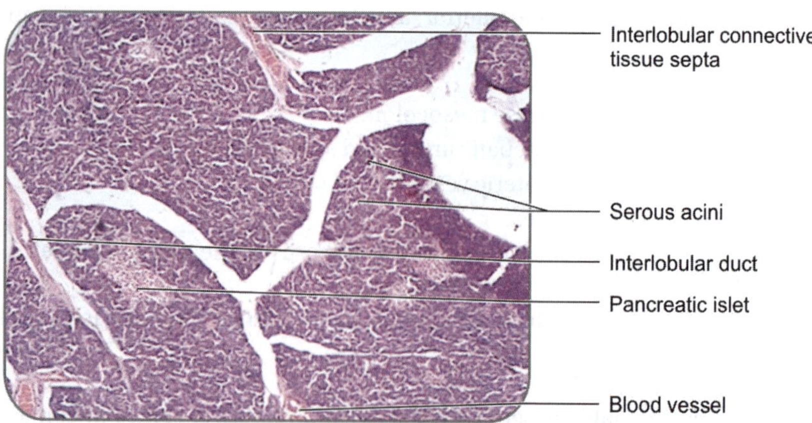

Fig. 8.29A: Photomicrograph of histology of pancreas.

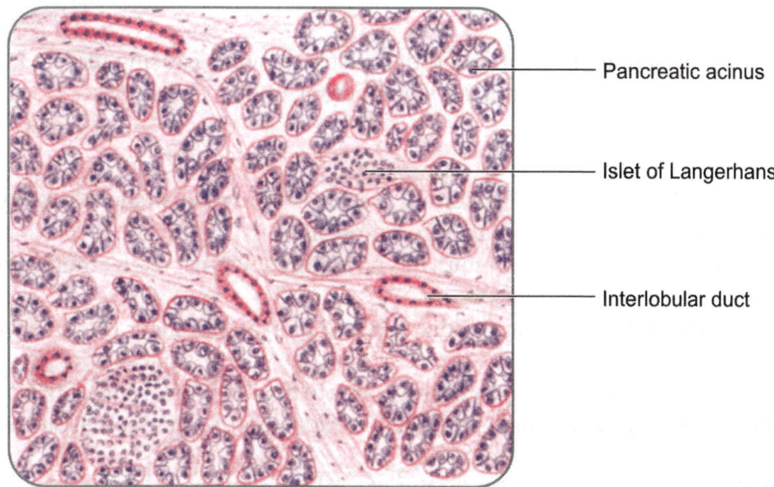

Fig. 8.29B: Diagrammatic representation of histology of pancreas.

Applied Anatomy

- Deficiency of insulin—diabetes mellitus.
- Deficiency of pancreatic enzymes causes digestive disturbances.
- Carcinoma is common over the head of pancreas. Pressure over the bile duct leads to persistence of obstructive jaundice which, in turn, gives pressure upon the portal vein and stomach, causing obstruction.
- **Developmental anomalies:**
  - Annular pancreas, encircling the 2nd part of duodenum leading to duodenal obstruction.
- Accessory pancreatic tissue may be seen.
- Inversion of the pancreatic ducts, wherein the accessory duct is larger than the main duct.

APPLIED ANATOMY

Tongue

- Injury to the hypoglossal nerve leads to paralysis of tongue muscles.
- Carcinoma of tongue is common.

Parotid Gland

- **Mumps:** Infectious disease in parotid gland caused by specific virus.
- During parotidectomy (removal of gland) care should be taken not to injure facial nerve.

Esophagus

- In portal hypertension, the veins at the lower end of esophagus dilate (esophageal varices). Rupture of these varices causes vomiting of blood (hematemesis).
- During esophagoscopy the normal constrictions of esophagus to be noted.
- In mediastinal syndrome, there will be compression of esophagus leading to dysphagia (difficulty in swallowing).

Stomach

Gastric ulcer: Increased acid secretion erodes gastric mucosa causing ulcer. Major cause is chronic inflammation due to *Helicobacter pylori* colonization.

Small and Large Intestine

- **Duodenal cap:** The first part of duodenum is seen as triangular shadow in X-rays.
- **Peptic ulcer:** First part of duodenum is common site.
- After barium meal, in X-rays the jejunum has no features, ileum looks feathery, large intestine shows characteristic haustrations.
- **Appendicitis:** Inflammation of appendix, referred pain at umbilicus (both supplied by T10 segment).
- **McBurney's point:** Base of appendix corresponds to the junction of lateral 1/3rd and medial 2/3rds of the line joining umbilicus to right anterior superior iliac spine. Site of maximum tenderness.
- **Prolapse of rectum:** Rectum protrudes out of anal canal.
- Per rectal examination is done in males to check the abnormalities in accessory genital organs.
- **Hemorrhoids/Piles:** Dilatation of veins in rectum and anal canal.
- **Anal fistula:** A narrow tunnel communicating between the internal opening in anal canal and external opening in the skin near the anus.

Spleen

- **Splenomegaly:** Enlargement of spleen which occurs in diseases like typhoid, malaria, leukemias and carcinoma.
- **Splenectomy:** Surgical removal of spleen.
- **Splenic puncture:** A needle can be passed into the spleen through the 8th or 9th intercostal space in the midaxillary line.

Liver

- **Hepatitis:** Inflammation of liver.
- **Cirrhosis of liver:** Liver tissue is replaced by fibrous tissue and shrinks.

Gallbladder

- **Cholecystography:** Radiological procedure used to visualize gallbladder.
- **Cholecystitis:** Inflammation of gallbladder.
- **Gallstones:** Bile contains enough chemicals to dissolve the cholesterol excreted by liver. But if liver excretes more cholesterol than bile can dissolve, the excess cholesterol may form into crystals and eventually into stones.
- **Cholecystectomy:** Removal of gallbladder.

Pancreas

- Deficiency of insulin secreted by pancreas leads to diabetes mellitus.
- Carcinoma is common over the head of pancreas. Pressure over the bile duct leads to persistence of obstructive jaundice which in turn gives pressure upon the portal vein and stomach causing obstruction.
- **Developmental anomalies of pancreas:** Annular pancreas, accessory pancreatic tissue, accessory pancreatic duct may be larger than main duct.

SUMMARY

Tongue

Features	*Details*
Functions	Taste, speech, mastication, deglutition
External features	Root, tip, ventral surface, dorsal surface, 2 lateral borders
Dorsal surface	Covered by mucous membrane with papillae in anterior 2/3rds and lingual tonsil in posterior 1/3rd
Ventral surface	Smooth
Muscles	Intrinsic (superior longitudinal, inferior longitudinal, transverse, vertical), extrinsic (genioglossus, hyoglossus, styloglossus, palatoglossus)
Blood supply	Lingual artery, venae comitantes, deep lingual vein, lingual vein
Lymphatic drainage	Submental nodes, submandibular nodes, jugulo-omohyoid nodes
Nerve supply	Motor—hypoglossal except palatoglossus by pharyngeal plexus, Sensory—general (lingual-anterior 2/3rds, glossopharyngeal—posterior 1/3rd), special (chorda tympani—anterior 2/3rds, glossopharyngeal—posterior 1/3rd), posterior most part—vagus

Salivary Glands

Features	*Parotid gland*	*Submandibular gland*	*Sublingual gland*
Situation	Near external acoustic meatus	Digastric triangle	Floor of mouth
Capsule	Investing layer of deep cervical fascia	Connective tissue	Connective tissue
External features	Apex, surfaces (Base or superior, superficial, anteromedial, posteromedial), borders (anterior, posterior, medial)	Superficial, deep parts	-
Structures in gland	Arteries (External carotid, maxillary, superficial temporal), veins (Maxillary, superficial temporal, retromandibular), facial nerve with its branches	-	-
Duct	Opens into vestibule of mouth opposite upper second molar tooth	Opens into floor of mouth	Opens into floor of mouth
Blood supply	External carotid artery, external jugular vein	Facial and lingual arteries, facial and lingual veins	Facial and lingual arteries, facial and lingual veins
Nerve supply			
Parasympathetic	Glossopharyngeal → otic ganglion → auriculotemporal	Facial → chorda tympani → submandibular ganglion → lingual	Facial → chorda tympani → submandibular ganglion → lingual

Features	Parotid gland	Submandibular gland	Sublingual gland
Sympathetic	Plexus around external carotid artery	Plexus around facial artery	Plexus around facial artery
Sensory	Auriculotemporal nerve	Lingual nerve	Lingual nerve

Different Parts of Digestive System

Organs	External features	Blood supply	Nerve supply
Pharynx	Parts (Nasopharynx, oropharynx, laryngopharynx), muscles (Constrictors–superior, middle, inferior), longitudinal (Stylopharyngeus, palatopharyngeus, salpingopharyngeus)	External carotid and maxillary arteries, facial and internal jugular veins	Motor (Pharyngeal plexus except stylopharyngeus by glossopharyngeal nerve), sensory (Glossopharyngeal nerve)
Esophagus	25 cm long, extends from cricoid cartilage to stomach, constrictions (From incisor teeth 6 inches, 9 inches, 11 inches, 15 inches)	Arteries (Inferior thyroid, esophageal branches, left gastric), veins (Brachiocephalic, azygos, left gastric)	Parasympathetic (Recurrent laryngeal, esophageal), sympathetic (Middle cervical ganglion, upper 4 thoracic ganglia)
Stomach	Situation: Epigastric, umbilical, hypochondriac regions. Two orifices: Cardiac, pyloric, Two curvatures: Lesser, greater, Two surfaces: Anterior (liver, diaphragm), posterior (diaphragm, left kidney, left suprarenal, pancreas, transverse mesocolon, splenic flexure of colon, splenic artery)	Arteries: Left gastric, right gastric, left gastroepiploic, right gastroepiploic, short gastric Veins: Superior mesenteric, portal, splenic Lymphatic: Pancreaticosplenic, left gastric, right gastroepiploic, splenic, hepatic, pyloric nodes	Sympathetic: T6–T10 spinal segments Parasympathetic: Vagus
Duodenum	Shortest of small intestine. 10 inches long. Extent: Pylorus to duodenojejunal flexure 4 parts: First/superior, second/vertical/descending, third/horizontal, fourth/ascending	Arteries: Superior and inferior pancreatico-duodenal Veins: Splenic, superior mesenteric, portal Lymphatics: Pancreatico-duodenal	Sympathetic: T9, T10 spinal segments Parasympathetic: Vagus
Jejunum	Forms upper 2/5ths of small intestine. Suspended from fold of mesentery, 1–2 arterial arcades, longer and few vasa recta Extent: Duodenojejunal flexure to proximal ileum. Thick and more vascular walls	Artery: Superior mesenteric Vein: Superior mesenteric Lymphatics: Superior mesenteric nodes	Sympathetic: T9, T10 spinal segments Parasympathetic: Vagus

Organs	*External features*	*Blood supply*	*Nerve supply*
Ileum	Forms upper 3/5ths of small intestine. Suspended from fold of mesentery, 3–6 arterial arcades, short and more vasa recta Extent: Distal jejunum to ileocecal junction. Thick and more vascular walls	Artery: Superior mesenteric Vein: Superior mesenteric Lymphatics: Superior mesenteric nodes	Sympathetic: T9, T10 spinal segments Parasympathetic: Vagus
Large intestine	Extent: Ileocecal junction to anus. 1.5 cm long Parts: Cecum and appendix, ascending colon, transverse colon, descending colon, sigmoid colon, rectum, anal canal Taenia coli: Thickened longitudinal muscle coats haustrations/ sacculations: Out-pocketing of wall Appendices epiploicae: Small bags of fat	Arteries: Superior mesenteric till right 2/3rds of transverse colon, inferior mesenteric for the rest Veins: Superior and inferior mesenteric Lymphatics: Epicolic and paracolic nodes	Sympathetic: T11–L1 spinal segments up to right 2/3rds of transverse colon, rest by L1, L2 spinal segments Parasympathetic: Vagus up to right 2/3rds, rest by pelvic splanchnic
Cecum	Blind pouch in right iliac fossa. Types: Conical (appendix at apex), funicular (appendix in depression at the center), ampullary (appendix at one side)	• Arteries: Cecal branches of ieocolic • Veins: Superior mesenteric	Sympathetic: T11–L1 spinal segments Parasympathetic: Vagus
Appendix	• Arises in posteromedial wall of cecum. 9 cm long • Positions: Paracolic/11 O'clock, retrocecal/12 O'clock, splenic/2 O'clock, sacral/promontoric/3 O'clock, pelvic/4 O'clock, midinguinal/6 O'clock	• Artery: Appendicular Veins: Appendicular, ileocolic, superior mesenteric • Lymphatic: Ileocolic nodes	• Sympathetic: T9, T10 spinal segments • Parasympathetic: Vagus
Rectum	• Extent: Sigmoid colon to anorectal junction, 12 cm long, • Curvatures: 2 anteroposterior, 3 lateral	• Artery: Superior and middle rectal, median sacral • Veins: Superior and middle rectal • Lymphatic: Internal iliac nodes	Sympathetic: L1, L2 spinal segments Parasympathetic: S2–S4
Anal canal	• 3.8 cm long, 3 parts • Upper part: 15 mm, mucous membrane thrown into folds (anal columns), attached at lower ends by anal valves (pectinate line), anal sinus is in between anal columns, Middle part: 15 mm, dense venous plexus	• Artery: Superior and inferior rectal • Veins: Internal and external rectal venous plexus • Lymphatic: Internal iliac and superficial inguinal nodes	Sympathetic: L1, L2 spinal segments Parasympathetic: S2–S4

Organs	*External features*	*Blood supply*	*Nerve supply*
	• Lower part: 8 mm, skin with glands and hair • White line of Hilton: Junction between mucous membrane (middle part) and skin (lower part) Sphincters: External, internal		
Spleen	• Lies in left hypochondrium • 2 ends: Anterior, posterior • 3 borders: Superior, intermediate, inferior • 2 surfaces: Diaphragmatic (pleura, lung, 9, 10, 11 ribs), visceral (gastric, renal, colic, pancreatic)	Artery: Splenic artery Vein: Splenic veins Lymphatics: Pancreaticosplenic nodes	Celiac plexus
Liver	Largest gland in the body, secretes bile, helps in metabolism. Surfaces: Anterior, posterior, right, superior, inferior Lobes: Right, left, caudate, quadrate Porta hepatis: Portal vein, hepatic artery, right and left hepatic duct, hepatic plexus of nerves Ligaments: Falciform, right triangular, left triangular, coronary	Arteries: Hepatic artery, portal vein Veins: Hepatic sinusoids → interlobar veins → sublobar veins → hepatic veins → inferior vena cava Lymphatics: Hepatic, paracardial, celiac nodes	Sympathetic: Hepatic plexus Parasympathetic: Vagus
Pancreas	Partly exocrine and endocrine gland Extent: Duodenum to spleen Parts: Head, neck, body, tail Ducts: Main pancreatic (duct of Wirsung), accessory pancreatic duct opens into major and minor duodenal papilla respectively	Arteries: Branches of splenic, superior and inferior pancreaticoduodenal Veins: Splenic vein Lymphatics: Pancreaticosplenic, celiac, superior mesenteric nodes	Sympathetic: Splanchnic nerves Parasympathetic: Vagus

QUESTIONS

Long Essays

- Name parts of GIT. Describe stomach/duodenum/intestines/cecum and appendix in detail.
- Name the salivary glands. Describe parotid/submandibular gland in detail.

Short Essays

- Extrahepatic biliary apparatus
- Gallbladder
- Pancreas
- Stomach

- Liver
- Submandibular/Parotid gland
- Tooth
- Tongue
- Pharnyx.

Short Answers

- Name parts of pancreas
- Parts of large intestine
- Parts of stomach
- Name muscles of pharynx
- Parts of pharynx
- Parts of small intestine
- Functions of liver
- Functions of spleen
- Differences between small and large intestines
- Meckel's diverticulum.

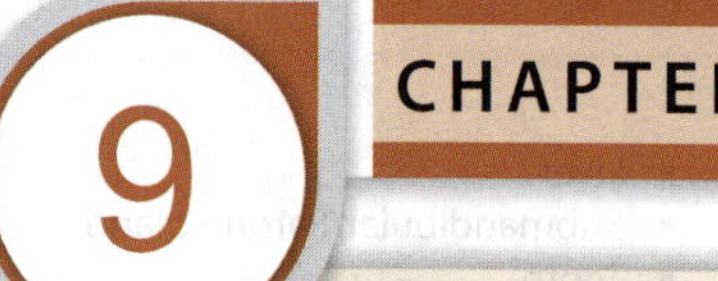

Urinary System

LEARNING OBJECTIVES

The student should be able to:

- Name the parts of urinary system, describe details of kidney, ureter, urinary bladder, male and female urethra.
- Histology of kidney, ureter and urinary bladder.

INTRODUCTION

- The parts of urinary system are a pair of kidneys and ureters and a urinary bladder and urethra.
- The organs of the urinary system excrete and eliminate the urine from the body. The production and excretion of urine are important since they are one of the mechanisms which maintain homeostasis in the body.

KIDNEYS (FIG. 9.1)

- Kidneys are a pair of excretory organs. They remove the waste products of metabolism and excess of water and salts from the blood and maintain its pH.
- **Situation:** They are retroperitoneal organs lying in the posterior abdominal wall, one on either side of the vertebral column, behind the peritoneum.
- The left kidney is slightly at a higher level than the right since the massive liver occupies the right hypochondrium.
- **Shape and size:** Bean shaped and has two poles: Upper and lower, two borders: Medial and lateral and two surfaces: Anterior and posterior.
- 11 cm long, 6 cm broad and 3 cm thick.

Coverings

- Each kidney is invested by the following layers from within outwards.
- The fibrous capsule is formed by the condensation of the fibrous connective tissue on the periphery of the organ. Normally it can be easily stripped off, but in diseased conditions, it becomes adherent to the kidney.
- Perirenal fat consists of collection of fatty tissue around the kidney.

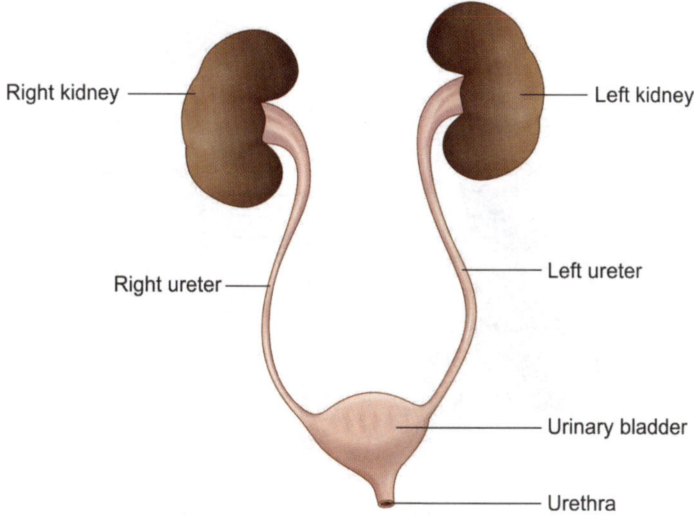

Fig. 9.1: Parts of urinary system.

- Renal fascia consists of an anterior layer and a posterior layer.
- Pararenal fat consists of fatty tissue. It is more posteriorly placed and forms a cushion for the kidneys.

Relations of the Kidneys

- **Upper pole** to the suprarenal gland. The lower pole lies about one inch above the iliac crests.
- **Lateral border** is convex. The **medial border** is concave. In the middle, the medial border presents a hilum through which the renal vein, lymphatics and ureter emerges out. The renal artery and renal plexus of nerves enter the hilum. From before backwards, the structures are arranged as renal vein, renal artery and ureter. The hilum leads into renal sinus.
- **Anterior surface (Fig. 9.2): Right kidney:** Right suprarenal gland, liver, 2nd part of the duodenum, hepatic flexure of the colon, small intestine; **Left kidney:** Left suprarenal gland, spleen, stomach, pancreas, splenic vessels, splenic flexure of the colon, descending colon, jejunum.
- **Posterior surface (Fig. 9.3):** Both the kidneys have same relations: The diaphragm, psoas major, quadratus lumborum, transversus abdominis, subcostal vessels, subcostal, iliohypogastric and ilioinguinal nerves. The right kidney is related to 12th ribs and the left kidney to the 11th and 12th ribs.

Structure of the Kidney

Macroscopic Structure (Fig. 9.4)

- Coronal section of a kidney shows an outer reddish-brown cortex and an inner pale medulla.
- The renal medulla is madeup of conical masses called the pyramids.
- Their apices form the renal papillae which project into the minor calyces.
- Each papilla is formed by the fusion of 2–4 pyramids.
- The renal cortex is granular in appearance.
- A pyramid and the overlying cortex are said to form one lobe of the kidney.

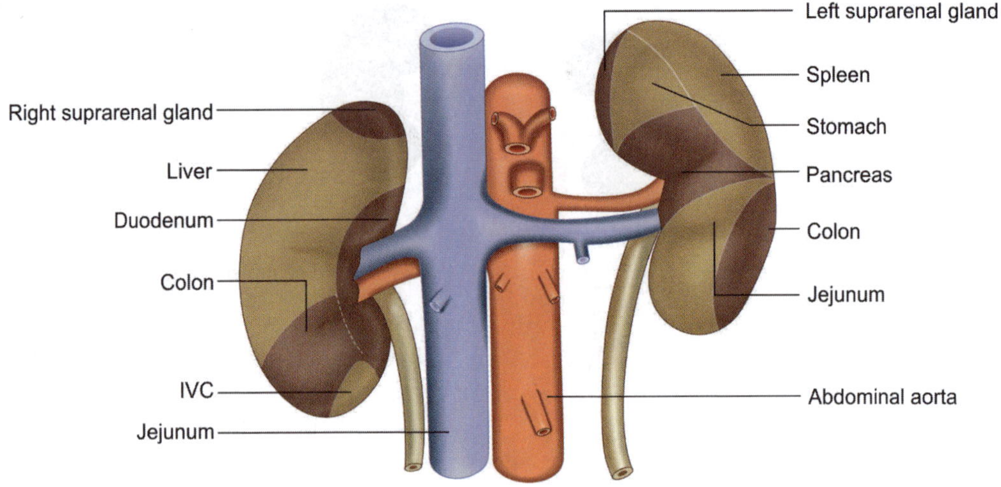

Fig. 9.2: Anterior relations of kidney.

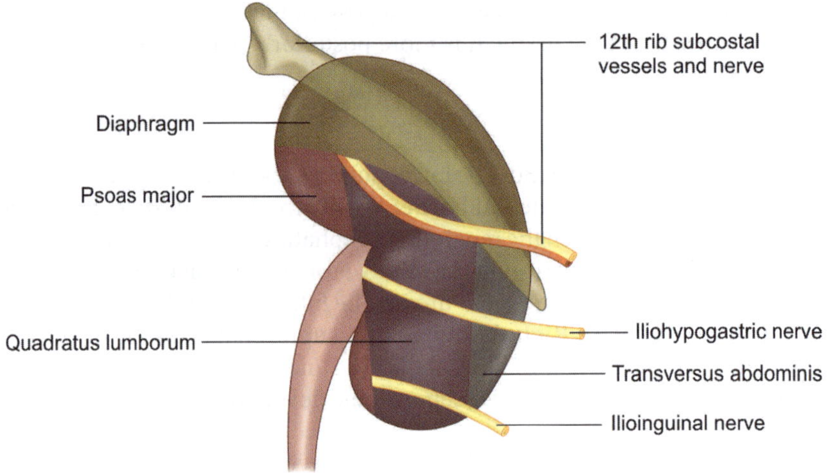

Fig. 9.3: Posterior relations of kidney.

Microscopic Structure (Figs. 9.5A and B)

- Each kidney is made up of masses of individual excretory units, the nephrons.
- A nephron consists of a Bowman's capsule, a proximal convoluted tubule, and a distal convoluted tubule, all three of which are located in the renal cortex.
- The proximal convoluted tubules are lined by tall pyramidal cells. The cytoplasm stains deeply with eosin and basal part of the cells are striated. The nuclei are large, spherical and are at the base of the cells. The free borders of the cells have microvilli—brush border appearance.
- The distal convoluted tubules are smaller in size, their lining cells are flatter and the lumen larger. The brush border and eosinophilic cytoplasm is absent.

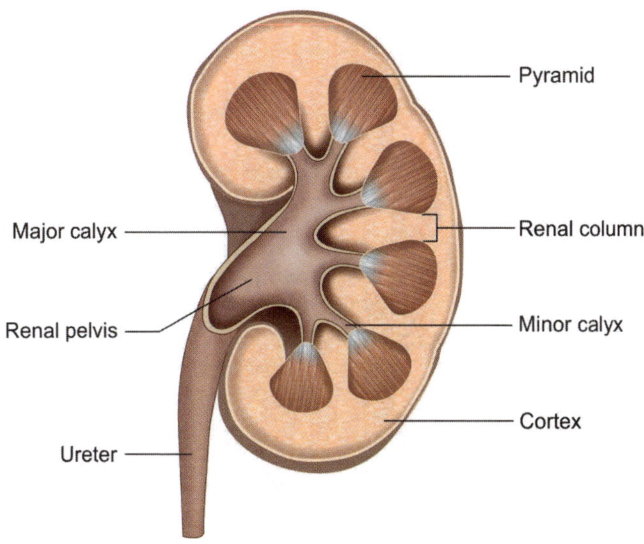

Fig. 9.4: Macroscopic structure of kidney.

- The two convoluted tubules are connected by the loop of Henle, which lies in the renal medulla.
- The descending limb of Henle's loop is thin and lining epithelium is flat. The ascending limb is thicker and the lining cells are cuboidal.
- Distal convoluted tubules empty into collecting tubules, which also lie in the medulla and which empty into the kidney's central cavity, the pelvis.
- The Bowman's capsule consists of a capillary bed called a glomerulus.
- The distal convoluted tubule lies between afferent and efferent arterioles at the vascular pole of glomerulus.
- Between the tubule and vascular pole there is a collection of small cells (macula densa).

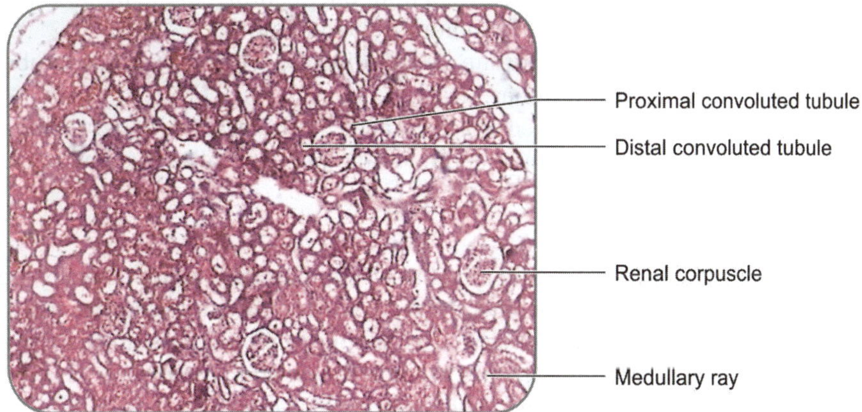

Fig. 9.5A: Photomicrograph of histology of kidney.

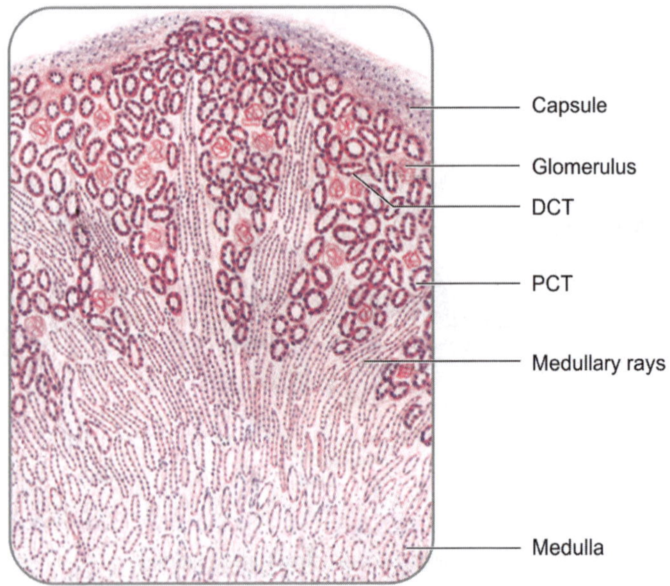

Fig. 9.5B: Diagrammatic representation of histology of kidney.

- The muscle cells of afferent arterioles of this region are large, rounded and epithelioid in type and have large spherical nuclei. The cytoplasm is granular, and the cells are called juxtaglomerular cells.

Process of Excretion

- The nephrons filter out urea and any other substances above their kidney threshold level from the blood.
- The nephrons reabsorb water as well as sugars, amino acids, and salts from the filtrate in their lumen, returning these materials to the blood.
- Sugars, amino acids, and salts are returned from the nephrons to the blood via an active transport mechanism in the form of a sodium/potassium pump.
- The collecting tubules collect the filtrate, called urine, from distal convoluted tubules and channel it into the pelvis of the kidney.
- From each kidney the urine is carried by a duct called the ureter to the urinary bladder which stores urine until it is emptied to the exterior via another duct called the urethra.

Blood Supply

- Renal artery, a branch from the abdominal aorta supplies the kidneys. Usually, one renal artery supplies each kidney. At the hilus, the renal artery divides into anterior and posterior divisions. Further, segmental arteries arise, each supplies one vascular segment. Five vascular segments have been noted—apical, upper, middle, lower and posterior.
- Renal veins, one on each side drain into the inferior vena cava.
- Left renal vein receives left gonadal vein, left suprarenal vein.

Lymphatic Drainage

Lateral aortic nodes.

Nerve Supply

Renal plexus. It contains sympathetic fibers which are chiefly vasomotor.

Developmental Anomalies of Kidneys

- Congenital polycystic kidney due to nonunion of the secretory and collecting parts.
- Horseshoe-shaped kidney due to fusion of the lower poles, rarely upper poles.

Applied Anatomy

Hydronephrosis–Stagnation of urine in kidneys. Glomerulonephritis, inflammation.

URETERS

- The ureters are a pair of narrow, thick-walled muscular tubes which convey urine from the kidneys to the urinary bladder.
- **Situation:** Lie posterior to the peritoneum, close to the posterior abdominal wall in the upper part and to the pelvic wall in the lower part.
- **Size:** Each ureter is about 25 cm long (10 inches) and 3 mm in diameter.
- **Course:** Begins within the renal sinus from the renal pelvis. It runs downwards along the medial margin of the kidney. It passes on the psoas major muscle, enters the pelvis by crossing in front of the termination of common iliac artery. It turns medially to reach the base of the urinary bladder. It enters the bladder wall obliquely and opens into the bladder at the lateral angle of its trigone.

Constrictions of the Ureter

- At the pelvi-ureteric junction.
- At the brim of the lesser pelvis.
- At its passage through the bladder wall.

Blood Supply

Branches from the renal artery, aorta, vesicular, middle rectal vessels.

Nerve Supply

- **Sympathetic:** T10-L1.
- **Parasympathetic:** S2-3 nerves.

Microscopic Structure (Figs. 9.6A and B)

- **Mucosa:** Epithelium consists of transitional epithelium. The lumen is star shaped with 4–6 folds. The lamina propria has connective tissue.
- **Muscularis externa:** It has an inner circular and outer longitudinal layer of smooth muscles.
- **Adventitia:** It has no peritoneal covering and is lined by fibrosa.

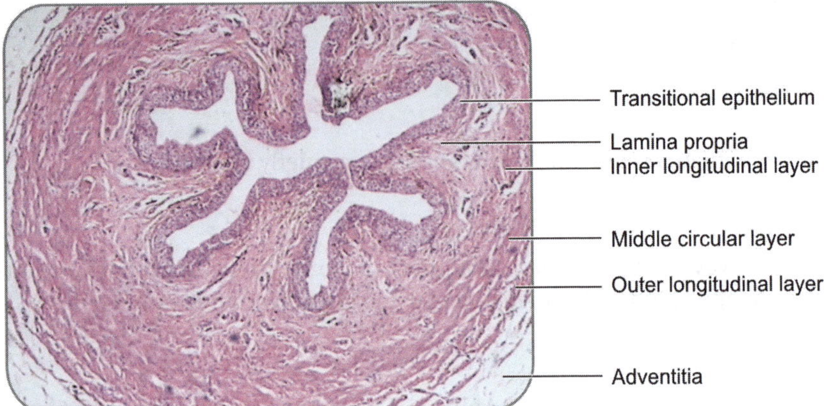

Fig. 9.6A: Photomicrograph of histology of ureter.

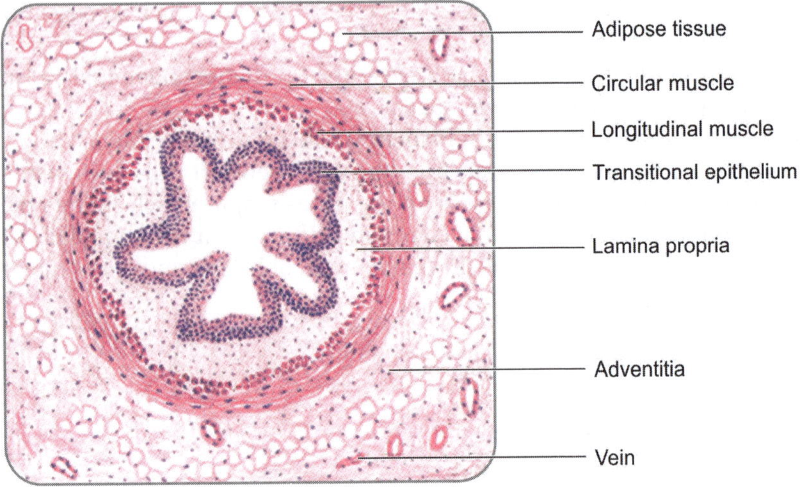

Fig. 9.6B: Diagrammatic representation of histology of ureter.

Applied Anatomy

- Renal colic is the term used for severe pain due to a ureteric stone which causes spasm of the ureter.
- A ureteric stone is liable to become impacted at one of the sites of normal constrictions of the ureter, causing hydronephrosis.

URINARY BLADDER (FIG. 9.7)

- The urinary bladder is a hollow muscular organ which acts like a reservoir of urine, to collect urine and discharge it out periodically.
- **Shape:** An empty bladder resembles a four-sided pyramid. It has an apex, a base, a neck, three surfaces—one superior and two inferolateral. A full bladder is ovoid in shape.

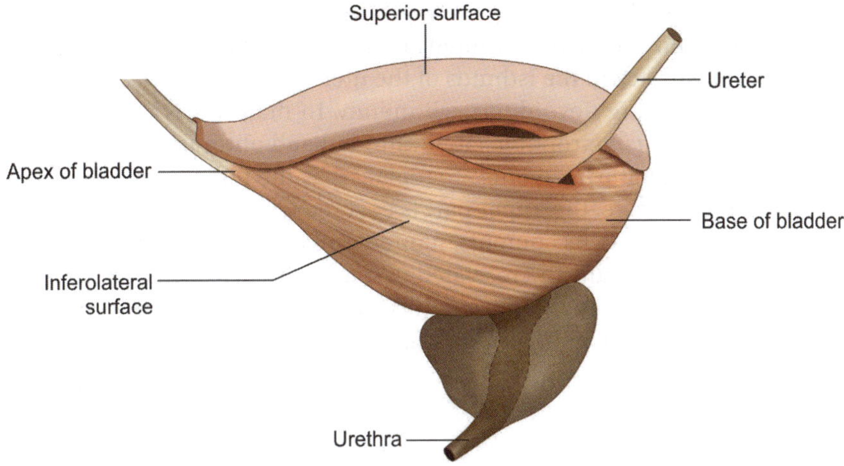

Fig. 9.7: Urinary bladder.

- **Situation:** An empty bladder is situated within the true pelvis. When it gets filled, it rises up to the abdominal cavity. In fetus and in newborn, even the empty bladder is abdominal in position as the pelvic cavity is not large enough to accommodate it.
- **Capacity:** The normal capacity of the bladder is about 200–300 cc.

Relations (Fig. 9.8)

- Apex is connected to the umbilicus by the median umbilical ligament which represents the obliterated embryonic urachus.
- Neck lies 3–4 cm behind the lower part of the pubic symphysis. It is pierced by the internal urethral orifice. In males, it rests on the base of the prostate.

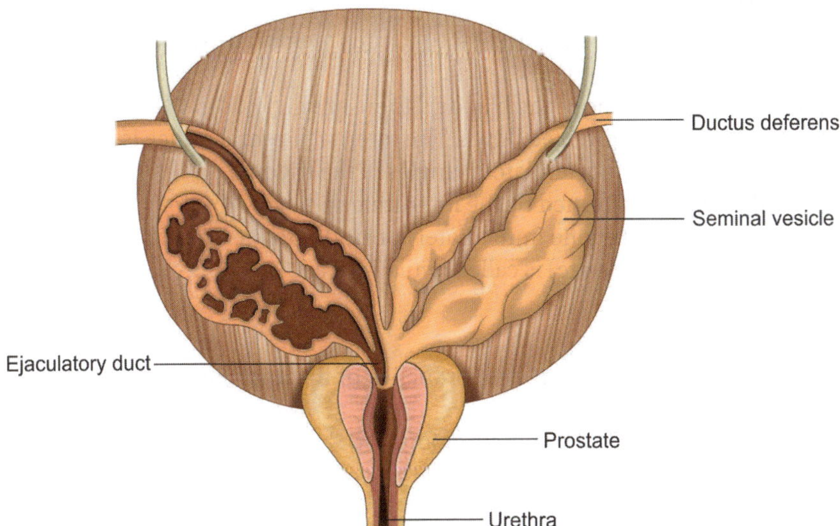

Fig. 9.8: Posterior relations of urinary bladder.

- Superior surface: In males, it is completely covered by peritoneum and is in contact with the sigmoid colon and coils of the terminal ileum. In females, the peritoneum is reflected from the superior surface to the isthmus of the uterus to form the vesicouterine pouch.
- Inferolateral surfaces are devoid of peritoneum. In males, it is related to the pubis, puboprostatic ligaments, retropubic fat, levator ani and obturator internus muscles. In females, the puboprostatic ligaments are replaced by the pubovesical ligaments.
- **Posterior surface:** In male, the upper part is covered with peritoneum and is related to the rectovesical pouch and its contents, namely coils of terminal ileum. The lower part is not covered by peritoneum and is related to seminal vesicles and vasa deferentia. The Denonvilliers fascia intervenes between these and the rectum. In the female, whole of this surface is not covered with peritoneum and is directly related to the anterior wall of the vagina.

Ligaments

True and false.

True ligaments: Help to support the bladder.
- Lateral true ligament
- Posterior true ligament
- Medial puboprostatic ligaments (in females, pubovesical ligaments)
- Lateral puboprostatic ligaments
- Median umbilical ligament.

False ligaments: Peritoneal folds.
- Median umbilical fold
- Two lateral umbilical folds
- Lateral false ligaments
- Posterior false ligaments.

Interior of the Bladder

- In an empty bladder, the greater part of the mucous membrane shows irregular folds due to its loose attachment to the muscular coat.
- In the posterior wall (trigone of the bladder) there are no folds in the mucosa.
- The apex of the trigone is directed down. The internal urethral orifice is situated here.
- The ureters open into the posterolateral angles of the trigone.
- The base of the trigone is formed by the interureteric ridge.
- A slight elevation on the trigone immediately posterior to the urethral orifice (produced by the median lobe of the prostate) is called uvula vesicae.

Blood Supply

- Superior and inferior vesical arteries (branches of the anterior trunk of the internal iliac artery).
- Vesical venous plexus drain the venous blood.

Lymphatics

Drain into the external iliac lymph nodes.

Nerve Supply

- Vesical plexus of nerves. It is made up of the inferior hypogastric plexus and contains both sympathetic and parasympathetic nerves.
- Sympathetic fibers (T12-L2) are inhibitory to the detrusor muscle and motor to sphincter vesicae. They are chiefly vasomotor.
- Parasympathetic fibers (S2,3,4) are motor to the detrusor muscle and inhibitory to the sphincter vesicae. If these are destroyed, normal micturition is not possible.
- **Sensory:** Pain sensations are carried mainly by the parasympathetic fibers.
- Somatic (pudendal nerve - S2, 3, 4) supplies the sphincter urethrae which is voluntary.

Microscopic Structure (Figs. 9.9A and B)

- **Mucosa:** It is lined by transitional epithelium. Lamina propria has connective tissue with very few mucous glands. Muscularis mucosa is absent.
- **Submucosa** is absent.
- **Muscularis externa** consists of longitudinal, circular and obliquely arranged muscles, specially called detrusor.
- **Adventitia** is lined by peritoneum in certain areas (serosa) and is nonperitoneal in certain areas (fibrosa).

Applied Anatomy

- A distended bladder may be ruptured by injuries of the lower abdominal wall.
- **Urinary incontinence** is due to loss of the voluntary initiation and voluntary inhibition of micturition.
  - In cases where excitatory pathways are affected, it is depressed leading to the retention of urine followed by overflow incontinence.
  - In cases where inhibitory pathways are affected, it is exaggerated leading to the precipitancy of micturition.
  - Lesions of sympathetic motor pathway produce dribbling incontinence due to the paralysis of sphincter mechanism.
  - Lesions of parasympathetic motor pathways leads to retention of urine.

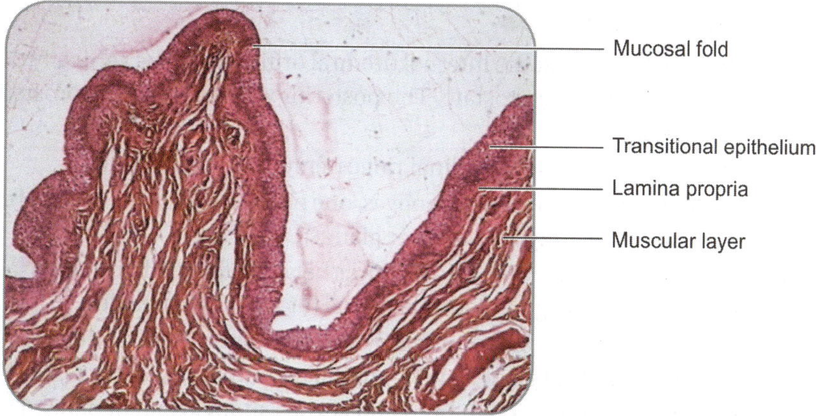

Fig. 9.9A: Photomicrograph of histology of urinary bladder.

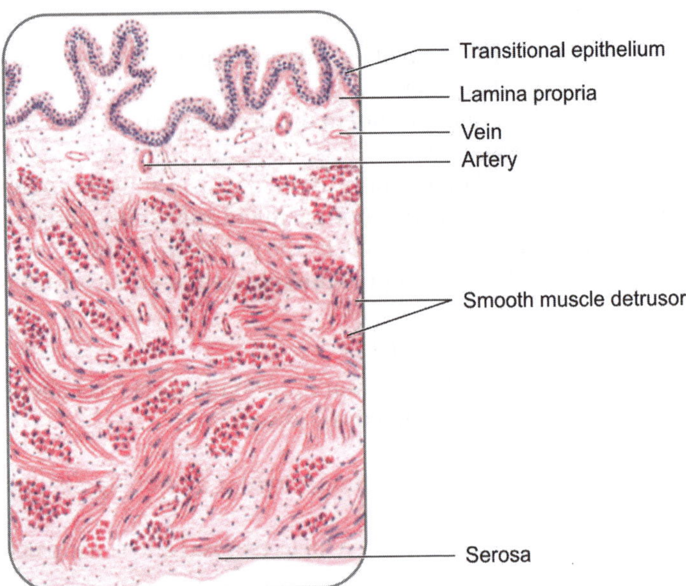

Fig. 9.9B: Diagrammatic representation of histology of urinary bladder.

- **Ectopia vesicae** is a developmental anomaly wherein the anterior wall of the urinary bladder is absent. The trigone and the ureters can be seen on the surface.
- **Cystoscopy** is done to see the interior of the bladder.

URETHRA

Male Urethra

Male urethra is 18–20 cm long. It extends from the internal urethral orifice (at the neck of the urinary bladder) to the external urethral orifice at the tip of the penis.

Parts of Male Urethra (Fig. 9.10)

- **Prostatic part:** 3 cm. It begins at the internal urethral orifice and runs vertically downwards through the anterior part of the prostate. The posterior wall (floor) of the prostatic urethra presents the following features:
  - A median urethral crest is a longitudinal ridge of mucous membrane.
  - The prostatic sinuses are two vertical grooves, one on each side of the urethral crest. Each sinus presents 20–30 openings of prostatic glands.
  - Prostatic utricle is a blind sac, directed upwards between the median and posterior lobes of the prostate. It is homologous with the uterus (or vagina) of females.
- **Membranous part:** 2 cm. It is surrounded by the sphincter urethrae (external urethral sphincter). Numerous urethral glands open into the membranous urethra.
- **Spongy part:** 15 cm. It passes through bulb and corpus spongiosum of penis. The ducts of the bulbourethral glands open here.

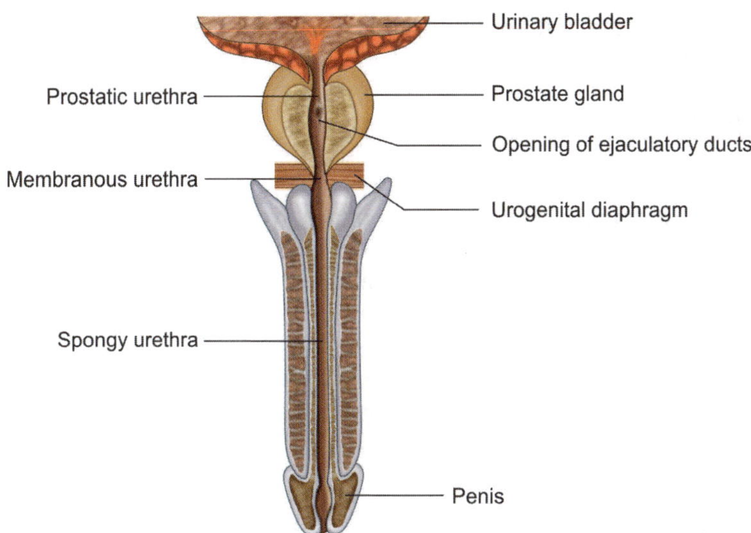

Fig. 9.10: Parts of male urethra.

Sphincters

- **Internal urethral sphincter:** It is involuntary and is supplied by sympathetic nerves. It is made up of collection of smooth muscle fibers and collagen and elastic tissue.
- **External urethral sphincter:** It is voluntary; made-up of striated muscle (sphincter urethrae) fibers and supplied by pudendal nerve (S2,3,4).

Blood Supply

The urethra is supplied by the inferior vesical, middle rectal and internal pudendal vessels.

Lymphatics

Drain into the external iliac and superficial inguinal nodes.

Applied Anatomy

- **Catheterization of bladder:** While passing a catheter into the bladder through the urethra, the curvatures of the urethra should be kept in consideration.
- **Rupture** of the urethra causes extravasation of urine.
- Infection of the urethra is called **urethritis.**
- **Hypospadias** is a common anomaly where urethra opens on undersurface of penis.
- **Epispadias** is a rare condition in which urethra opens on dorsum of the penis.

Female Urethra

- The female urethra is 4 cm long. Developmentally, it corresponds to the upper part of the prostatic urethra in males.
- It begins at the internal urethral orifice, at the neck of the urinary bladder.
- It runs downwards and traverses the urogenital diaphragm and ends at the external urethral orifice.

- In a female urethra, the paraurethral glands are found, one on each side. These glands correspond to the male prostate.

APPLIED ANATOMY

Kidney

- **Developmental anomalies of kidney:** Congenital polycystic kidney (nonunion of collecting and secretory parts), horseshoe-shaped kidney (fusion of lower poles).
- **Hydronephrosis:** Swelling of kidney due to failure of drainage of urine.
- Urinalysis is the examination and analysis of urine.
- **Urolithiasis:** Stones in kidney.
- Urinary tract infections may occur in the urethra (urethritis), the urinary bladder (cystitis), the prostate gland (prostatitis), and the kidney (pyelonephritis).

Ureter

- **Renal colic:** Severe pain due to ureteric stone which causes spasm of ureter.
- Ureteric stone is liable to become impacted at one of the sites of normal constrictions of the ureter.

Urinary Bladder

- Distended bladder can be ruptured by injuries of the lower abdominal wall.
- **Urinary incontinence:** Involuntary leakage of urine.
- **Ectopia vesicae:** Urinary bladder can be seen on the surface due to the absence of lower anterior abdominal wall.
- **Cystoscopy:** Is a procedure to look inside the bladder using a thin camera called a cystoscope.
- During catheterization of bladder, the curvatures of urethra should be kept in mind.

Urethra

- Rupture of urethra causes extravasation of urine.
- **Urethritis:** Infection of urethra.
- **Hypospadias:** Urethra opens on undersurface of penis.
- **Epispadias:** Urethra opens on dorsum of penis.

SUMMARY

Organs	*External features*	*Blood supply*	*Nerve supply*
Kidney	• Maintains homeostasis of body • **Coverings:** Fibrous capsule, perirenal fat, renal fascia, pararenal fat. • **Surfaces:** Anterior (right-right suprarenal gland, liver, duodenum, colon, small intestine; left-left suprarenal gland, spleen, stomach, pancreas, splenic vessels, colon, jejunum), posterior (diaphragm, psoas major, quadratus lumborum, transverse abdominis, subcostal vessels and nerves, iliohypogastric and ilioinguinal nerves)	• Arteries: Right and left renal • Veins: Right and left renal • Lymphatics: Lateral aortic nodes	• **Sympathetic:** Renal plexus • **Parasympathetic:** Vagus

Organs	*External features*	*Blood supply*	*Nerve supply*
Ureter	• Muscular tube • Conveys urine from kidney to urinary bladder • **Constrictions:** Pelviureteric junction, brim of lesser pelvis, passage through bladder wall	• **Arteries:** Branches from renal, aorta, vesicular, middle rectal • **Veins:** Lymphatics	• **Sympathetic:** T10 – L1 • **Parasympathetic:** S2 – S3
Urinary bladder	• Hollow muscular organ, stores urine • **Surfaces:** Superior—male (peritoneum, sigmoid colon, coils of ileum), female (peritoneum, vesicouterine pouch); inferolateral-male (pubis, puboprostatic ligaments, retropubic fat, levator ani, obturator internus), female (pubis, pubovesical ligament, retropubic fat, levator ani, obturator internus); posterior —male (peritoneum, rectovesical pouch, coils of ileum, seminal vesicle, vas deferens), female (peritoneum, vagina). • True ligaments (lateral, posterior, medial and lateral puboprostatic, median umbilical) • False ligaments (median umbilical fold, lateral umbilical fold, lateral, posterior)	• **Arteries:** Superior and inferior vesical • **Veins:** Vesical venous plexus • **Lymphatics:** External iliac nodes	• **Sympathetic:** T12 – L2 • **Parasympathetic:** S2–S4

QUESTIONS

Long Essays

- List the different parts of the urinary system and give the functions of each.
- Name the different parts of the urinary system. Describe the kidney in detail.
- Draw a section of the kidney showing the salient features.
- Write in detail the structure of a nephron.
- Name the different parts of the urinary system. Describe the bladder in detail.
- Describe the kidney and its applied importance.

Short Essays

- Kidney
- Capsules of kidney
- Histology of kidney
- Anomalies of kidney
- Proximal convoluted tubule
- Urinary bladder
- Interior of the urinary bladder
- Name the ligaments of urinary bladder
- Prostatic urethra/female urethra.

Short Notes

- Arterial segments of the kidney
- Constrictions of the ureter
- Parts of male urethra
- Sphincters of urethra.

CHAPTER 10

Reproductive System

LEARNING OBJECTIVES

The student should be able to:

- Name the parts of male reproductive system, details of testis, epididymis, vas deferens, prostate—gross and histology.
- Name the parts of female reproductive system, details of uterus, fallopian tubes, ovary—gross and histology.
- Mammary gland—gross.

MALE REPRODUCTIVE SYSTEM

- Male genital system is made up of testes, vas deferens, seminal vesicles and ejaculatory ducts.
- Accessory sex organs are prostate and bulbourethral glands.
- Male external genitalia are made up of scrotum and penis.

Testis

- Testes are a pair of ellipsoid bodies suspended by spermatic cord into the scrotum.
- Each testis lies obliquely such that the upper pole is tilted forwards and laterally.
- **Testis has two poles or ends:** Upper and lower, two borders: Anterior and posterior, two surfaces: Medial and lateral.
- Upper end of testis is covered by epididymis and is connected to it by ducts called efferent ductules. Lower end is related to tail of epididymis and connected to it by areolar tissue.
- Anterior border is smooth and convex. Posterior border is broad and flat and the spermatic cord is attached to its upper part.
- Medial surface is smooth and convex.
- Lateral surface is overlapped by epididymis and separated from it by a fold of processus vaginalis by a space called sinus of epididymis (this is useful for side determination).

Coverings of Testis

Testis is covered by three layers. From outside inwards, they are:

1. **Tunica vaginalis:** It has two layers, the outer **parietal** layer and the inner **visceral** layer. The visceral layer covers the testis and the epididymis except at the posterior border and is continuous with the parietal layer forming a closed sac. This sac is a site of collection of fluid; the condition is called **hydrocele**.

2. **Tunica albuginea:** It is a thick fibrous layer that covers the whole of the testis. It is thickened at the posterior border to form the mediastinum testis that sends septae inside the testis to divide it into lobules. About 200 to 300 lobules are present in each testis.
3. **Tunica vasculosa:** It is a vascular membrane that covers each lobule of the testis.

Macroscopic Structure of Testis (Fig. 10.1)

- Each lobule of the testis has one to three seminiferous tubules and some interstitial cells of Leydig.
- Total number of tubules in the testis is 400–600.
- Seminiferous tubules have a coiled part in the front and a straight part at the back.
- The straight parts join at the level of mediastinum testis to form a plexus of tubules called the rete testis.
- From the rete testis, efferent ductules arise and enter the head of the epididymis.
- Each seminiferous tubule has two kinds of cells, the spermatogenic cells (which produce sperms) and the Sertoli cells (supporting cells).
- Sertoli cells provide nutrition to the developing sperms and phagocytose the residual bodies.
- The **interstitial cells of Leydig** are situated outside the seminiferous tubules and secrete testosterone. This is the hormone responsible for maintenance of the sexual organs of a male.

Blood Supply

- Testicular artery which is a branch of abdominal aorta.
- A plexus of veins called the pampiniform plexus finally forms one vein which drains into the inferior vena cava on the right side and the renal vein on the left side.
- The plexus helps to absorb the heat produced by the testicular arteries and hence the temperature of the scrotum is less than the abdominal cavity which is necessary for production of sperms.

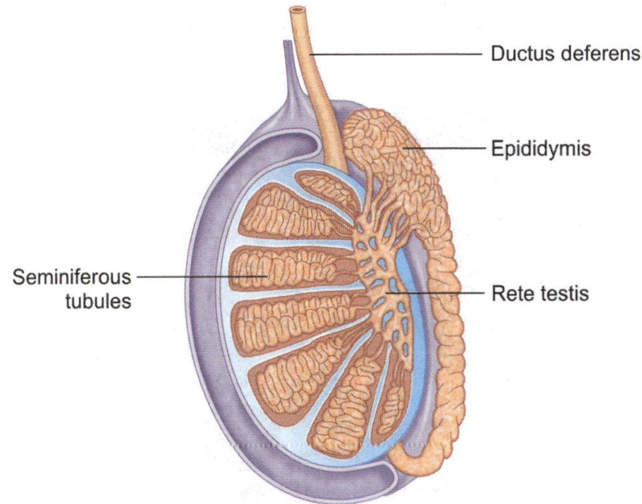

Fig. 10.1: Parts of testis.

Lymphatic Drainage

Drains into the pre- and the para-aortic group of lymph nodes.

Nerve Supply

- Sympathetic nerves of the renal and aortic plexuses.
- The preganglionic fibers are derived from T10 and T11 segments of spinal cord.

Descent of Testis

- In fetal life, testis is formed at the level of the iliac fossa at the 4th month.
- It descends down slowly so that it reaches the deep inguinal ring at the 7th month, the inguinal canal in the 8th month and then in the scrotal sacs by the end of 9th month that is just before birth. This is called the descent of testis.

Microscopic Structure of Testis (Figs. 10.2A and B)

- The testis is made up of coiled tubes called the seminiferous tubules.
- These are separated from each other by connective tissue that has blood vessels and nerves.
- The wall of each tubule is made up of an outer layer of fibrous tissue that also contains muscle. The contraction of this layer helps in the propulsion of spermatozoa.
- Between the lumen of the tubule and the outer layer are rows of cells that are of various types. In these are the supporting cells called the Sertoli cells and the spermatozoa in various stages of development. Each sperm is formed by a process called spermatogenesis.
- The primordial cells are the spermatogonia. They lie in the most basal layer. The spermatogonia is divided by mitosis to form primary spermatocytes (2n). They are large cells with a prominent central oval nucleus. They form the second layer of cells. These undergo the first meiotic division to form secondary spermatocytes (n). They are smaller than the primary and form the third layer of cells. The secondary spermatocytes undergo the second meiotic division to form the spermatids (n). These are immature sperms, and they undergo a process called spermiogenesis to form sperms.
- Each sperm has a head, a body and a tail. The head lies embedded in the Sertoli cells such that the lumen of the seminiferous tubule shows tails of the sperms.

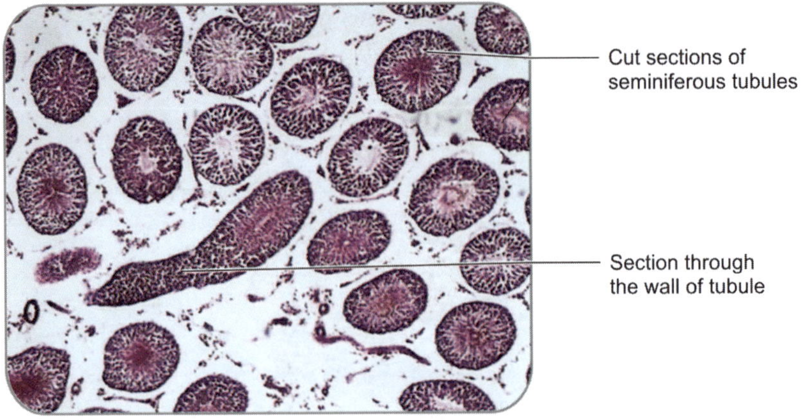

Fig. 10.2A: Photomicrograph of histology of testis.

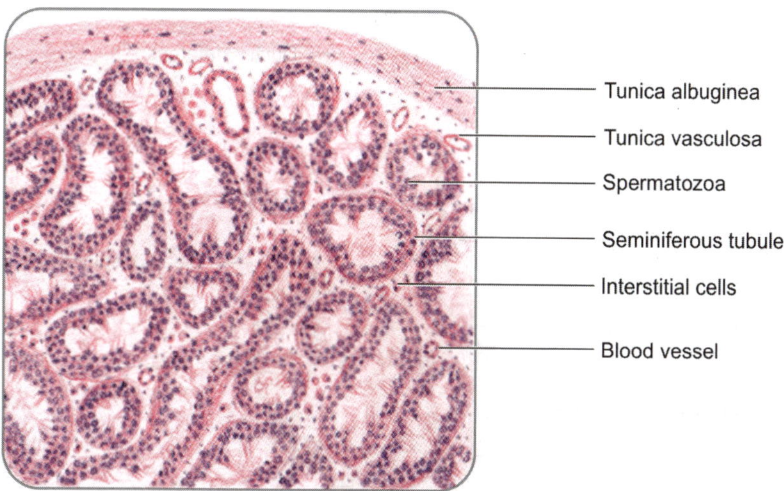

Fig. 10.2B: Diagrammatic representation of histology of testis.

- Sertoli cells are large cells with a basal nucleus. The spermatogonia in the various stages of development lie closely associated with the Sertoli cells in the layers one above the other. The mature sperms lie embedded in the Sertoli cell apex. Hence, the Sertoli cells support the sperms, provide nutrition to them and remove the waste products formed after spermatogenesis.
- Lying in between the seminiferous tubules in the connective tissue are cells that secrete testosterone. These are called interstitial cells of Leydig and are round cells with round nuclei.

Applied Anatomy

- **Hydrocele:** This is the collection of fluid in the sac formed by the visceral and parietal layers of the processus vaginalis.
- **Hernia:** Contents of the abdomen may descend into the testis if the processus vaginalis remains patent. This is called inguinal hernia.
- **Varicocele:** The pampiniform plexus of veins becomes dilated and enlarged to give rise to a condition called varicocele. It is more common on the left side as the left testicular vein is longer than the right, the left vein may be compressed by a loaded colon in iliac fossa and also because the left testicular vein enters the renal vein at a right angle.
- **Cryptorchidism:** This is a condition where the testis fails to descend and lies in the abdominal cavity only. These patients are sterile. An undescended testis is a frequent site of carcinoma.
- **Ectopic testis:** An ectopic testis is one that deviates from its normal path of descent so that it lies at an abnormal site.

Epididymis (Fig. 10.3)

- This is a comma shaped organ that lies along the lateral part of the posterior surface of the testis.
- It is made up of a head, a body and a tail. The head is connected to the testis by the efferent ductules. The tail continues as the ductus deferens.
- The epididymis transports sperms from the testis to the vas deferens.

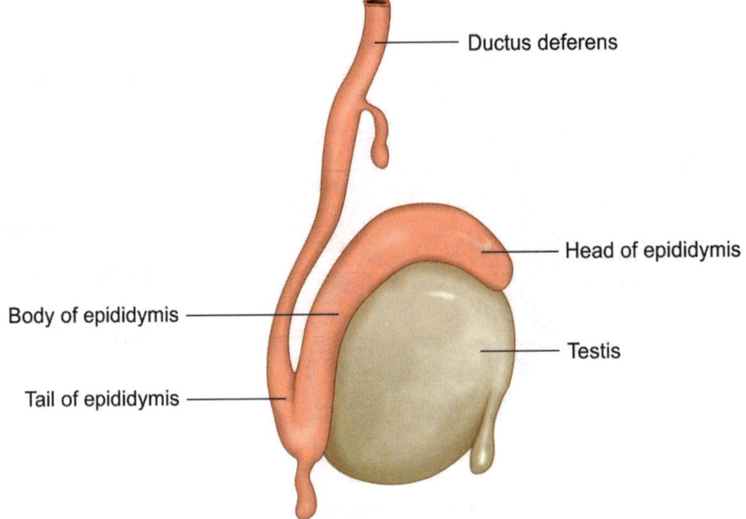

Fig. 10.3: Parts of epididymis.

Microscopic Structure (Figs. 10.4A and B)

- The epididymis is made up of tubules separated by smooth muscle.
- The tubules are lined by columnar epithelium with stereocilia.

Vas Deferens

- The vas deferens or the ductus deferens is a thick cord-like tubular structure and is about 45 cm long.
- It starts from the tail of the epididymis and enters the spermatic cord.
- At the level of the deep inguinal ring, it becomes subperitoneal and then reaches the urinary bladder.
- At the base of prostate, it joins with duct of seminal vesicle to form ejaculatory duct.
- Bilateral ligation (tying) of the ductus deferens is done in vasectomy, a family planning procedure.

Histology

- The wall of the ductus deferens is made up of three layers.
- The innermost mucosa, thrown into folds, is lined by simple columnar epithelium.
- The middle layer is made up of smooth muscle arranged in three layers—inner longitudinal, middle circular and outer longitudinal.
- The outermost layer is connective tissue.

Seminal Vesicle

- They are a pair of pyramidal organs present between the base of the bladder and the ampulla of rectum.
- Secrete a viscid, yellowish white alkaline fluid that forms bulk of the semen.

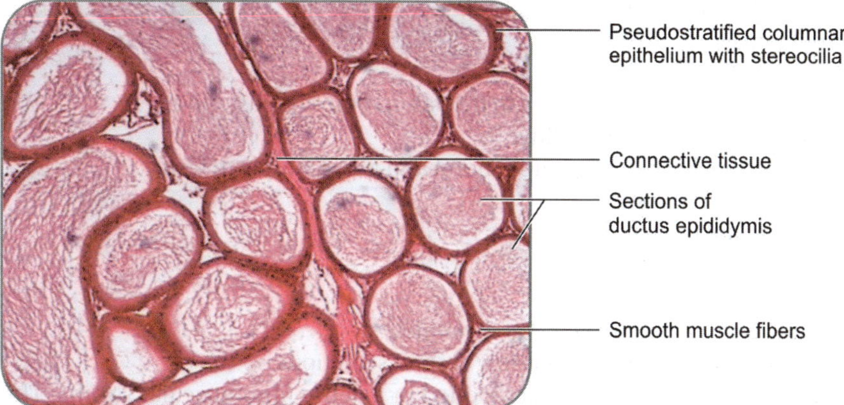

Fig.10.4A: Photomicrograph of histology of epididymis.

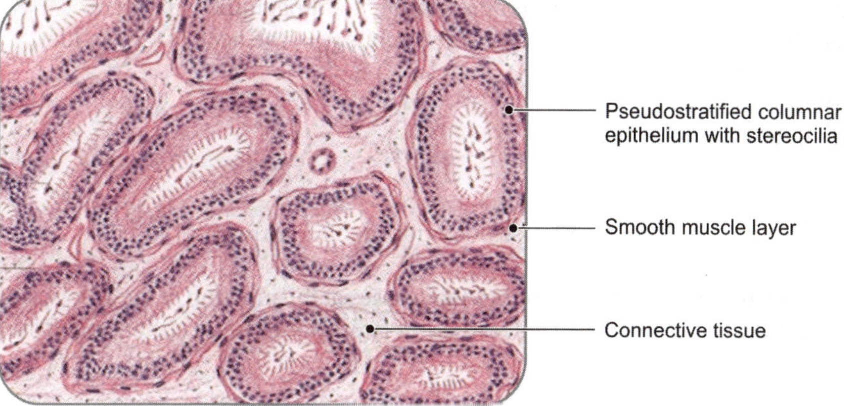

Fig. 10.4B: Diagrammatic representation of histology of epididymis.

Ejaculatory Ducts

- There are two ejaculatory ducts, each formed by the union of vas deferens and the duct of seminal vesicle.
- Each duct opens into the prostatic urethra at the colliculus seminalis on the sides of the prostatic utricle.
- They are responsible for the transport of sperms from the testis to the exterior.

Spermatic Cord

- The spermatic cord is a tubular sheath that contains the vas deferens and the vessels and nerves of the testis and epididymis.
- It is about 7.5 cm long and extends from the deep inguinal ring to the upper border of the testis.
- It suspends the testis in the scrotum.

- **Contents of the cord are:**
  - Vas deferens
  - Pampiniform plexus of veins
  - *Arteries:* Testicular artery, artery to the vas and the cremasteric artery
  - Lymphatics of testis and epididymis.
  - *Nerves:* Genital branch of genitofemoral and nerve supply to testis
  - Loose connective tissue
  - Remains of the processus vaginalis.

Prostate Gland (Fig. 10.5)

- The prostate is an accessory gland of the males.
- It adds to the seminal fluid by secreting certain secretions.
- It is made up of glandular tissue embedded in a dense fibromuscular stroma. This makes the prostate firm in consistency.
- It lies in the lesser pelvis, below the neck of the urinary bladder behind the lower border of the pubic symphysis and in front of the ampulla of rectum.
- **It has the following parts:**
  - Apex that is directed downwards and rests on the urogenital diaphragm.
  - Base that is directed upwards and is continuous with the neck of the bladder.
  - Anterior surface.
  - Posterior surface.
  - Two inferolateral surfaces.

Lobes

- The prostate has five lobes—anterior, posterior, median (or medial) and right and left lateral lobes.
- The prostate is traversed by the urethra that passes at the junction of the anterior 1/3rd and posterior 2/3rd of the prostate. Hence, the two lateral lobes lie on either side of the urethra.

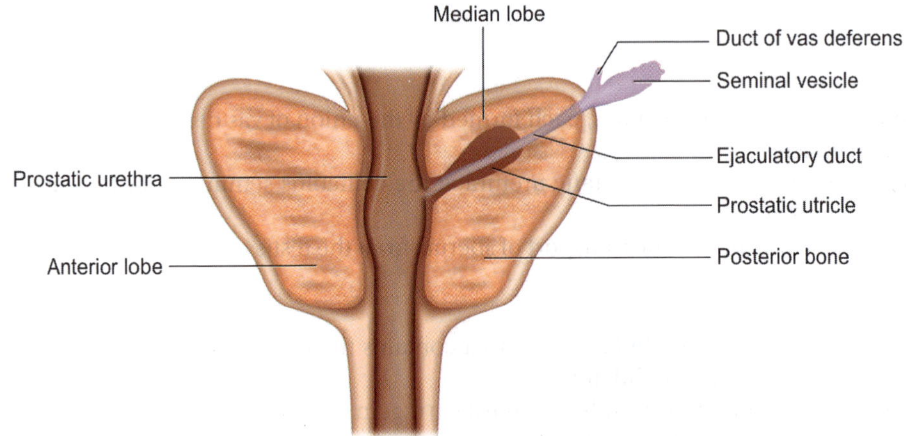

Fig. 10.5: Lobes of prostate gland.

- The anterior lobes connect the lateral lobes in front of the urethra and the posterior lobes connect the lateral lobes behind the urethra.
- The median lobe lies just behind the upper part of urethra in front of the opening of the ejaculatory ducts in the urethra.

Capsules

- **True capsule:** It is formed by the condensation of the peripheral part of the gland. It contains no venous plexus.
- **False capsule:** It lies outside the true capsule and is derived from the pelvic fascia.
- The venous plexus that drains the prostate lies between the two capsules.

Structures within the Prostate

- Prostatic urethra that lies at the junction of anterior 1/3rd and posterior 2/3rd.
- The prostatic utricle is a blind sac that opens into the prostatic urethra.
- Opening of the two ejaculatory ducts on either side of the prostatic utricle.

Blood Supply

- Inferior vesical, middle rectal and the internal pudendal arteries.
- The veins form a rich plexus between the two capsules of the gland.
- It communicates with the vesical plexus and the vertebral venous plexus.

Lymphatic Drainage

Drain into the internal iliac and the sacral nodes.

Nerve Supply

- Inferior hypogastric plexus.
- It is supplied by both parasympathetic and sympathetic nerves derived from L3, L4, L5 and the upper sacral segments.

Age Changes in the Prostate

- At birth the prostate is small in size and made up of mainly stroma in which a small amount of duct system is present.
- At puberty, the gland greatly increases in size due to growth of glandular tissue. Hence, the amount of stromal connective tissue decreases.
- As the age advances, the size of the gland either increases or decreases and degenerate bodies called the amyloid bodies appear.

Microscopic Structure (Figs. 10.6A and B)

- The prostate is made up of 30–50 compound tubuloalveolar glands embedded in fibromuscular tissue and covered by a capsule.
- The capsule contains numerous veins and nerve fibers.
- Each gland is lined by columnar epithelium which is thrown into numerous folds in the lumen.

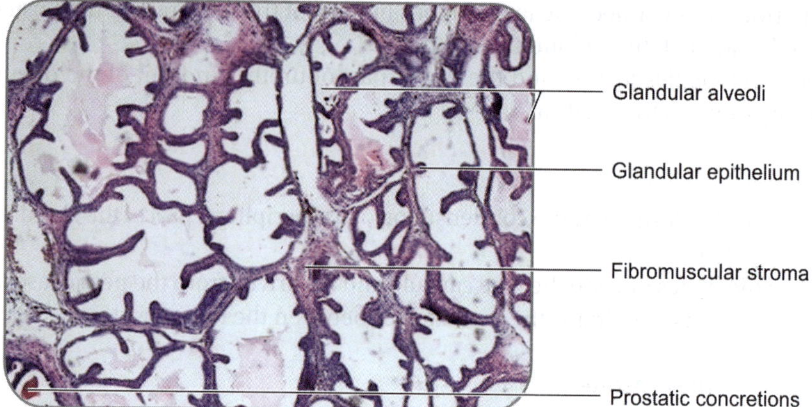

Fig. 10.6A: Photomicrograph of histology of prostate gland.

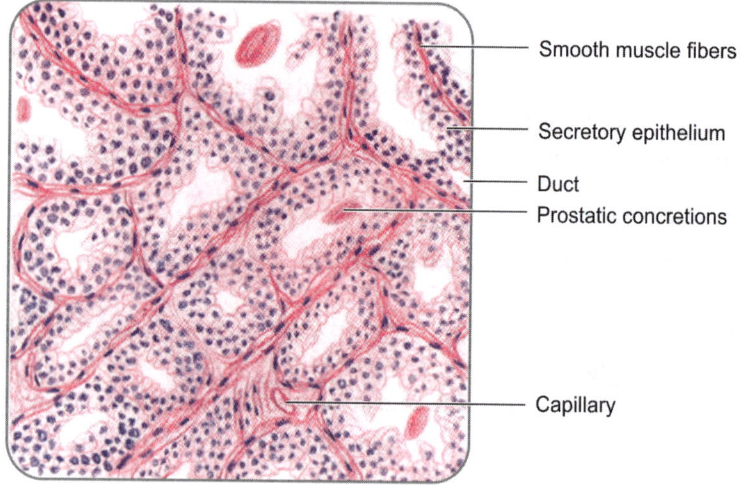

Fig. 10.6B: Diagrammatic representation of histology of prostate gland.

- Small rounded bodies are found in the lumen of each gland. They are called amyloid bodies and are found in a greater number in old age.
- The fibromuscular tissue is made up of collagen fibers and smooth muscle.
- Secretion of each gland goes to excretory ducts lined by double layered epithelium. The basal layer is cuboidal and the superficial layer is columnar. These ducts lie in the fibromuscular tissue.

Applied Anatomy

- **Senile enlargement of the prostate:** It is also called benign prostatic hyperplasia (BPH) which occurs due to enlargement of the median lobe of the prostate. Due to this the patient complains of increased frequency of urination and other urinary complaints due to distortion of the urethra.

- Carcinoma of the prostate is more common in the posterior lobe. As the venous plexus of the prostate is connected to the vertebral venous plexus by valve less veins, carcinoma spreads to the vertebral bodies.
- Removal of an enlarged prostate is called prostatectomy. In these cases, the prostate is scooped out leaving the two capsules behind (due to the venous plexus present between the two capsules). This is called enucleation.

Scrotum

- Scrotum is a pouch that lies in the lower part of the anterior abdominal wall and contains the testis and the lower parts of the spermatic cords.
- It protects the testis from injury and maintains the temperature of the testis lower than the abdominal temperature, which is necessary for spermatogenesis.

Layers of the Scrotum

- Outermost skin.
- **Dartos muscle:** This is the modification of the superficial fascia.
- **External spermatic fascia:** It is derived from the aponeurosis of the external oblique muscle of the abdomen.
- **Cremasteric muscle and its fascia:** It is derived from the internal oblique muscle.
- **Internal spermatic fascia:** It is derived from the fascia transversalis.
- Parietal layer of the tunica vaginalis.

Cremasteric Reflex

- The genital branch of the genitofemoral nerve supplies both the cremasteric muscle and the medial side of the thigh.
- Due to this, stroking of the medial side of the thigh leads to contraction of the cremastetric muscle and elevation of the testis. This is called cremasteric reflex.

Penis

- The penis is the copulatory organ of the male. It is made up of a root and a body.
- The root is made of three parts; one crus on either side dorsally and a median bulb of the penis. Each crus is covered by the ischiocavernosus muscle and the bulb is covered by the bulbospongiosus muscle.
- When traced forwards in the body, the two crura form the corpora cavernosa of the penis and the bulb forms the corpus spongiosum.
- The corpora cavernosa is made up of cavernous spaces filled by blood during erection. The blood comes from the helicine arteries that are branches of the deep artery to the penis and the blood is drained into the deep dorsal vein of the penis. Hence, erection is a purely vascular phenomenon. The corpus spongiosum is traversed by the spongy urethra.
- The body of the penis shows an expanded portion at the end called the glans penis which is covered by a fold of skin called the prepuce. Circumcision is a surgery where the prepuce is removed.

Blood Supply

- Deep artery of penis, artery to bulb and the dorsal artery of the penis. These are the branches of the internal pudendal artery.

- Superficial system of veins drain into great saphenous vein through superficial dorsal vein. The corpora are drained by the deep dorsal veins that drain into the prostatic venous plexus.

Lymphatic Drainage

Superficial and the deep groups of the inguinal lymph nodes.

Nerve Supply

- Somatic nerves that convey pain are derived from the pudendal nerves (dorsal nerve of penis).
- Parasympathetic nerves come from S2, S3 and S4 segments of the spinal cord. They are vasodilators.
- The sympathetic supply is from the L1 segment through the superior hypogastric plexus. These nerves are vasoconstrictor.

FEMALE REPRODUCTIVE SYSTEM

Female reproductive system is made up of a pair of ovaries, a pair of uterine tubes, uterus, vagina and external genitalia (labia majora, labia minora, clitoris and vestibule).

Ovaries

- The ovaries are female gonads situated in the ovarian fossa on the lateral pelvic wall.
- In young girls before the onset of ovulation the ovaries have a smooth surface and are pinkish in color. After the onset of puberty, the surface becomes uneven, and the color changes from pink to gray.
- The position of the ovary is variable. In a woman who has not borne any children, they are vertical in position such that they have an upper pole and a lower pole. In multipara, they become horizontal so that the upper pole faces laterally and the lower pole medially.

Parts of Ovary

- **Upper pole:** It is also called the tubal pole and is related to the uterine tube.
- **Lower pole:** It is also called the uterine pole and is related to the lateral angle of uterus by a ligament called the ligament of ovary.
- **Anterior (mesovarian) border:** It is straight and attached to the broad ligament by a fold of peritoneum called the mesovarium. It is also called the hilum of the ovary from where vessels enter the ovary.
- **Posterior (free) border:** It is convex and related to the ureter and uterine tube.
- **Lateral surface:** It is related to the ovarian fossa which is lined by the parietal peritoneum.
- **Medial surface:** It is covered by the uterine tube and separated from it by a bursa called the ovarian bursa.

Blood Supply

- Ovarian artery which is a branch of the abdominal aorta, uterine artery.
- The veins emerge at the hilus and form a pampiniform plexus of veins that drains into a single ovarian vein near the pelvic inlet. This drains into the inferior vena cava on the right side and the left renal vein on the left side.

Lymphatic Drainage

Drain into the lateral aortic and the preaortic group of lymph nodes.

Nerve Supply

- The ovarian plexus has both sympathetic and parasympathetic nerves.
- The sympathetic nerves T10 and T11 are afferent for pain as well as vasomotor.
- Parasympathetic S2, 3, 4 are vasodilators.

Microscopic Structure (Figs.10.7A and B)

- The ovary is covered by cuboidal epithelium called germinal epithelium. This is modified mesothelium and does not form germ cells.
- The ovary is covered by a thick capsule below the cuboidal epithelium called **tunica** albuginea.
- Below this the substance of the ovary is divided into a cortex and a medulla. The cortex contains the developing follicles and the medulla has the blood vessels supplying the ovary.

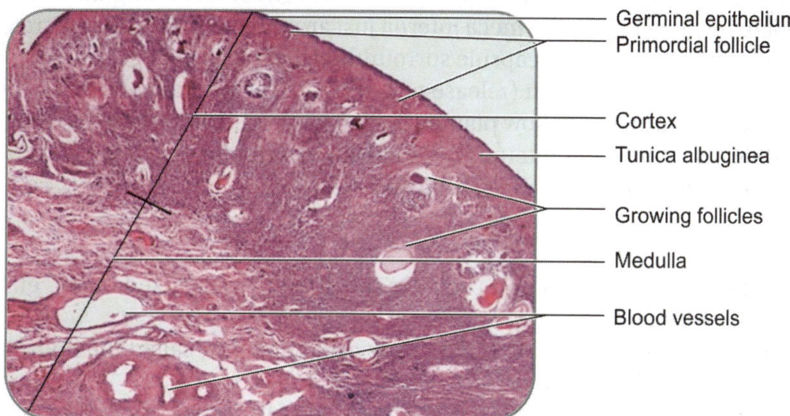

Fig. 10.7A: Photomicrograph of histology of ovary.

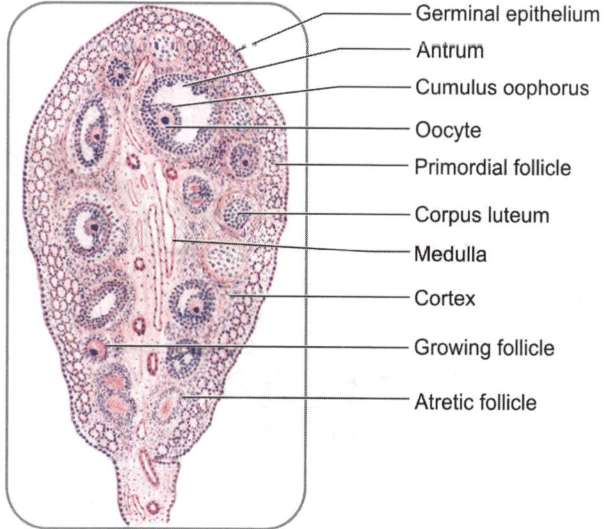

Fig. 10.7B: Diagrammatic representation of histology of ovary.

The cortex has the following follicles:

- **Primordial follicles:** These are present just below the tunica albuginea and are the smallest in size and the largest in number. They consist of the ovum lined by a single layer of squamous epithelium.
- **Primary follicles:** The lining epithelium that surrounds the ovum changes from squamous to columnar.
- **Secondary follicles:** The stromal cells around the ovum now collect around the ovum to form layers of cells called follicular cells and now the ovum becomes a secondary follicle.
- **Graafian follicle:** Between the follicular cells that surround the ovum, a cavity appears in the cells that pushes the ovum to the periphery. This is called the antrum and is filled by fluid. The ovum now lies in a fluid filled cavity and it is most mature and ready for ovulation. This structure is called the Graafian follicle. The stromal cells surrounding the Graafian follicle differentiate into two layers, the theca interna just around the follicle that secretes estrogen and theca externa that is like a capsule surrounding the follicle.
- **Corpus luteum:** After ovulation (release of ovum into the peritoneal cavity), the follicular cells enlarge; accumulate a yellow pigment called lutein and start secreting progesterone.
- **Corpus albicans:** The corpus luteum after some time degenerates to leave fibrous scar tissue forming a structure called the corpus albicans.

Uterus (Fig. 10.8)

- It is the organ which protects and provides nutrition to a fertilized ovum, enabling it to become a fully formed fetus.
- It is piriform in shape. It is divided into upper expanded part called the body and a lower cylindrical part called the cervix.
- The junction of the two parts is constricted. The body forms the upper 2/3rd and the cervix forms the lower 1/3rd of the organ.

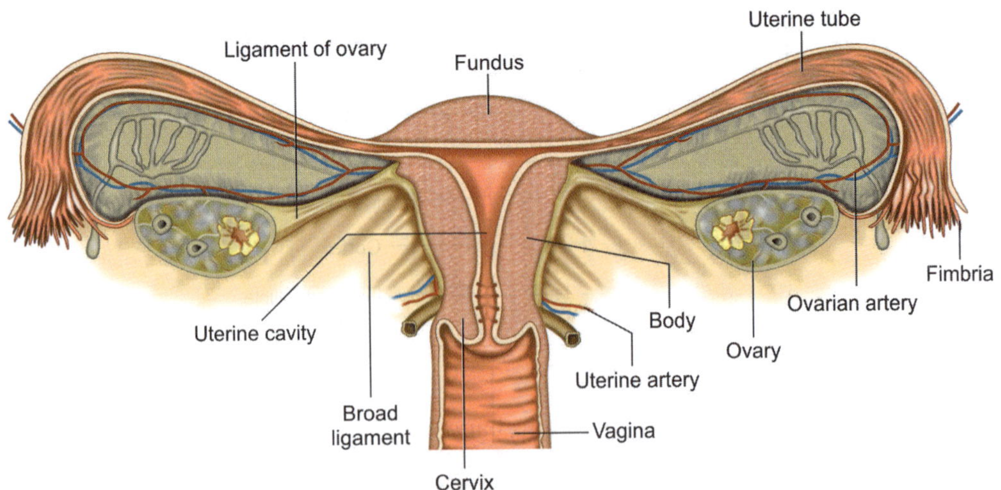

Fig. 10.8: Parts of female reproductive system.

- Normally the long axis of uterus forms an angle of 90° with the vagina. This angle opens forwards and is called the angle of anteversion.
- The uterus is also slightly bended on itself at an angle of 120° called the angle of anteflexion.
- Superiorly, the uterus communicates on each side with the uterine tubes and inferiorly with the vagina.

Body of Uterus

The body has:

- A fundus which is the free upper end of the uterus. It is dome shaped and covered with peritoneum on all sides. Implantation takes place at the posterior wall of the fundus.
- The anterior surface is related to the urinary bladder and covered with peritoneum.
- The posterior surface is related to the coils of the small intestine and is also covered by peritoneum.
- There are two lateral borders which are related to a fold of peritoneum called the broad ligament. At the upper end is the attachment of the uterine tubes on either side.

Cervix of Uterus

- The cervix is cylindrical in shape and projects into the upper part of the vagina on its anterior wall. This divides the cervix into a supravaginal part and the vaginal part.
- The cavity of the cervix is called the cervical canal. It opens into the vagina at an opening called the external os. In a nulliparous woman, the os is small and circular but in a multiparous woman, it becomes oval.
- Similarly, the cavity of the body of the uterus communicates with the cervical canal at the internal os.

Ligaments of Uterus

Broad Ligament

- It is a large fold of peritoneum that lies on the lateral borders of the body of uterus.
- They attach the uterus to the lateral pelvic wall.
- Each broad ligament has two layers and covers the uterus like a sleeve.
- The superior border is free; the inferior and lateral borders are attached to the pelvic wall, the medial border is attached to the lateral border of uterus.
- Anterior surface and posterior surface become continuous at the superior border.
- **The broad ligament contains the following structures:**
  - Uterine tube
  - Round ligament of the uterus
  - Ligament of the ovary
  - Uterine vessels
  - Ovarian vessels
  - Nerve plexuses supplying the ovary, the uterus and the vagina.
  - Lymph nodes and lymph vessels
  - Dense connective tissue.

Round ligament of the uterus: It is a fibrous band that lies in the broad ligament below the attachment of the uterine tube. It passes through the deep inguinal ring, traverses the inguinal canal and ends in the labium majus. It keeps the fundus directed forwards and maintains the angle of anteversion.

Transverse cervical ligaments: These are fan shaped condensations of the pelvic fascia on either side of the cervix. They connect the lateral wall of the cervix to the lateral pelvic wall and form a sling that supports the uterus.

Uterosacral ligaments: These are also condensations of the pelvic fascia that connect the cervix to the sacrum. They pull the cervix backwards. Thus, they balance the forward pull of round ligament.

Pubocervical ligaments: These are condensations of the pelvic fascia and connect the cervix to the posterior surface of pubis.

Blood Supply

Uterine artery and partly by the ovarian artery. The veins drain into the internal veins through the plexuses formed by uterine, ovarian and vaginal veins.

Lymphatic Drainage

The upper part of the uterus drains into the aortic group of lymph nodes. The rest of the uterus drains into the external iliac group of lymph nodes.

Nerve Supply

Uterus is supplied by the parasympathetic, S2,3,4 and sympathetic T12, L1 nerves.

Supports of Uterus (Fig. 10.9)

The uterus is a mobile organ that is prevented from sagging down by the following supports:

Primary Supports

Muscular

- **Pelvic diaphragm:** It is a muscular diaphragm that supports the pelvic organs and resists any increase in intra-abdominal pressure. Some of the fibers of the pubococcygeus part

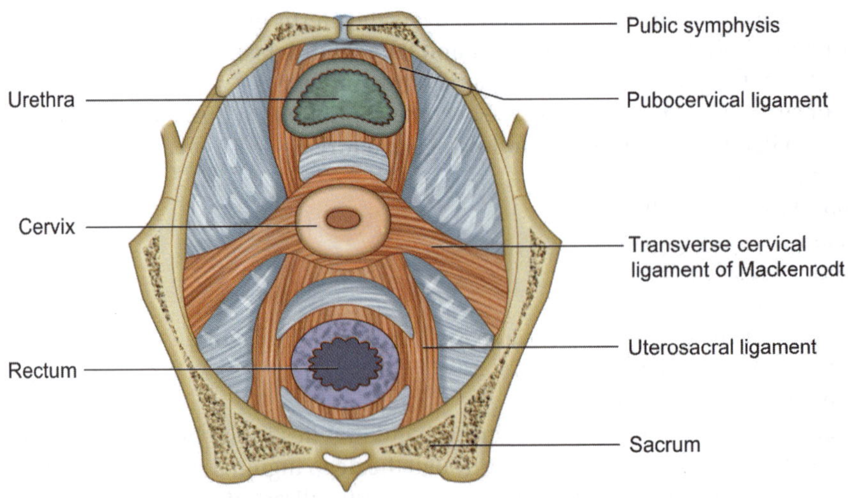

Fig. 10.9: Supports of uterus.

of levator ani are inserted in the vagina and hence support the vagina and indirectly the uterus.

- **Perineal body:** It helps to support the pelvic diaphragm and hence indirectly supports the uterus.
- **Urogenital diaphragm:** A part of the diaphragm, i.e., the sphincter urethra muscle supports the vagina and hence supports the uterus.

Fibromuscular or mechanical

- **Uterine axis:** The anteverted position of the uterus prevents it from sagging down.
- **Pubocervical ligaments:** Support the cervix anteriorly.
- **Transverse cervical ligaments:** Support the cervix from the sides.
- **Uterosacral ligaments:** Support the cervix posteriorly.
- **Round ligament of uterus:** Keeps the uterus anteverted.

Secondary Supports

- Broad ligament
- **Uterovesical fold of peritoneum:** This fold lies between the uterus and the urinary bladder.
- **Rectovaginal fold of peritoneum:** This lies in between the rectum and the vagina. It is also called the pouch of Douglas.

Microscopic Structure (Figs. 10.10A and B)

The uterus is made up of three layers:

1. **Endometrium:** It is the innermost layer lined by simple columnar epithelium. The epithelium dips into the underlying connective tissue in the form of glands called the uterine glands. The endometrium is divided into an upper 2/3rd called the functional layer (it is shed off during menstruation) and the lower 1/3rd called the basal layer (it is retained during menstruation). The uterine glands become more coiled as the uterus reaches the secretory phase. The endometrium is richly supplied by blood vessels. They have thicker walls than elsewhere in the body and are called coiled arteries.
2. **Myometrium:** It is the middle layer. It is made up of smooth muscle bundles running in all directions and separated by connective tissue which has a rich supply of blood vessels.

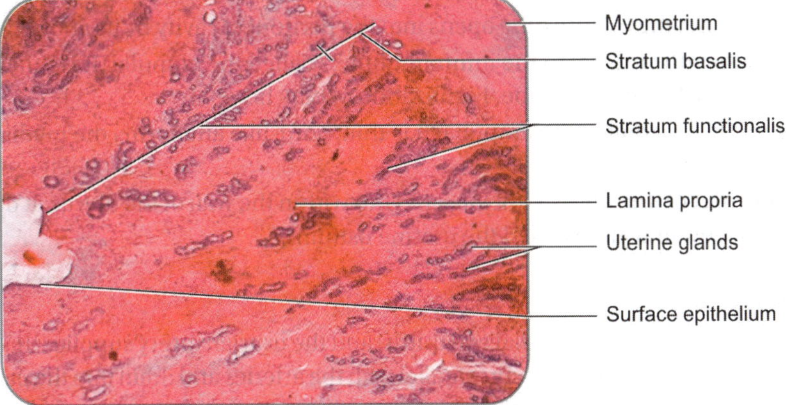

Fig. 10.10A: Photomicrograph of histology of uterus.

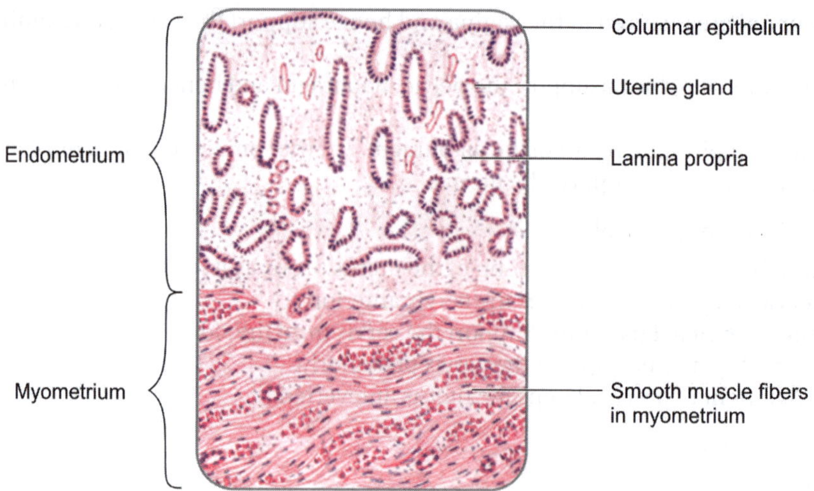

Fig. 10.10B: Diagrammatic representation of histology of uterus.

3. **Perimetrium:** It is the outermost layer of uterus made up of peritoneum and connective fibrous tissue.

Uterine Tubes/Fallopian Tubes

- These are ducts that convey ova from the ovary to the uterus.
- Spermatozoa introduced into the vagina travel through the uterus to the fallopian tubes. Fertilization normally takes place in the lateral part of the tube.

Parts of the Tube

- Each uterine tube is about 10 cm in length.
- The lateral end of the tube is shaped like a funnel and is called the infundibulum. It bears a number of finger-like processes called fimbria. One of them is the largest and is attached to the tubal pole of the ovary and is called the ovarian fimbria.
- At the lateral end, the uterine tube opens into the peritoneal cavity by its abdominal ostium.
- The part of the tube medial to the infundibulum is called the ampulla. It is thin walled and forms the lateral 2/3rd of the tube. Fertilization occurs here.
- The isthmus lies medial to the ampulla. It is thin, cord-like and forms the medial one third of the fallopian tube.
- The uterine part of the tube is 1 cm long and lies within the wall of the uterus. It opens in the uterine cavity by an ostium called the uterine ostium.

Blood Supply

The uterine artery supplies the medial two thirds, and the ovarian artery supplies the lateral one third of the fallopian tube. The veins run parallel with the arteries and drain into the pampiniform plexus of the ovary and into the uterine veins.

Lymphatic Drainage

Most of the tube drains into the lateral aortic and the preaortic group of lymph nodes. The isthmus drains into the superficial inguinal group of lymph nodes.

Nerve Supply

The sympathetic nerves T10 to L2 are vasomotor and stimulate peristalsis. However, peristalsis is under mainly hormonal control. Parasympathetic S2, 3, 4 are vasodilator and inhibit peristalsis.

Microscopic Structure (Figs. 10.11A and B)

The fallopian tube has the following layers:

- **Epithelium:** It is lined by ciliated columnar epithelium thrown into many primary, secondary and tertiary folds.
- **Muscularis externa:** This is made up of smooth muscle arranged in two layers, inner circular and outer longitudinal.
- **Serosa:** Made up of fibrous tissue and mesothelium.

Vagina

- The vagina is a fibromuscular canal that is used for copulation.
- It extends from the vulva below to the uterus above and lies behind the bladder and urethra and in front of the rectum and anal canal.
- Its anterior and posterior walls are normally in contact except at its upper end where the cervix projects into the vagina. The cervix and the upper end of vagina are separated by a sulcus called fornix which is deep posteriorly.
- The fornix present on the posterior wall is related to the rectouterine pouch which is the most dependent part. The pus or blood tends to collect here. The fluid can be drained by inserting the needle into rectouterine pouch through the posterior fornix.

Mammary Gland

- Mammary gland is a modified sweat gland situated in the pectoral region.
- It is rudimentary in males. In females it starts enlarging at puberty.

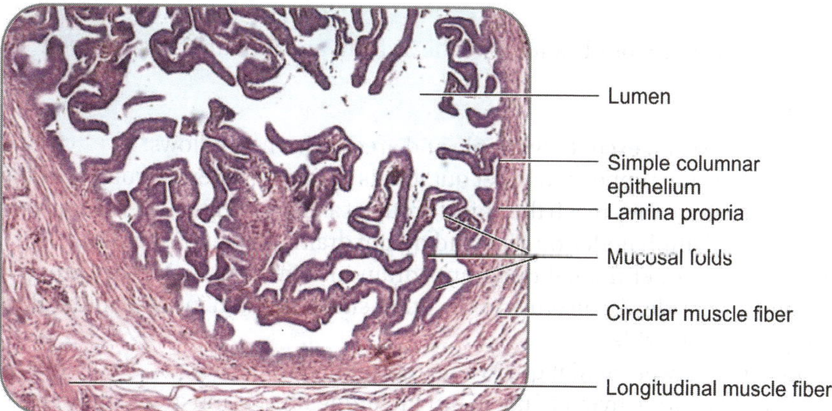

Fig. 10.11A: Photomicrograph of histology of uterine tube.

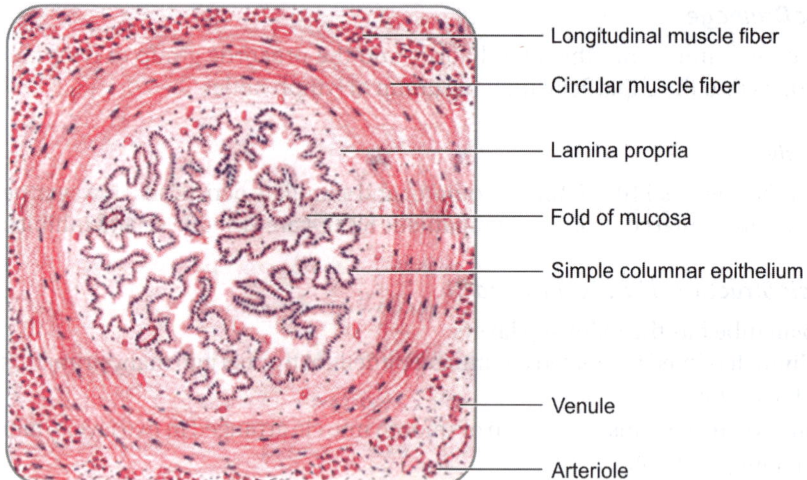

Fig. 10.11B: Diagrammatic representation of histology of uterine tube.

- It is conical in shape, extending from the lateral margin of the sternum to the midaxillary line transversely and from the 2nd to the 6th rib vertically.
- The gland rests on the pectoralis major which is covered by the pectoral fascia.

Structure

The gland is covered by the skin and shows a conical projection in the middle called the nipple. Surrounding the nipple is a circular area of skin called the areola which contains sebaceous glands.

Blood Supply

Lateral thoracic, internal thoracic and the 3rd, 4th and 5th intercostal arteries. The veins drain into the internal thoracic, axillary and intercostal veins.

Nerve Supply

Anterior and lateral cutaneous branches of the 3rd, 4th and 5th intercostal nerves.

Lymphatic Drainage

Lymphatics from the skin, except the nipple and areola, drain as follows:

- Lymphatics from outer upper and lower quadrants drain into anterior group of axillary lymph nodes and from there they reach the apical group of axillary lymph nodes. Some reach apical group of axillary lymph nodes directly and do not drain into anterior group.
- Lymphatics from upper medial quadrants drain into internal mammary group of lymph nodes of the same side. Some cross to the other side and drain into the internal mammary group of the opposite side.
- Lymphatics from lower medial quadrants drain into subperitoneal plexus of lymphatics. Lymphatics from parenchyma of the gland including nipple and areola drain into pectoral group of lymph nodes.

Applied Anatomy

- Very common site for carcinoma. Removal of the gland is called mastectomy.
- Mastitis is inflammation of mammary gland.

Blood Supply

Vaginal branches of internal iliac and the uterine arteries. The veins drain into internal iliac veins.

Lymphatic Drainage

Upper 2/3rd: Internal and external iliac nodes; lower 1/3rd: Upper superficial inguinal nodes.

APPLIED ANATOMY

Male Reproductive System

Testes

- **Hydrocele:** Collection of fluid between visceral and parietal layer of processus vaginalis.
- **Hernia:** Abdominal contents may descend into testis if processus vaginalis is patent.
- **Varicocele:** Dilatation of pampiniform plexus.
- **Cryptorchidism:** Failure of descent of testes, lies in the abdominal cavity and is frequent site of carcinoma.
- **Ectopic testis:** Testis lies at an abnormal site deviating its normal path.

Prostate

- **Benign prostatic hyperplasia:** Enlargement of prostate.
- Carcinoma in prostate may spread to vertebral bodies due to the communication between prostatic venous plexus and vertebral venous plexus.
- **Prostatectomy:** Removal of prostate.

Female Reproductive System

Ovary

- **PCOD (polycystic ovarian disorder):** Obesity, irregular menstruation, acne, hirsutism.
- **Oophoritis:** Inflammation of ovary.
- **Krukenberg's syndrome (secondary ovarian cancer):** Cancer cells migrate from other tissues like breast.

Fallopian Tube

- **Tubectomy:** Fallopian tube cut between two ligated points.
- **Salpingitis:** Inflammation of the fallopian tube.
- Tubal implantation is the common type of ectopic pregnancy.

Uterus

- **Prolapse of uterus:** Uterus descends into vagina due to weakness of ligaments of uterus.
- **Myoma or fibroid:** Tumor in myometrium of uterus.
- **Hysterectomy:** Surgical removal of uterus.

SUMMARY

Male Reproductive System

Testes

- **Parts:** Two poles (upper, lower), two borders (anterior, posterior), two surfaces (medial, lateral)
- **Epididymis:** Overlaps on lateral surface and connected to testis by efferent ductules
- **Coverings:** Tunica vaginalis, tunica albuginea, tunica vasculosa
- **Blood supply:** Arteries-testicular artery, veins-pampiniform plexus of veins → testicular vein
- **Nerve supply:** Sympathetic—renal and aortic plexus from T10 and T11 spinal segments.

Prostate

- Accessory gland, secretions add to seminal fluid
- **Components:** Glandular tissue, fibromuscular stroma
- **Parts:** Apex, base, surfaces (anterior, posterior, two inferolateral)
- **Lobes:** Anterior, posterior, median, right and left lateral
- **Coverings:** False capsule, true capsule and venous plexus between two
- **Structures within prostate:** Urethra, prostatic utricle, two ejaculatory ducts
- **Blood supply:** Arteries-inferior vesical, middle rectal, internal pudendal; veins-prostatic venous plexus
- **Nerve supply:** Sympathetic—L3, L4, L5 spinal segments; parasympathetic—upper sacral spinal segments.

Female Reproductive System

Ovaries

- **Situation:** Ovarian fossa on lateral pelvic wall.
- **Parts:** Two poles (upper and lower in nulliparous woman, lateral and medial in multiparous woman), two borders (anterior/mesovariam, posterior/free), two surfaces (lateral, medial).
- **Blood supply:** Arteries-ovarian artery, uterine artery; veins-ovarian vein.
- **Nerve supply:** Sympathetic—T10, T11 spinal segments; parasympathetic—S2, S3, S4 spinal segments.

Uterus

- Muscular organ which protects and nourishes the embryo.
- **Parts:** Fundus, body, cervix.
- **Anteversion:** Long axis of uterus forms an angle of 90° with long axis of vagina.
- **Anteflexion:** Long axis of body of uterus forms an angle of 120° with long axis of cervix.
- **Ligaments:** Broad ligament, round ligament of uterus, transverse cervical ligament, uterosacral ligament, pubocervical ligament.
- **Supports of uterus:** Primary supports-muscular (pelvic diaphragm, perineal body, urogenital diaphragm), fibromuscular/mechanical (uterine axis, pubocervical ligaments, transverse cervical ligaments, uterosacral ligaments, round ligament of uterus); secondary supports-broad ligament, uterovesical fold of peritoneum, rectovaginal fold of peritoneum.
- **Blood supply:** Arteries-uterine artery, ovarian artery; veins-uterine, ovarian, vaginal veins
- **Nerve supply:** Sympathetic—T12, L1 spinal segments; parasympathetic—S2, S3, S4 spinal segments

Uterine Tube

- **Pair of ducts:** Convey ova from the ovary to uterus.
- **Parts:** Fimbria, infundibulum, ampulla, isthmus, uterine part.
- **Blood supply:** Arteries-uterine artery, ovarian artery; veins-pampiniform plexus of ovary, uterine vein.
- **Nerve supply:** Sympathetic-T10 to L2 spinal segments; parasympathetic—S2, S3, S4 spinal segments.

QUESTIONS

MALE REPRODUCTIVE SYSTEM

Long Essay

Name the parts of male genital system and describe the testis.

Short Essays

- Male urethra
- Testis—gross anatomy
- Testis—histology.

Short Answers

- Name the coverings of testis
- Components of male reproductive system
- Structure of testis
- Contents of spermatic cord
- Name accessory male reproductive organs
- Prostatic urethra
- Parts of epididymis and its lining epithelium
- Vasectomy
- Vas deferens—origin and termination
- Prostate—importance
- Prostate—histology.

FEMALE REPRODUCTIVE SYSTEM

Long Essays

- Name the parts of female reproductive system. Describe the anatomy of uterus.
- Name the organs of female reproductive system. Describe the ovary.

Short Essays

- Microscopic structure of ovary
- Microscopic structure of uterus
- Microscopic structure of fallopian tube
- Graafian follicle
- Mammary glands
- Ligaments of uterus
- Fallopian tube
- Lymphatic drainage of breast.

Short Answers

- Name the parts of uterus giving function of each part.
- Name the parts of fallopian tubes and lining epithelium. Which is the widest part?
- Position of uterus in the body
- Where does fertilization occur?

CHAPTER

Endocrine System

LEARNING OBJECTIVES

The student should be able to:

- Name all endocrine glands, describe details of pituitary gland, thyroid gland, parathyroid gland, suprarenal gland (gross and microscopic structure).

INTRODUCTION

- Endocrine tissues are highly vascular.
- The secretions of endocrine glands are called hormones. Hormones travel through blood to the target cells whose functioning they may influence profoundly.
- A hormone acts on cells that bear specific receptors for it.
- The endocrine organs along with autonomic nervous system coordinate and control the metabolic activities and internal environment of the body.
- The endocrine glands are pituitary, pineal, thyroid, parathyroid, pancreas, suprarenal gland, testis/ovary.

PITUITARY GLAND

The pituitary gland (hypophysis cerebri) is a small endocrine gland, ovoid in shape, and is suspended from the base of the brain by a stalk.

Situation

The gland lies in the hypophyseal fossa of the sphenoid bone. The fossa is roofed by the diaphragma sellae.

Dimensions

It measures 8 mm anteroposteriorly and 12 mm transversely. It weighs about 500 mg.

Relations

- **Superiorly:** Diaphragma sellae, optic chiasma, tuber cinereum, infundibular recess of the 3rd ventricle.

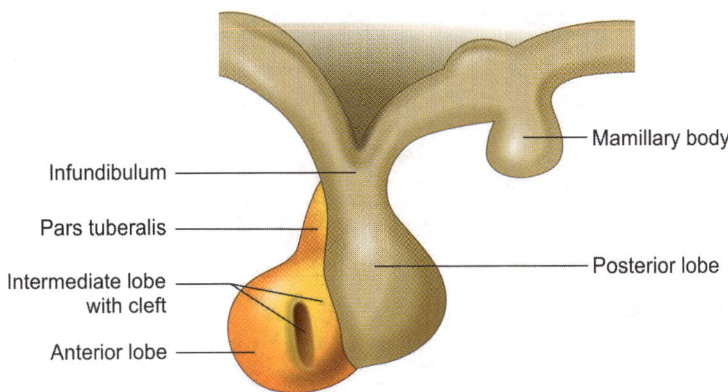

Fig. 11.1: Parts of pituitary gland.

- **Inferiorly:** Hypophyseal fossa of the sphenoid bone, sphenoidal air sinuses.
- **On each side:** Cavernous sinus with its contents.

Subdivisions (Fig. 11.1)

The pituitary gland has two parts, adenohypophysis and neurohypophysis.

Adenohypophysis

Adenohypophysis is divided into:
- **Pars anterior/anterior lobe:** Largest part of the gland.
- **Pars intermedia:** Thin strip, separated from anterior lobe by an intraglandular cleft.
- **Pars tuberalis:** Is an upward extension of anterior lobe that surrounds the infundibulum.

Neurohypophysis

Neurohypophysis is divided into:
- Posterior lobe.
- Infundibular stem containing neural connections of posterior lobe with hypothalamus.
- Median eminence continuous with the infundibular stem.

Blood Supply

Superior hypophyseal artery and inferior hypophyseal artery (branches from the internal carotid artery). Veins drain into the neighboring dural venous sinuses.

Microscopic Structure (Figs. 11.2A and B)

The anterior lobe consists of thick, irregular cords of cells, separated by sinusoids (lined by reticuloendothelial cells).
- The cells are of two types—chromophils (50%) and chromophobes (50%). The chromophils are acidophils (43%) and basophils (7%). Chromophobes are much smaller in size. They represent the nonsecretory phase of the other types (precursors of other types of cells).
- The posterior lobe is made up of a large number of nonmyelinated nerve fibers (forming the hypothalamo-hypophyseal tract) and modified neuroglial cells, called the pituicytes.
- The middle lobe is made up of colloid-filled vesicles lined with cuboidal epithelium.

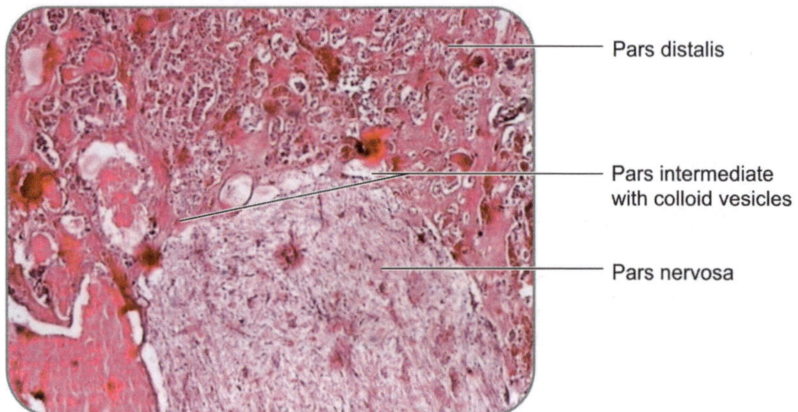

Fig. 11.2A: Photomicrograph of histology of pituitary gland.

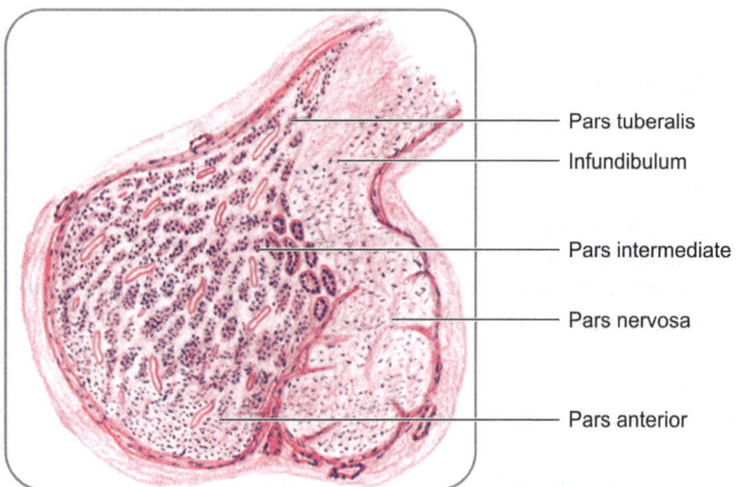

Fig. 11.2B: Diagrammatic representation of histology of pituitary gland.

Applied Anatomy

Pituitary tumors give rise to the following symptoms:

General Symptoms

- The sella turcica becomes enlarged in size.
- Pressure over the optic chiasma causes bitemporal hemianopia.
- A large tumor may press upon the third ventricle, causing a rise in the intracranial pressure.

Specific Symptoms

- Acidophil adenoma causes acromegaly in adults and gigantism in the young patients.
- Basophil adenoma causes Cushing's syndrome.
- Chromophobe adenoma causes effects of hypopituitarism.
- Posterior lobe damage causes diabetes insipidus.

THYROID GLAND (FIG. 11.3)

- Thyroid gland is an endocrine gland, yellowish brown in color, richly vascular.
- It maintains the metabolic rate, stimulates somatic and psychic growth and plays an important role in calcium metabolism.

Parts

- Consists of right and left lobes that are connected together by an isthmus.
- The lobes are conical in shape, presenting an apex, a base, three surfaces—medial, anterolateral and posterolateral and three borders—anterior, posterior and lateral. The isthmus connects the lower parts of the lobes. It has two surfaces—anterior and posterior and two borders—superior and inferior.

Situation

It is situated in the front and sides of the lower part of the neck opposite the levels C5, C6, C7 and T1 vertebrae. Each lobe extends from the middle of the thyroid cartilage to the fourth or fifth tracheal ring.

Capsules

- The true capsule is the peripheral condensation of the connective tissue of the gland.
- The false capsule is derived from deep fascia.
- A dense capillary plexus is present deep to the true capsule. To avoid hemorrhage during operations, the thyroid is removed with the true capsule.

Relations

- The anterolateral surface of the lateral lobes are covered with sternothyroid, sternohyoid and overlapped by the sternocleidomastoid.
- The posterolateral surface is related to the carotid sheath and its contents (internal jugular vein, common carotid artery, and vagus nerve). The superior and inferior parathyroids lie on the posterior surface of the gland.

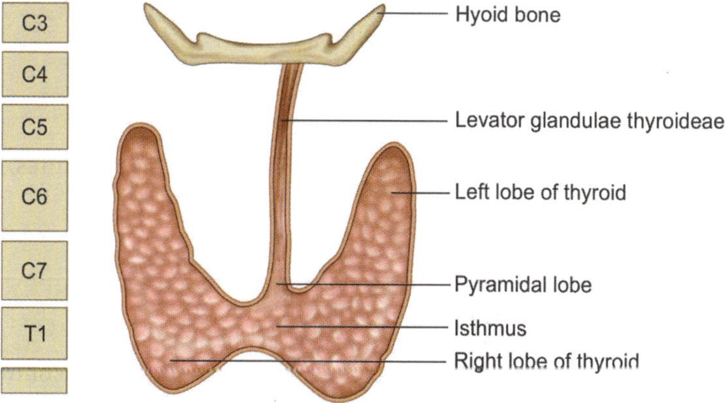

Fig. 11.3: Thyroid gland.

- The medial surface is related to 2 tubes (trachea and esophagus), 2 nerves (external and recurrent laryngeal nerves), 2 muscles (cricothyroid and inferior constrictor) and 2 cartilages (thyroid and cricoid).
- Anterior surface of the isthmus is covered by skin, superficial fascia and the deep fascia.
- The posterior surface is resting on the 2nd, 3rd and 4th tracheal rings.
- From the upper border of the isthmus, a small conical projection called the pyramidal lobe is often seen to arise, if present, the pyramidal lobe may be connected to the body of the hyoid bone by a fibromuscular band called the levator glandulae thyroideae.
- From the lower border of the isthmus, a pair of inferior thyroid veins emerge out.

Blood Supply

The thyroid gland is supplied by superior thyroid artery (branch of external carotid artery), inferior thyroid artery (branch of thyrocervical trunk) and rarely by thyroidea ima artery (from brachiocephalic trunk or the arch of aorta). Accessory thyroid arteries arising from the tracheal and esophageal arteries also supply the thyroid gland. Superior thyroid vein ends in the internal jugular vein or the common facial vein, middle thyroid vein into the internal jugular vein, inferior thyroid veins into left brachiocephalic vein. A fourth thyroid vein (of Kocher) may be present and drains into the internal jugular vein.

Lymphatic Drainage

Deep cervical nodes.

Nerve Supply

Parasympathetic fibers are from the vagi and their recurrent laryngeal branches; sympathetic fibers from middle and inferior cervical sympathetic ganglia.

Microscopic Structure (Figs.11.4A and B)

- The gland is made up of numerous follicles called thyroid follicles.
- Each thyroid follicle has a basement membrane and a single layer of cuboidal cells.
- **The follicles are made up of two types of secretory cells:** Follicular cells lining the follicles, secreting tri-iodothyronine and tetra-iodothyronine and parafollicular cells lie between the follicular cells and basement membrane which secrete thyrocalcitonin.
- The follicles are filled with pink staining colloid.

Applied Anatomy

- The enlargement of the thyroid gland is goiter.
- Benign tumors of the gland displace or compress the neighboring structures, like the carotid sheath, trachea, etc.

PARATHYROID GLAND

- The parathyroid glands are two pairs, superior and inferior.
- Each is yellowish orange in color and is the size of a split pea.
- Each gland weighs about 50 grams. They secrete parathormone (which controls the calcium and phosphorus metabolism).

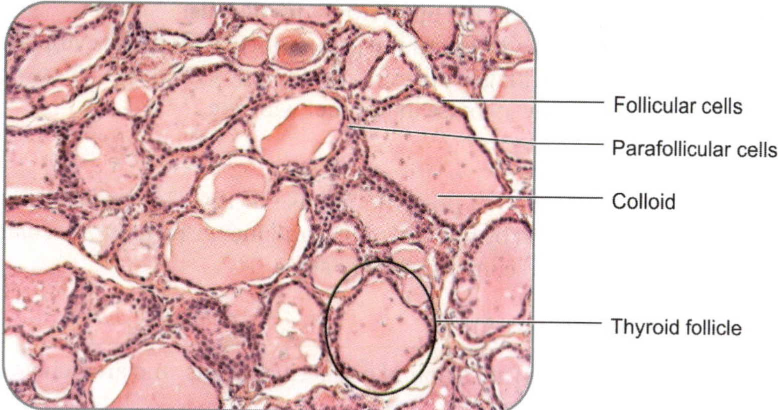

Fig. 11.4A: Photomicrograph of histology of thyroid gland.

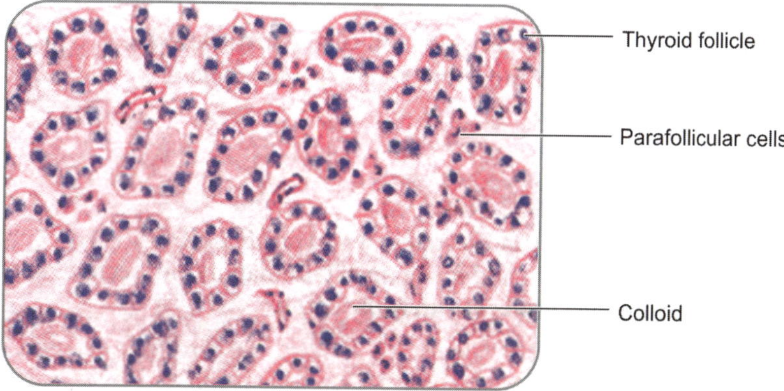

Fig. 11.4B: Diagrammatic representation of histology of thyroid gland.

Situation

- The superior parathyroid is more constant in position at the posterior border of the lobe of thyroid.
- The inferior parathyroids are variable in position. It may lie within or behind and outside the thyroid capsule or within the substance of the lobe.

Blood Supply

Inferior thyroid arteries. Veins and lymphatics go to those of the thyroid.

Nerve Supply

Branches from the middle and superior cervical sympathetic ganglia.

Histology

- A thin fibrous connective tissue capsule surrounds the gland.
- It sends septae inwards into the gland.

- **The parenchyma of the gland is made up of two types of cells:**
  - Chief cells: Polygonal cells with central nucleus, scanty, acidophilic cytoplasm.
  - Oxyphil cells: Larger cells with granular and acidophilic cytoplasm. These have smaller and darker nucleus and they increase in number with age.

Applied Anatomy

Accidental removal of parathyroid is possible in case of thyroidectomy. This results in hypoparathyroidism, characterized by hypocalcemia, and increased neurovascular irritability producing carpopedal spasms and convulsions—tetany.

SUPRARENAL GLAND (FIG. 11.5)

Suprarenal glands (adrenal glands) are a pair of endocrine glands, and are richly vascular.

Situation

Posterior abdominal wall behind the peritoneum over the upper pole of the kidneys.

Measurements

- About 50 mm in height, 30 mm in breadth and 10 mm in thickness.
- It is 1/3rd of the kidney at birth and about 1/13th of it in adults.
- **Weight:** About 5 gram.

Subdivisions

Outer cortex and an inner medulla.

- Cortex is mesodermal in origin and secretes steroid hormones.
- Medulla is of neural crest origin and made up of chromaffin cells, secretes adrenaline and noradrenaline. The medulla forms 1/10th of the cortex.

Right Suprarenal Gland

- Triangular in shape
- Has an apex, a base, 2 surfaces (anterior and posterior) and 3 borders (anterior, medial and lateral).

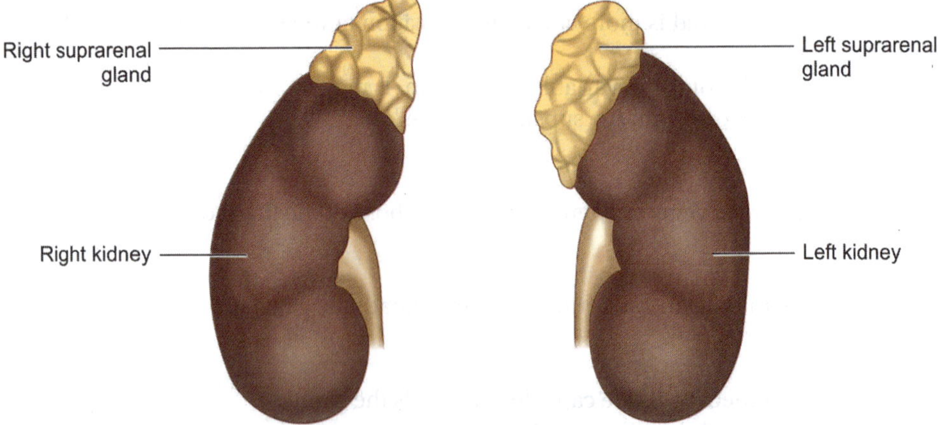

Fig. 11.5: The suprarenal glands.

Relations

- **Base:** Upper pole of right kidney.
- **Anterior surface (Fig. 11.6):** Inferior vena cava, liver and duodenum.
- **Posterior surface:** Crus of the diaphragm.
- **Anterior border:** A hilum just below the apex, where the suprarenal vein emerges.
- **Medial border:** Right celiac ganglion, right inferior phrenic artery.

Left Suprarenal Gland

- Semilunar in shape
- It presents two ends (upper narrow end and lower rounded end), two borders (medial and lateral) and two surfaces (anterior and posterior).

Relations

- **Anterior surface (Fig. 11.6):** Cardiac end of the stomach, splenic artery, pancreas.
- Near the lower end is the hilum where the suprarenal vein emerges.
- **Posterior surface:** Kidney, left crus of the diaphragm.
- **Medial border:** Left celiac ganglion, left phrenic artery and the left gastric artery.

Blood Supply

Superior suprarenal (branch of the inferior phrenic), middle suprarenal (branch of abdominal aorta) and inferior suprarenal (branch of renal artery). Right suprarenal vein drains into inferior vena cava and left suprarenal vein drains into left renal vein.

Lymphatic Drainage

Drains into the lateral aortic nodes.

Nerve Supply

The suprarenal medulla has a rich nerve supply through the preganglionic sympathetic plexus. The chromaffin cells form the postganglionic sympathetic neurons.

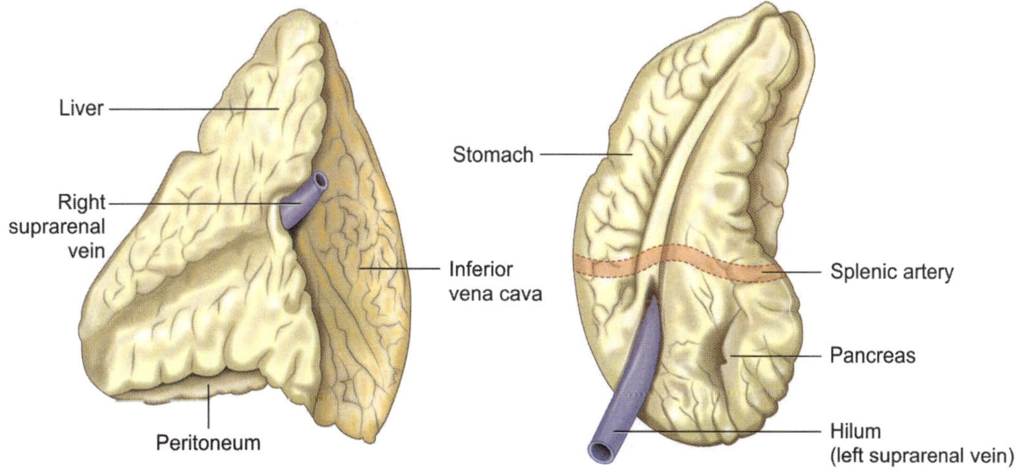

Fig. 11.6: Anterior surface of right and left suprarenal glands.

Microscopic Structure (Figs. 11.7A and B)

The gland is covered by a thin fibrous capsule.

Outer *cortex* shows three zones:

1. Outermost zona glomerulosa made of polyhedral cells arranged in curves. These cells have deeply stained rounded nuclei with scanty cytoplasm.
2. Middle zona fasciculata made up of large polygonal cells, with basophilic cytoplasm and lipid droplets. They are arranged in long columns with sinusoids between them.
3. Inner zona reticularis with rounded cells, arranged in branching and anastomosing cords to form a network.

Inner medulla is made up of irregular collection of large epithelial cells with large venous sinusoids between them. The adrenal medulla belongs to the chromaffin cell system. The cells of this system stain yellow when treated with some salts of chromium.

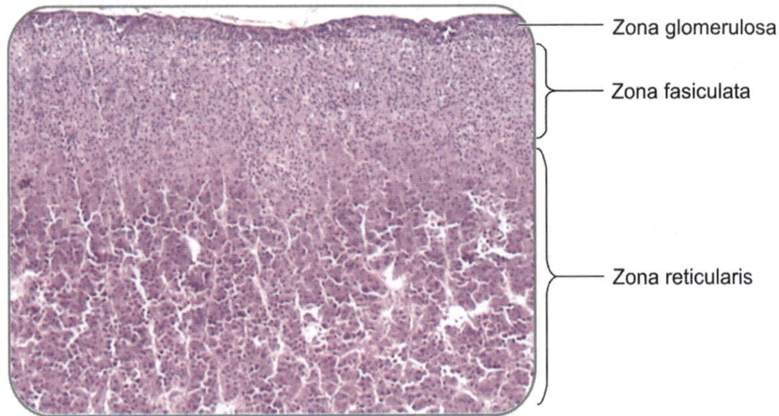

Fig. 11.7A: Photomicrograph of histology of suprarenal gland.

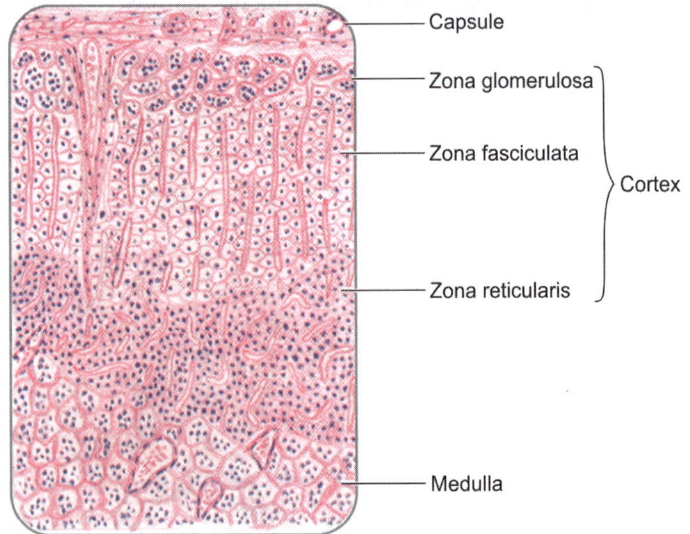

Fig. 11.7B: Diagrammatic representation of histology of suprarenal gland.

Applied Anatomy

- Carcinoma of the suprarenal cortex, Cushing's syndrome (hypogonadism, hirsutism, diabetes and obesity), in women virilism, in men feminization due to excess formation of the opposite sex hormone.
- Insufficiency of the cortex may result in Addison's disease—hypotension, pigmentation of the skin, anemia and muscular weakness.

APPLIED ANATOMY

Pituitary Gland

- **Pituitary tumors may compress the surrounding structures leading to the following symptoms:** Enlarged sella turcica, bitemporal hemianopia, increased intracranial pressure.
- Acidophil adenoma leads to acromegaly in adults and gigantism in children.
- Basophil adenoma leads to Cushing's syndrome.
- Chromophobe adenoma leads to hypopituitarism.
- Posterior lobe damage causes diabetes insipidus.

Thyroid Gland

- **Goiter:** Enlargement of thyroid.
- Thyroid tumors compress the surrounding structures.
- During thyroidectomy, by mistake parathyroid can also be removed leading to hypoparathyroidism.

Suprarenal Gland

- **Female pseudohermaphroditism:** External genitalia of female fetus resemble that of male due to excess production of androgens in suprarenal gland.
- Deficiency of aldosterone leads to Addison's disease (hypotension, pigmentation of skin, anemia, muscular weakness).
- Excess production of sex steroids leads to feminization of male and masculinization of female.
- Excess production of glucocorticoid leads to Cushing's syndrome (hypogonadism, hirsutism, diabetes, obesity).

SUMMARY

Features	*Pituitary gland*	*Thyroid gland*	*Suprarenal gland*
Situation	Hypophyseal fossa	Neck opposite to C5 to T1 vertebrae	Upper pole of kidneys
Gross features	• **Parts:** Adenohypophysis (pars anterior, pars intermedia, pars tuberalis); neurohypophysis (posterior lobe, infundibulum, median eminence) • **Relations:** Superior (diaphragm sellae, optic chiasma, tuber cinereum, infundibular recess); inferior (hypophyseal fossa, sphenoidal air sinus); lateral (cavernous sinus)	• **Coverings:** True and false capsules, venous plexus deep to true capsule Parts: Right and left lobes, isthmus • **Relations:** Anterolateral (sternohyoid, sternothyroid, sternocleidomastoid); posterolateral (carotid sheath, superior and inferior parathyroids); medial (trachea, esophagus, external and recurrent laryngeal nerves, cricothyroid and inferior constrictor muscles, thyroid and cricoid cartilages)	• **Relations:** Right suprarenal (base—upper pole of right kidney; anterior surface-inferior vena cava, liver, duodenum; posterior surface—crus of diaphragm; medial border—right celiac ganglion, right inferior phrenic artery) left suprarenal (anterior surface—stomach, splenic artery, pancreas; posterior surface—kidney, left crus of diaphragm; medial border—left celiac ganglion, left phrenic artery, left gastric artery)
Blood supply	• **Arteries:** Superior and inferior hypophyseal • **Veins:** Neighboring dural venous sinuses	• **Arteries:** Superior and inferior thyroid arteries • **Veins:** Superior, middle and inferior thyroid veins	• **Arteries:** Superior, middle and inferior suprarenal arteries • **Veins:** Right and left suprarenal veins

QUESTIONS

Long Essays

- Mention the different types of glands on the basis of their mode of secretions. Give examples.
- Name the endocrine glands. Describe briefly the pituitary gland.
- Describe any one endocrine gland in detail.
- What is a gland? Distinguish between endocrine and exocrine glands.
- Briefly describe the thyroid gland. Write a note on its applied aspects.

Short Essays

- Where is the adrenal gland located? What does it secrete?
- Name one condition affecting the thyroid gland.
- Give the endocrine secretions of the ovary. What are its functions?
- Enumerate the endocrine glands. Mention one hormone for each.
- Anterior lobe of pituitary.
- Blood supply of the thyroid gland.
- Suprarenal/thyroid/pancreas.

Short Note

- Name the parts of the pancreas/pituitary and its functions.

CHAPTER

Nervous System

LEARNING OBJECTIVES

The student should be able to:

- Describe neuron and its classification.
- Classify nervous system.
- Describe meninges with dural folds, layers of meninges.
- Describe lateral, third and fourth ventricles and cerebrospinal fluid.
- Brief on cerebrum, cerebellum, midbrain, pons, medulla oblongata, spinal cord with spinal/peripheral nerve (gross and histology).
- Describe upper and lower motor neurons.
- Describe basal nuclei, internal capsule.
- Describe blood supply of brain.
- Name the cranial nerve, their functions, nuclear origin, course, exit through foramina in skull, their branches.
- Describe sympathetic and parasympathetic nervous system.
- Brief on brachial, lumbar plexus, ansa cervicalis, median, radial, ulnar, femoral, obturator, sciatic, cutaneous nerve supply of dorsum of hand and foot.

INTRODUCTION

Neuroanatomy is the study of the structural aspects of the nervous system. The nervous system is made up of specialized tissue that has the special property to conduct impulses rapidly from one part of the body to another. The specialized cells that constitute the functional units of the nervous system are called neurons.

The nervous system is divided into the central and peripheral nervous systems.

Central Nervous System

- This comprises brain and spinal cord. The brain consists of cerebrum, cerebellum, midbrain, pons, and medulla oblongata.
- The midbrain, pons and medulla together form the brainstem.
- Within the brain and spinal cord, neurons are supported by a special connective tissue called the neuroglia.
- Nervous tissue, composed of neurons and neuroglia, is richly supplied with blood.

Peripheral Nervous System

- This is made up of peripheral nerves and associated ganglia.
- Peripheral nerves attached to the brain are called cranial nerves; and those attached to the spinal cord are called the spinal nerves.

NEURON

- A neuron consists of a cell body/soma/perikaryon.
- The cell consists of a mass of cytoplasm surrounded by a cell membrane.
- Cytoplasm contains a large central nucleus, numerous mitochondria, lysosomes, centrioles and a Golgi complex.
- Cytoplasm shows the presence of a granular material that stains intensely with basic dyes, the Nissl substance which is the distinctive feature.
- Under EM, the Nissl substance is composed of rough endoplasmic reticulum, abundant presence of these indicates the high level of protein synthesis in the neuron.
- The proteins are needed for maintenance and repair, and for production of neurotransmitters and enzymes.
- Neurofibrils consist of microfilaments and microtubules.
- Some neurons contain pigment granules (e.g. neuromelanin in neurons of the substantia nigra).
- Aging neurons contain a pigment lipofuscin (made up of residual bodies derived from lysosomes).

Processes of Neurons

The processes arising from the cell body of neuron are of two kinds, i.e. dendrite and axon. Dendrites carry nerve impulses to the cell body while axons carry nerve impulses away from the cell body. Difference between axons and dendrites is shown in **Table 12.1**.

Myelin Sheath

- A sheath known as myelin sheath covers the axons; these axons are termed as myelinated axons.
- There are axons that are devoid of myelin sheaths called unmyelinated axons.
- Schwann cells provide this myelin sheath for the axons lying outside the central nervous system.

Table 12.1: Difference between axons and dendrites.

Axon	*Dendrite*
• Single long process. • They extend a considerable distance away from the cell body (longest a meter long)	• Numerous short branching
• Devoid of Nissl substance. This Nissl-free zone extends for a short distance into the cell body; this part of the cell body is called the axon hillock. • The part of the axon just beyond the axon hillock is called the initial segment	• Nissl substance extends into this
• Impulse travels away from the cell body	• Impulse travels towards the cell body

- Oligodendrocytes provide this myelin sheath for the axons lying within the central nervous system.
- Presence of a myelin sheath increases the velocity of conduction. It also reduces the energy expended in the process of conduction.

Formation of Myelin Sheath

- An axon lying near a Schwann cell invaginates into cytoplasm of Schwann cell.
- In this process the axon comes to be suspended by a fold of the cell membrane of the Schwann cell, this fold is called the mesaxon.
- In some situations, the mesaxon becomes greatly elongated and comes to be spirally wound around the axon, which is thus surrounded by several layers of cell membrane.
- Lipids are deposited between adjacent layers of the membrane. These layers of the mesaxon, along with the lipids, form the myelin sheath.
- Outside the myelin sheath a thin layer of Schwann cell cytoplasm persists to form an additional sheath called the neurilemma.
- Each Schwann cell provides the myelin sheath for a short segment of the axon. At the junction of any two such segments, there is a short gap in the myelin sheath. These gaps are called the nodes of Ranvier.
- The nodes of Ranvier are of importance since the impulse jumps from one node to the other; this type of conduction is termed as saltatory conduction.
- The part of the nerve fiber between two nodes of Ranvier is called the internode.

Types of Neurons (Fig. 12.1)

- There are different sizes and shapes of neuronal cell bodies.
- The shape of the cell body depends upon the number of processes arising from it.
- **Multipolar neuron:** The most common type, where the cell body gives off several processes.
- **Bipolar neurons:** These have only one axon and one dendrite.
- **Unipolar neurons:** The neurons have only a single process.
- **Pseudounipolar neurons:** After a short course, the process of the unipolar neuron divides into two, of which one forms the axon and the other forms the dendrite with different functions.

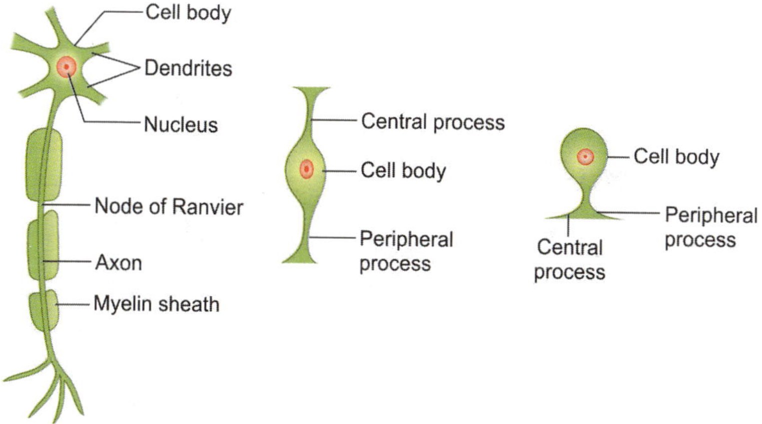

Fig. 12.1: Multipolar, bipolar and pseudounipolar neurons.

NEUROGLIA/SUPPORTING CELLS

In addition to the neurons, the nervous system contains several types of supporting cells. They are:

- **Neuroglial cells:** Found in parenchyma of the brain and spinal cord. Different types of neuroglial cells are astrocytes, oligodendrocytes, microglia.
- **Ependymal cells:** Lining the ventricular system.
- **Schwann cells:** Forming sheaths for axons of peripheral nerves.
- **Satellite cells:** Surrounding neurons in peripheral ganglia.

Functions of Neuroglia

- Provides mechanical support to neurons.
- Due to their nonconducting nature they serve as insulators and prevent neuronal impulses from spreading in unwanted directions.
- Help in neuronal function by playing an important role in maintaining a suitable metabolic environment for the neurons.
- They are responsible for repair of damaged areas of nervous tissue.
- Oligodendrocytes provide myelin sheath to nerve fibers within the CNS.
- Ependymal cells are concerned in exchanges of material between the brain and the CSF.
- Signals arising in Schwann cells can influence the growth of axons and their diameter; therefore they are essential for repair of damaged peripheral nerves.

MENINGES (FIG. 12.2)

The brain and the spinal cord are covered by three membranes or meninges.
They are: (i) Dura mater, (ii) Arachnoid, and (iii) Pia mater from superficial to deep.

Dura Mater

It is a thick opaque inelastic membrane which is made up of outer endosteal and inner meningeal layer.

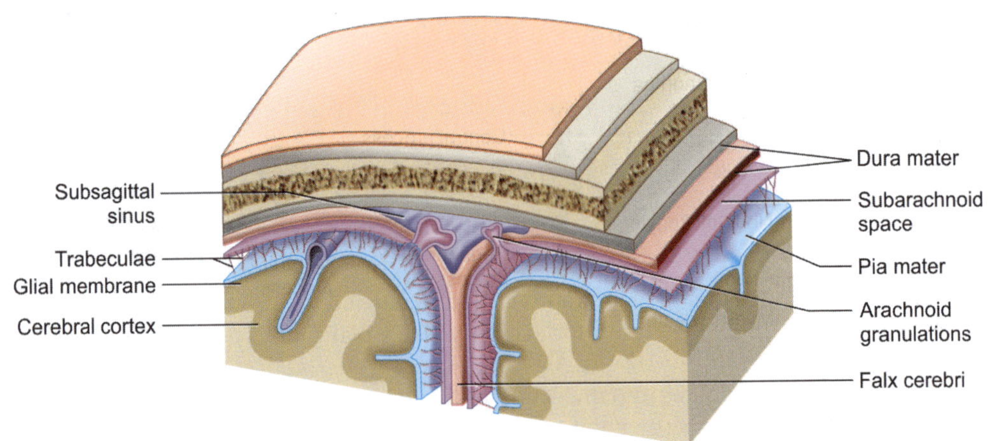

Fig. 12.2: Meninges.

The outer and the inner layers of the dura mater are firmly adherent to each other except in certain places where they separate to form spaces lined by endothelium and filled with blood. Such spaces are called dural venous sinuses.

These sinuses differ from the veins in the following aspects:

- They are irregular in outline.
- They have no smooth muscle fiber in their walls.
- They have no valves hence the blood can flow in either direction in the sinuses.
- The inner meningeal layer gets reduplicated and forms certain folds called the dural folds.
- They are the falx cerebri, falx cerebelli, tentorium cerebelli and diaphragma sellae.

Falx cerebri: It is a sickle shaped-fold which dips into the longitudinal fissure between the two cerebral hemispheres thus separating them. The upper border contains the superior sagittal sinus and the lower border contains inferior sagittal sinus.

Falx cerebelli: This separates the two cerebellar hemispheres and contains the occipital sinus.

Tentorium cerebelli: A horizontal dome-shaped fold which passes into the gap between the cerebellum and hinder part of cerebrum, thus separating the cerebellar hemispheres from the posterior lobes of cerebrum. It meets the inferior layer of falx cerebri on its superior aspect and between them is enclosed the straight sinus.

Diaphragma sellae: A circular fold of dura mater which overhangs the pituitary fossa and is attached to the four clinoid processes.

Arachnoid Mater

- It is a translucent avascular membrane situated between the dura mater and the pia mater.
- It covers the brain loosely and does not dip into the sulci and fissures except the longitudinal fissure.
- There is a thin space between the dura and the arachnoid mater known as the subdural space, which contains a thin film of lymph like fluid.
- Subarachnoid space is the space between the arachnoid and the pia mater, which contains the CSF, larger blood vessels of the brain and a delicate vascular subarachnoid tissue.
- The subarachnoid space communicates with the ventricular system of the brain as well as the central canal of the spinal cord.
- Cisternal puncture is done by introducing a needle anterosuperiorly through the posterior atlanto-occipital membrane between the posterior arch of the atlas and the posterior margin of the foramen magnum.
- Nodular elevations called arachnoid granulations which drain cerebrospinal fluid into superior sagittal sinus are seen on the surface of the arachnoid mater in the regions of the superior sagittal and the transverse sinuses. They enlarge with age and may even absorb the overlying bones causing pits.

Pia Mater

- It is a thin, vascular, transparent membrane which dips into the sulci and fissures of the brain.
- As the blood vessels pierce the brain surface, they take a pial sheath around them into the brain.
- The pia mater also invaginates into the ventricles by the choroid plexuses and helps in the formation of the CSF and is termed the tela choroidea of the ventricles.

SPINAL CORD

- **Situation:** In the upper 2/3rd of the vertebral canal.
- **Extent:** From the level of foramen magnum, where it is continuous with medulla oblongata to the lower border of L1, where it ends in a conical extremity called conus medullaris.
- Early in development, the lower end of the spinal cord corresponds to the lower sacral level. At birth and in infants the lower limit of the cord is at L3 or L4 level.
- Its average length is about 45 cm.
- **Shape:** It is cylindrical and flattened.
- It presents cervical enlargement opposite the attachments of roots of brachial plexus, and lumbar enlargement opposite the attachments of lumbosacral plexus.

Coverings

The spinal cord is surrounded by three meninges, which are continuous with those of the brain. They are dura mater, arachnoid mater and pia mater.

Dura Mater

Dura mater is a thick opaque, fibrous membrane which is continuous with inner meningeal layer of dura of brain. The extradural/epidural space (space between dura mater and vertebral column) contains some areolar tissue, fat and plexus of veins. The subdural space (space between dura mater and arachnoid mater) contains a thin film of lymph-like fluid.

Arachnoid Mater

A translucent delicate avascular membrane. The subarachnoid space (between arachnoid mater and pia mater) contains the cerebrospinal fluid.

Pia Mater

It is a thin, transparent vascular membrane, closely adherent to the surface of the spinal cord. Below the conus medullaris, the pia mater is continued as a slender filament, the filum terminale.

External Features

The surface of the spinal cord presents:

- An anterior median fissure
- A posteromedian sulcus
- A pair of posterolateral and anterolateral sulci

Internal Features (Fig. 12.3)

In a section of the spinal cord:

- It shows a central 'H'-shaped gray matter—made of nerve cell bodies.
- A peripheral white matter made of nerve fiber tracts.
- The gray matter presents a pair of anterior (ventral) horns made of large motor cells and a pair of posterior (dorsal) horns made of smaller sensory cells.
  Lateral gray horn is found in the thoracic and upper lumbar regions (T1 to L2) only and contains cells of origin of the sympathetic system. Parasympathetic fibers arise from middle sacral region (S2, S3, S4).

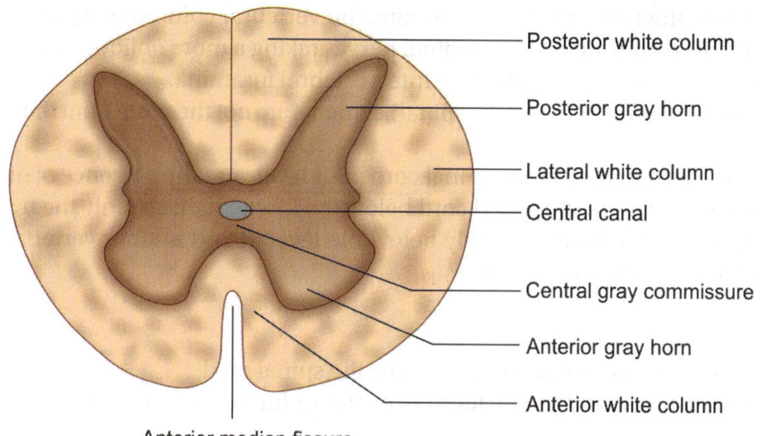

Fig. 12.3: Parts of spinal cord.

- The horns of two sides are connected by a transverse gray commissure in which the central canal of the spinal cord is situated.
  The central canal contains the *cerebrospinal fluid* and is lined by ciliated columnar cells.

Spinal Cord at Different Levels

Cervical Region

- It is large and oval in shape.
- The amount of white matter is more compared to gray matter.
- The anterior gray horn is thick.
- Posterior gray is slender and long.

Thoracic Region

- Section is small and circular.
- Anterior and posterior gray columns are slender.
- The lateral gray horn present.

Lumbar Region

- Section is large and circular.
- More of gray matter than white matter
- Both the anterior and posterior horns are wide and short.
- Lateral gray horn is present in the upper segments.

Sacral Region

- Section is very small.
- Small gray and white matters compared to other regions. Very little white matter compared to gray matter.

Relationships of the Spinal Segments to the Vertebral Column

In early stages of development, the lower end of the spinal cord and the vertebral column are at the same level, and all the spinal nerves pass horizontally and laterally to leave through the corresponding intervertebral foramina.

Later, due to a difference in the growth rate, the vertebral column elongates more rapidly than the cord. This results in the lower spinal nerves taking a more oblique course downwards and laterally to reach their corresponding intervertebral foramina.

Therefore, the vertebral level and the spinal segments are not the same from the lower cervical levels.

Because of the termination of the spinal cord at L1 level, and the presence of only the cauda equina below L1, injuries to the spinal cord below the L2 can damage only the nerve roots.

Lumbar puncture can be done safely below the level of 2nd lumbar vertebra to draw out cerebrospinal fluid for diagnostic purposes.

Blood Supply

- Anterior and posterior spinal arteries supply the spinal cord.
- Veins drain into the lateral sacral, lumbar, posterior intercostals and the vertebral veins.

Tracts of the Spinal Cord (Fig. 12.4)

Descending Tracts

Corticospinal, rubrospinal, tectospinal, vestibulospinal, reticulospinal and olivospinal tracts.

Corticospinal tract (pyramidal tract):

- **Origin:** From the motor area of the cortex.
- **Course:** Fibers descend through the corona radiata, internal capsule, cerebral peduncles, ventral part of pons, and pyramids of the medulla.
- Two-thirds of the fibers cross to opposite side at pyramidal decussation of medulla and descend in lateral white column of the spinal cord as lateral corticospinal tract.
- Uncrossed fibers descend in anterior white column of spinal cord as anterior corticospinal tract.
- **Termination:** Fibers end in anterior horn cells of spinal cord.
- **Function:** These are important motor pathways in spinal cord.

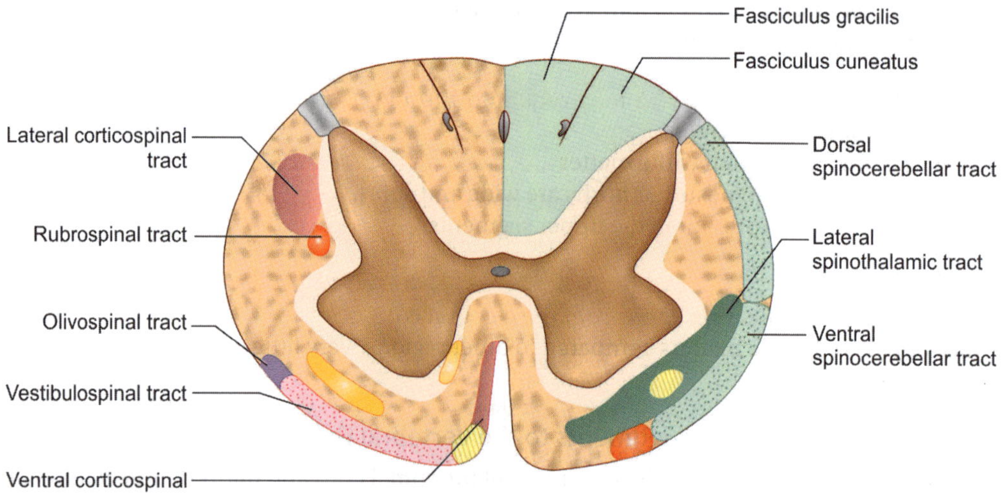

Fig. 12.4: Tracts of spinal cord.

Ascending Tracts

Lateral spinothalamic, ventral spinothalamic, spinocerebellar, spinoreticular fibers, spinovestibular, and spinotectal tracts.

Lateral spinothalamic tract

- **Origin:** From the dorsal root ganglia of the spinal nerves.
- **Course:** The fibers enter the spinal cord and ascend upwards.
- **Termination:** Fibers end in the thalamus.
- **Function:** The fibers carry pain and temperature sensations.

Ventral spinothalamic tract

- **Origin:** Cell bodies are situated in the dorsal root ganglia of the spinal nerves.
- **Course:** Nerve fibers enter the spinal cord. The axons cross the midline and ascend.
- **Termination:** The tract ends in the thalamus.
- **Function:** This tract carries touch and pressure impulses.

Spinocerebellar tract

There are two tracts: Anterior and posterior.

- Posterior tract contains uncrossed fibers and anterior tract has both crossed and uncrossed fibers. They are named according to the position they occupy in the spinal cord: Anterior or posterior part of the white matter.
- **Origin:** From dorsal root ganglion of spinal nerves.
- **Course:** Central processes of these cells enter the spinal cord through posterior roots of spinal nerves.
- Some of the axons ascend up in the gray column as the posterior spinocerebellar tract on the same side, and reach cerebellum through the inferior cerebellar peduncle.
- Rest of the axons cross to the opposite side and ascend upwards as the anterior spinocerebellar tract in the anterior part of the spinal cord. Some uncrossed fibers also ascend up in the anterior spinocerebellar tract. These reach cerebellum through the superior cerebellar peduncle.
- **Termination:** The fibers go to cerebellum through the superior or inferior cerebellar peduncles.
- **Function:** These tracts convey proprioceptive information to the cerebellum, providing it with afferent impulses necessary for its unconscious coordination.

Upper Motor Neurons

These are the neurons that come from the cerebral cortex (as corticospinal tracts) and end in the spinal cord and cranial nerve nuclei.

Lower Motor Neurons

These are the ventral horn cells and their processes that travel through a peripheral nerve to innervate a muscle.

The interruption of either of these neurons leads to paralysis, as shown in **Table 12.2.**

Table 12.2: Interruption in function of neurons.

Feature	*Upper motor neuron*	*Lower motor neuron*
Type of paralysis	Spastic	Flaccid
Tendon reflexes	Exaggerated	Absent
Muscle atrophy	Absent	Present
Clonus	Present	Absent
Rigidity	Present	Absent
Babinski's sign	Positive	Negative

BRAINSTEM (FIG. 12.5)

- The brainstem consists of midbrain, pons and medulla oblongata from above downwards.
- The midbrain is continuous above with the cerebral hemispheres. The medulla is continuous, below with the spinal cord.
- Posteriorly, the pons and the medulla are separated from the cerebellum by the cavity of fourth ventricle.
- The ventricle is continuous, below with the central canal, which traverses the lower part of the medulla, and becomes continuous with the central canal of the spinal cord.
- Cranially, the fourth ventricle is continuous with the aqueduct, which passes through the midbrain.
- The midbrain, pons and medulla are connected to the cerebellum by the superior, middle and inferior cerebellar peduncles, respectively.

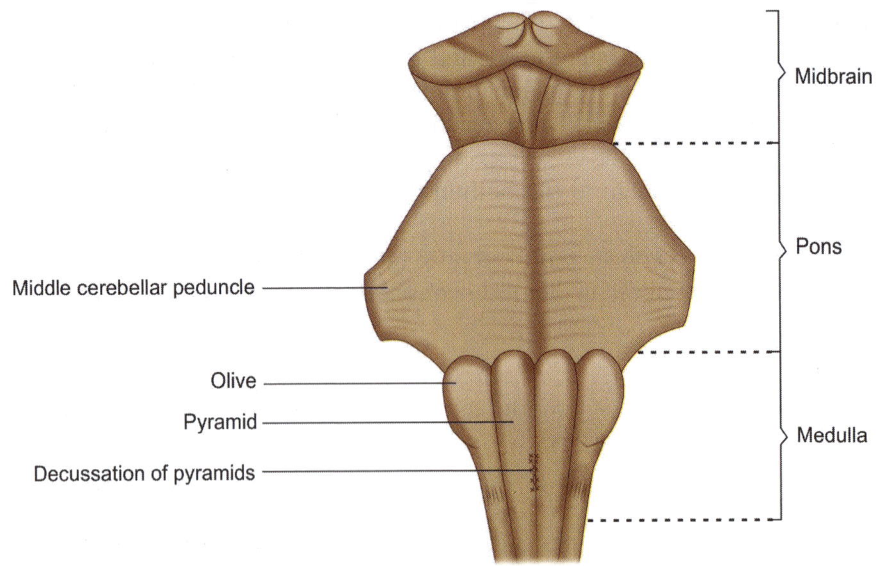

Fig. 12.5: The brainstem.

- The third and fourth cranial nerves emerge from the surface of the midbrain, the fifth from the pons, the sixth, seventh and eighth cranial nerves emerge at the junction of the pons and medulla. The ninth, tenth, eleventh and twelfth cranial nerves emerge from the surface of the medulla.

Medulla Oblongata

Lowermost part of the hindbrain.

Extent

Extent from lower border of pons as far as the level of foramen magnum where it is continued as spinal cord.

Shape

- Roughly conical, the upper end being broader than the lower end.
- Situated in posterior cranial fossa below pons.
- Covered by cranial meninges.
- Divided into a lower closed part, where there is a central canal and an upper open part where central canal opens into floor of fourth ventricle.

External Features

- **Anteromedian fissure:** It is a vertical fissure present in the middle of the ventral surface.
- **Posteromedian fissure:** It is a vertical fissure in the middle of the posterior fissure.
- **Anterolateral sulci:** They are the two longitudinal sulci situated one on each side of the anteromedian fissure. Rootlets of the hypoglossal nerve emerge out of the anterolateral sulci of the medulla.
- **Posterolateral sulci:** Present one on each side of the posteromedian sulcus. The rootlets of glossopharyngeal, vagus and the cranial accessory are attached to these grooves in that order from above downwards.
- **There are three regions on each half of the medulla:** Ventral, lateral and dorsal.
    1. *Ventral region:* It is present between the anteromedian fissure and the anterolateral sulcus and is termed as pyramid. It is seen as a pyramidal prominence, which is caused by the underlying pyramidal tract decussation. At the upper end of the pyramid the abducent nerve emerges out. On the superficial surface of the pyramid, arcuate nuclei and the anterior external arcuate fibers are seen.
    2. *Lateral region:* This part is situated between the anterolateral and the posterolateral sulci. In the upper part of this region there is an oval prominence called the olive produced by the underlying inferior olivary nucleus. At its upper end the two roots of the facial nerve are attached.
    3. *Dorsal region:* It is the part situated between the posterolateral sulci and the posteromedian fissure. In the closed part of the medulla this region presents two longitudinal columns separated by a faint groove. The medial column is called the fasciculus gracilis, which is caused by the underlying gracile tract or the tract of Goll. The lateral column called the fasciculus cuneatus is produced by the cuneate tract or tract of Burdach. These tracts end at their upper ends in tubercular elevations in the open part of the medulla called the gracile and the cuneate tubercles respectively. They are caused by the underlying gracile and cuneate nuclei.

- Lateral to the cuneate tubercle, in the open part of the medulla is a thick rounded structure called the inferior cerebellar peduncle, which connects the medulla with the cerebellum.
- The tracts of Goll and Burdach convey position sense, vibratory sense and two-point tactile discrimination. The tract of Goll receives fibers from the lower half of the body while the tract of Burdach receives fibers from the upper half.

Blood Supply

Vertebral, anterior and posterior spinal, posterior inferior cerebellar and basilar arteries.

Applied Anatomy

- **Vascular lesion:** Wallenberg's syndrome: Occlusion of the posterior inferior cerebellar artery involves 10th, 11th (bulbar part) and part of 5th cranial nerves. Nucleus ambiguus, tractus solitarius, spinal tract of V, hypoglossal nucleus, inferior cerebellar peduncle and the reticular formation are also affected.
- This leads to ipsilateral paralysis of pharynx and larynx causing dysphagia and dysarthria.
- Ipsilateral loss of taste on posterior 1/3rd of tongue.
- Ipsilateral Horner's syndrome (miosis, ptosis, enophthalmos, anhidrosis and sympathetic inactivity).
- Ipsilateral loss of pain and temperature on the face.
- Ipsilateral analgesia and ataxia and a tendency to fall on the same side.
- Contralateral dissociated hemianesthesia, where there is loss of pain and temperature but not touch and pressure since the lateral spinothalamic tract only is involved but not the medial lemniscus.
- **Anterior medullary syndrome:** Occurs due to the involvement of the pyramid of the medulla and the emerging 12th nerve roots. There are contralateral hemiplegia and ipsilateral paralysis of the tongue.
- **Arnold-Chiari malformation:** It is a congenital anomaly in which there is a herniation of tonsils of cerebellum and medulla oblongata into vertebral canal through foramen magnum. This causes obstruction to flow of CSF, which leads to internal hydrocephalus.
- Tumors of posterior cranial fossa where there is an increase in intracranial pressure, tend to push tonsils of cerebellum and medulla down through foramen magnum. The 9th, 10th, 11th and 12th cranial nerves are subjected to a stretch which may paralyze them. In such cases, lumbar puncture should not be done as sudden withdrawal of CSF may precipitate further herniation of medulla through foramen magnum, which will cause ischemia, and failure of vital (respiratory and cardiac) functions performed by medulla.

Pons

- Middle part of brainstem situated between midbrain and medulla oblongata.
- Roughly cubical in shape and has 2 surfaces (ventral and dorsal) and 2 borders (superior and inferior).
- **Ventral surface:** Presents a vertical groove in the center for the basilar artery. On each side of the groove is an eminence produced by the pyramidal tract. The middle cerebellar peduncle connects pons and cerebellum. It carries corticopontocerebellar fibers of opposite side. At the line of demarcation between pons and middle cerebellar peduncles, the roots of trigeminal nerve are attached.

- **Dorsal or tegmental part:** Serves to conduct ascending and descending tracts. The following cranial nerve nuclei are situated inside the pons:
  - Abducent nerve nucleus lies deep to facial colliculus on dorsal part of the lower pons.
  - Motor nucleus of facial nerve lies ventrolateral to abducent nerve nucleus.
  - Sensory and motor nucleus of trigeminal nerve.
  - Vestibular and ventral and dorsal cochlear nuclei.

Blood Supply

Multiple perforating pontine branches from the basilar, anterior, inferior and superior cerebellar arteries supply the pons.

Applied Anatomy

- **Foville's syndrome:** Contralateral hemiplegia, loss of sensory modalities in the opposite side with ipsilateral paralysis of the 6th and 7th cranial nerves.
- **Millard-Gubler syndrome:** Results due to lesion in the more ventral part of inferior pons, corticospinal tract and facial nerve fibers are involved.
- **Pontine hemorrhage:** In extensive bilateral hemorrhages the pupils become pinpoint due to involvement of ocular sympathetic fibers, bilateral paralysis of face and limbs.
- **Alternating trigeminal hemiplegia:** Occurs due to lesions of ventral pons involving the corticospinal tract and adjacent 5th nerve fibers. There is contralateral hemiplegia and ipsilateral paralysis of jaw muscles and loss of sensation over the ipsilateral face.
- **Pontocerebellar angle tumor (Acoustic neuroma):** Usually presses lateral part of pons involving the 8th nerve and resulting in tinnitus, progressive deafness and vertigo.

Midbrain

- A part of the brainstem, which connects the forebrain with the hindbrain.
- A short stout stem-like structure lodged in the tentorial notch.
- Consists of two halves called the cerebral peduncles, which are united across the midline in their dorsal parts, but separated by a notch ventrally.
- Each cerebral peduncle consists of crus cerebri ventrally and substantia nigra, a plate of darkly pigmented gray matter in the middle and tegmentum dorsally. The part dorsal to the aqueduct of Sylvius is called the tectum of the midbrain (colliculus).
- Oculomotor and trochlear nerve nuclei are seen at the midbrain.

Blood Supply

Branches of posterior cerebral arteries, posterior communicating arteries, anterior choroidal arteries and superior cerebellar arteries supply the midbrain.

Applied Anatomy

- **Hydrocephalus:** May be due to the result of a blockage of cerebral aqueduct.
- **Weber's syndrome:** Occurs due to a vascular lesion involving the crus cerebri and the third nerve involvement. There is ipsilateral oculomotor nerve paralysis and contralateral hemiplegia.
- **Benedikt's syndrome:** It is similar to Weber's, but the lesion includes the red nucleus and medial lemniscus causing in addition involuntary movements of the limbs of opposite side.
- **Parinaud syndrome:** Usually occurs due to pineal gland tumors pressing on the superior colliculi.

Cerebellum (Fig. 12.6)

- Cerebellum is the largest part of the hindbrain.
- **Functions:** Maintains equilibrium, muscle tone and coordination.
- **Situation:** It is present in the posterior cranial fossa, behind the pons and medulla and in front of the cavity of the fourth ventricle.
- **External features:** It consists of two expanded, laterally placed hemispheres, connected by a narrow worm-like structure called vermis, two surfaces—superior and inferior.
- **Fissures and lobes:** Three fissures—primary, posterolateral and horizontal.
- Primary and posterolateral fissures divide the cerebellum into three lobes. The part anterior to the primary fissure is the anterior lobe. Part in between the primary and posterolateral fissures is the posterior lobe, and the remaining part is the flocculonodular lobe.
- A horizontal fissure divides the cerebellum into upper and lower halves.

Structure

- It has a central core of white matter, arranged in the form of the branching pattern of a tree, known as arbor vitae cerebelli. The peduncles continue in the white matter. The white matter of both sides is connected by a thin lamina of white fibers called the superior and inferior medullary velum. It consists of fibers entering the cerebellum from outside, fibers carried to the cerebellar nuclei, fibers connecting the two cerebellar hemispheres and fibers connecting the cerebellum to other structures in the brain.
- Central white matter is covered by a thin layer of gray matter. This is called cerebellar cortex.
- In each half of the cerebellum, embedded inside the central white matter are masses of gray matter called nuclei of cerebellum. There are 4 pairs of nuclei—dentate, emboliform, globose and fastigial. The dentate nucleus is the largest of all. The nuclei give rise to afferent and efferent fibers from and to the cerebral cortex.

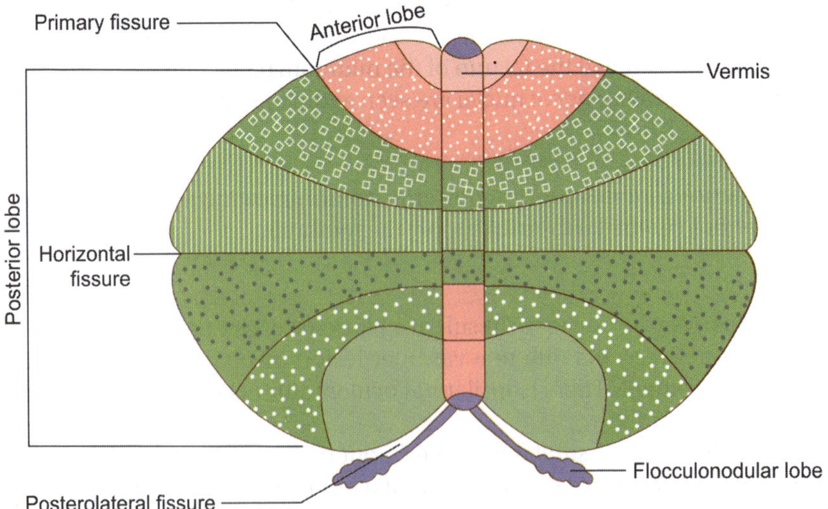

Fig. 12.6: Parts of cerebellum.

Cerebellar Peduncles

The fibers entering and leaving the cerebellum pass through thick bundles called cerebellar peduncles.

There are three pairs of cerebellar peduncles.

1. **Superior cerebellar peduncle:** Connects the cerebellum and the midbrain. It mainly contains fibers from the dentate nucleus.
2. **Middle cerebellar peduncle:** Connects the cerebellum and the pons and contains fibers from the pontine nuclei.
3. **Inferior cerebellar peduncle:** Connects the cerebellum and the medulla oblongata and connects the cerebellum to the spinal cord, thalamus, red nucleus and cranial nerve nulcei.

Histology (Figs. 12.7A and B)

The cerebellar cortex consists of three layers:

1. **Outer molecular layer:** A few scattered cells and rich plexus of nonmyelinated fibers.
2. **Middle Purkinje cell layer:** Single layer of large flask-shaped cells arranged at regular intervals. The dendrites of these cells fan out in the molecular layer. Axons run into the white matter of the cerebellum to reach the dentate nucleus. From the axons collaterals arise which make contact with the adjacent Purkinje cells. Basket cells, their axons run horizontally.
3. **Inner granular layer:** Contains a number of small rounded cells called granule cells, the nuclei occupying the entire cell bodies. The axons of these cells reach molecular layer where they bifurcate and run in a transverse direction.

Blood Supply

Superior cerebellar, anterior inferior cerebellar, posterior inferior cerebellar arteries.

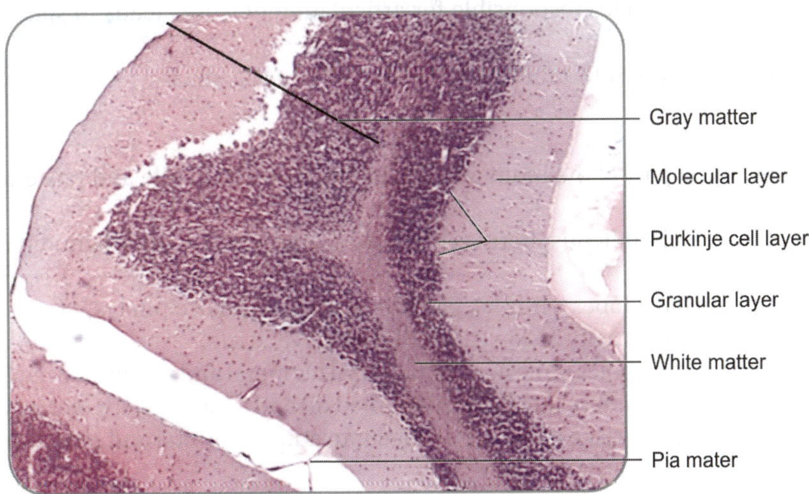

Fig. 12.7A: Photomicrograph of histology of cerebellum.

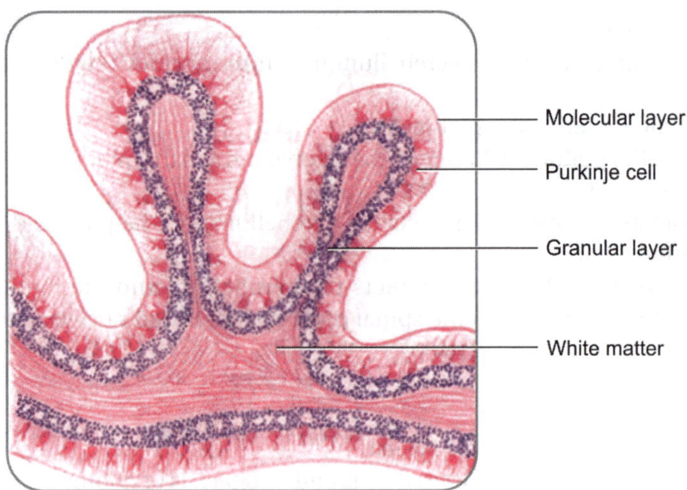

Fig. 12.7B: Diagrammatic representation of histology of cerebellum.

Applied Anatomy

- Any lesion in the cerebellum leads to an inability to maintain the equilibrium of the body while standing or walking. This is called ataxia.
- There is disorder in coordination of activity of different groups of muscles. The person is unable to stand with his feet close together, his body sways from side-to-side and the person may fall. He is not able to walk in a straight line. These findings are more pronounced when the person closes his eyes. This is called Romberg's sign.
- There is difficulty in performing rapid movements involving opposite group of muscles called dysdiadochokinesia.
- Incoordination of muscles responsible for articulation of words leads to speech defects called dysarthria.
- There are repeated jerky movements of eyeballs called nystagmus.

Cerebrum (Fig. 12.8)

- It forms the largest part of the brain and lies in the anterior, middle and posterior cranial fossae.
- Consists of two cerebral hemispheres separated incompletely by the longitudinal cerebral fissure.
- Each hemisphere has 4 lobes—frontal, parietal, temporal and occipital.
- Each hemisphere has a cavity inside called the lateral ventricle.
- Each hemisphere has 3 poles (anterior frontal, basal temporal and posterior occipital) and 3 borders (superomedial, inferolateral and inferomedial) and 3 surfaces (superolateral, medial and inferior). Inferior surface is further divided into anterior orbital and posterior tentorial surface by lateral sulcus.
- The surface of the cerebral cortex presents irregular elevations called the gyri and are separated by linear depressions called the sulci.

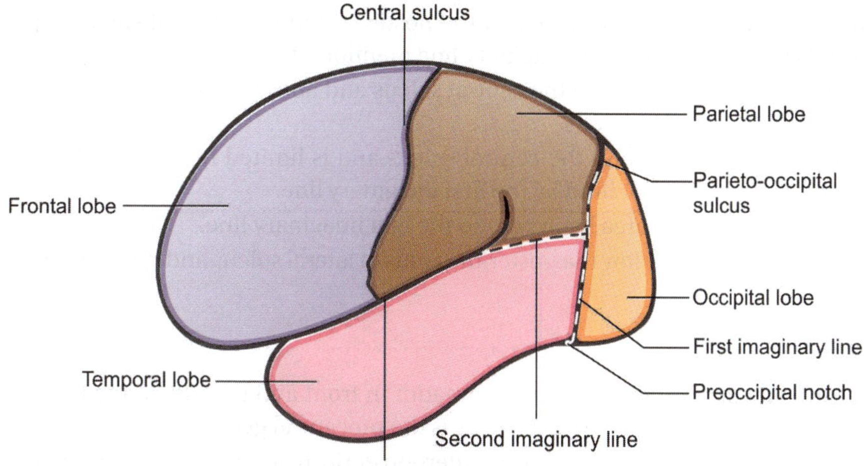

Fig. 12.8: Lobes of cerebrum.

Superolateral Surface (Fig. 12.9)

This is divided into various regions by sulci and gyri.

- **Posterior ramus of the lateral sulcus:** It begins near the temporal pole and runs backwards and slightly upwards.
- **Central sulcus:** It begins on the superomedial margin a little behind the midpoint between the frontal and occipital poles, and runs downwards and forwards to end a little above the posterior ramus of the lateral sulcus.
- Parieto-occipital sulcus from medial surface curves round the superolateral border and ends in the upper part of the superolateral surface.
- An imaginary line connecting parieto-occipital sulcus with preoccipital notch (a notch on inferolateral border 5 cm in front of occipital pole).

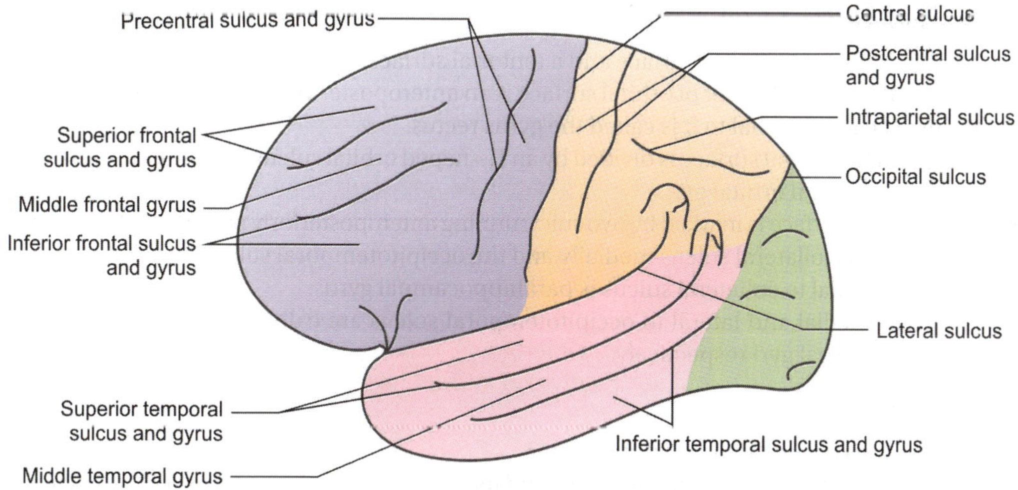

Fig. 12.9: Sulci and gyri on the superolateral surface of cerebral hemisphere.

- Another imaginary line is drawn when the posterior ramus of lateral sulcus is prolonged backwards to meet the vertical imaginary line mentioned.
- The frontal lobe lies anterior to the central sulcus and above the posterior ramus of lateral sulcus.
- The parietal lobe lies behind the central sulcus and is limited from below by the second imaginary line and from behind by the first imaginary line.
- The occipital lobe is the area lying behind the first imaginary line.
- The temporal lobe lies below the posterior ramus of lateral sulcus and the second imaginary line.

Frontal Lobe

- **Precentral sulcus:** Situated one finger breadth in front and parallel to the central sulcus. Between the precentral and central sulcus is the precentral gyrus.
- Superior and inferior frontal sulci run anteroposteriorly in the area in front of precentral sulcus and divided it into three parallel gyri called the superior, middle and inferior frontal gyri.
- Horizontal and vertical rami of lateral sulcus are seen in the lower part.

Temporal Lobe

- Superior and inferior temporal sulci run anteroposteriorly parallel to posterior ramus of lateral sulcus.
- They divide the lobe into superior, middle and inferior temporal gyri.

Parietal Lobe

- Postcentral sulcus is one finger breadth behind and parallel to central sulcus. Between it and central sulcus is postcentral gyrus.
- Intraparietal sulcus runs anteroposteriorly in the area behind postcentral sulcus. This sulcus divides the area into superior and inferior parietal lobules.

Inferior Surface (Fig. 12.10)

- It is divided into an orbital surface and a tentorial surface.
- Close to the medial border of orbital surface is an anteroposterior sulcus called the olfactory sulcus. The area medial to it is called the gyrus rectus.
- The rest of the orbital surface is divided by an H-shaped orbital sulcus into anterior, posterior, medial and lateral orbital gyri.
- The tentorial surface is marked by two sulci running anteroposteriorly parallel to one another.
- These are the collateral sulcus medially and the occipitotemporal sulcus laterally.
- The area medial to collateral sulcus is parahippocampal gyrus.
- The areas medial and lateral to occipitotemporal sulcus are called the medial and lateral occipitotemporal gyri respectively.

Medial Surface (Fig. 12.11)

- It shows the corpus callosum in the center.
- Lying superior to it is the cingulate sulcus and the area between the two is called the cingulate gyrus.

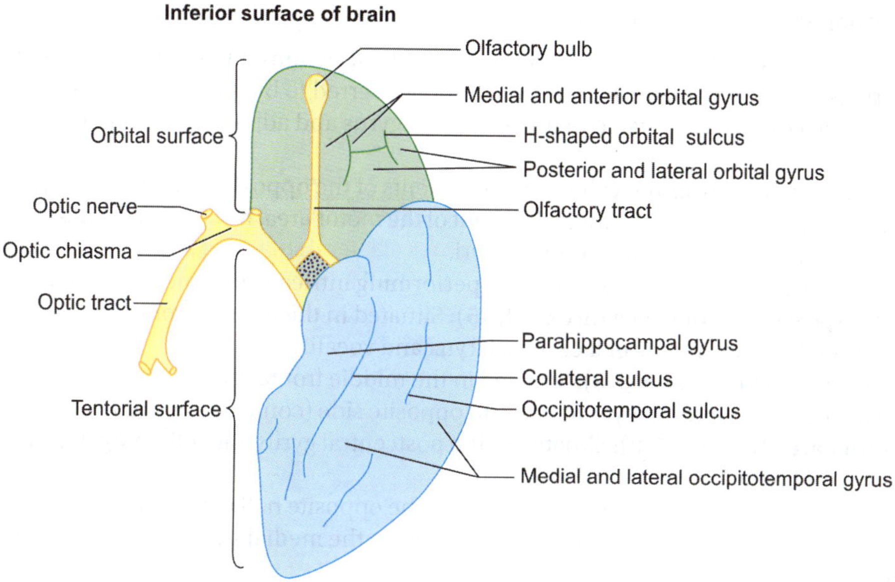

Inferior surface of brain

Olfactory bulb
Medial and anterior orbital gyrus
Orbital surface
H-shaped orbital sulcus
Posterior and lateral orbital gyrus
Optic nerve
Olfactory tract
Optic chiasma
Optic tract
Parahippocampal gyrus
Collateral sulcus
Tentorial surface
Occipitotemporal sulcus
Medial and lateral occipitotemporal gyrus

Fig. 12.10: Inferior surface of cerebrum.

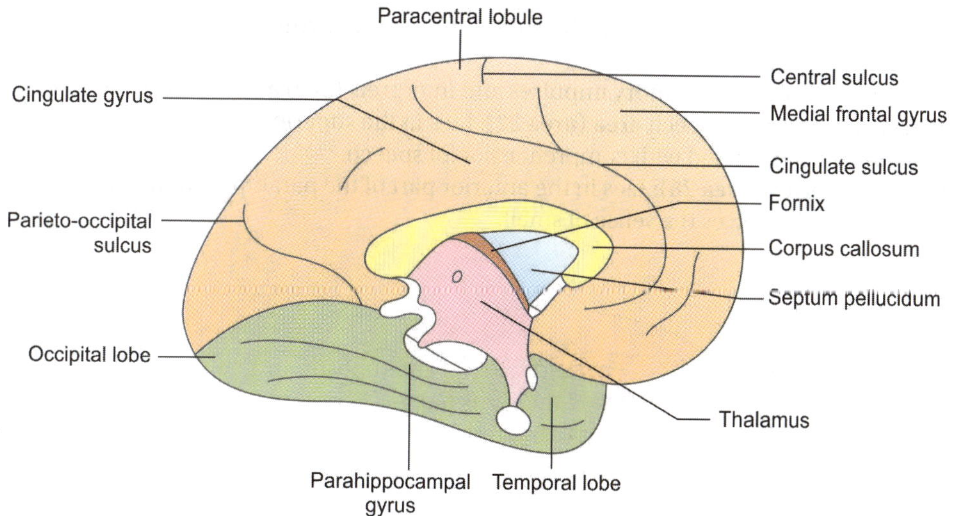

Fig. 12.11: Medial surface of cerebral hemisphere.

- The part of the medial surface of the hemisphere above the cingulate gyrus is divided into two parts.
- The larger anterior portion in front of the central sulcus is called the medial frontal gyrus.
- The smaller posterior portion is called the paracentral lobule.
- The cavity of the cerebral hemisphere is called the lateral ventricle and is situated on the medial surface. It is covered by septum pellucidum.

Functional Areas of the Cortex (Fig. 12.12)

Some areas of cerebral cortex can be assigned specific functions. They correspond to the sulci and gyri discussed previously. They are commonly referred to by Brodmann's numbers.

- **Motor area (areas 4):** Situated in the precentral gyrus and adjoining part of the paracentral lobule.
  - *Function:* It controls the voluntary movements of the opposite half of the body.
- **Premotor area (areas 6, 8):** Situated in front of the motor area. It occupies the posterior parts of superior, middle and inferior frontal gyri.
  - *Function:* This area is responsible for performing intricate and fine movements.
- **Motor speech area of Broca (areas 44, 45):** Situated in the inferior frontal gyrus.
- **Function:** For movements of face, lips, larynx and vocalization.
- **Frontal eye field (areas 6, 8, 9):** Situated in the middle frontal gyrus.
  - *Function:* Causes both eyes to move to opposite side (conjugate eye movements).
- **Sensory area (areas 3, 1, 2):** Situated in the postcentral gyrus and adjoining portions of the paracentral lobule.
  - *Function:* It controls the sensory supply of the opposite half of the body.
- **Visual area (area 17):** Seen in the occipital lobe on the medial surface above and below the calcarine sulcus.
  - *Function:* Receives visual sensations.
- **Psychovisual area (areas 18, 19):** Seen above and below the visual area.
  - *Function:* Interpretation of visual impulses.
- **Auditory area (area 41):** Lies in the superior temporal gyrus along the floor of posterior ramus of lateral sulcus.
  - *Function:* Receives auditory impulses and interprets them as sound.
- **Wernicke's sensory speech area (area 22):** Lies in the superior temporal gyrus.
  - *Function:* Associated with comprehension of speech.
- **Olfactory cortex (area 28):** Lies in the anterior part of the parahippocampal gyrus.
  - *Function:* Perceives the sense of smell.

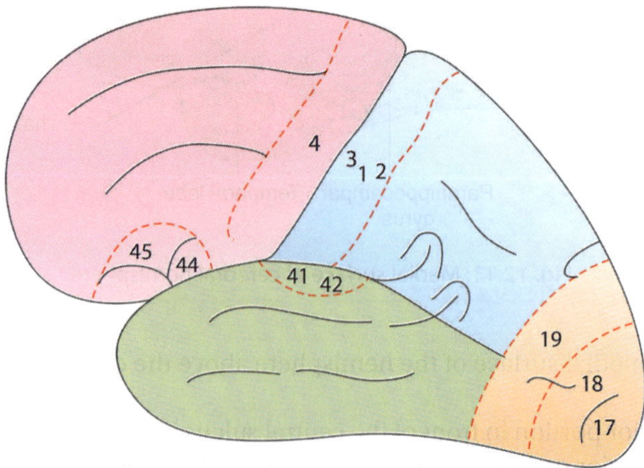

Fig. 12.12: Functional areas of the brain.

White Matter of the Cerebrum

Deep to the cerebral cortex is white matter of cerebrum. It is made up of mainly three types of fibers:

- Association fibers are fibers that interconnect different regions of the cerebral cortex.
- Projection fibers connect cerebral cortex to centers in the brainstem and spinal cord and vice-versa. The fibers coming to the cortex are called corticopetal fibers and the fibers going away from it are called corticofugal fibers.
- Commissural fibers interconnect identical areas of the two cerebral hemispheres.

Corpus Callosum (Fig. 12.13)

It is the commissural white fiber which connects both sides of the cerebrum.

- Parts from anterior to posterior aspect are rostrum, genu, body and splenium.
- The fibers of the genu connect the two frontal lobes and form a fork-like structure called forceps minor.
- Splenium connects the occipital lobes and forms fibers called forceps major.
- Some fibers of body and splenium form a flattened band called tapetum.

Internal Capsule (Fig. 12.14)

Internal capsule is a large collection of projection fibers that lies between the caudate nucleus and thalamus medially and the lentiform nucleus laterally. Above it is continuous with the corona radiata and below with the crus cerebri of midbrain. It is divided into five parts.

1. The anterior limb lies between the caudate nucleus medially and the anterior part of lentiform nucleus laterally. It contains fibers from the thalamus to frontal lobe of the cerebral cortex. It carries the frontopontine fibers to pontine nuclei from frontal lobe.
2. The posterior limb lies between the thalamus medially and the posterior part of lentiform nucleus laterally. It contains sensory fibers from the thalamus to the postcentral gyrus. It also carries corticospinal fibers from the cortex to the head, neck, upper limb, thorax and lower limb.
3. Genu is the bend where the anterior and posterior limbs meet. It carries the corticonuclear fibers to the cranial nerve nuclei.
4. The retrolentiform part lies behind the lentiform nucleus. It carries visual fibers from the thalamus to occipital lobe. It also has occipitopontine and parietopontine fibers.

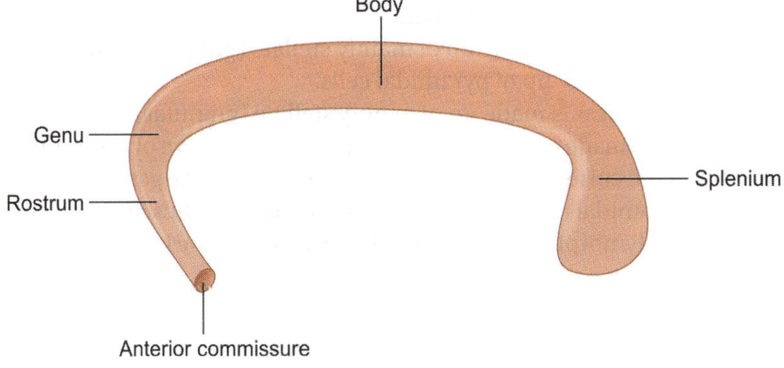

Fig. 12.13: Parts of corpus callosum.

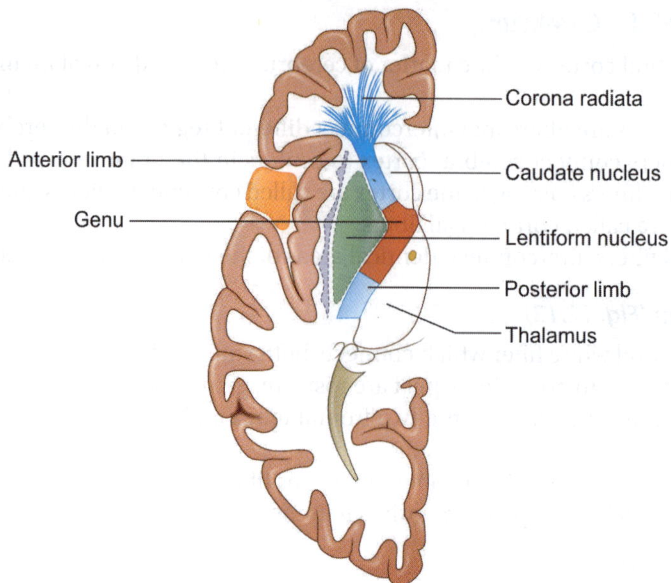

Fig. 12.14: Internal capsule and basal ganglia.

5. The sublentiform part lies below the lentiform nucleus. It carries acoustic fibers from the thalamus to the temporal lobe. It also carries the temporopontine fibers.

Basal Ganglia (Fig. 12.14)

They are masses of gray matter situated within the cerebral hemispheres.

- They consist of corpus striatum, claustrum, amygdaloid body. Corpus striatum consists of caudate and lentiform nuclei.
- **Functions:** It receives information from the cerebral cortex, thalamus and brainstem. It controls the muscle tone and helps to regulate and smoothens the voluntary motor activities of the body. It also controls group movements and expressions.

Histology of Cerebrum (Figs. 12.15A and B)

Cerebral cortex has six layers from superficial surface downwards:

1. Molecular layer is made up of mainly fibers.
2. The external granular layer is made up of mainly stellate (granular) cells.
3. The pyramidal layer is made up of pyramidal cells.
4. The internal granular layer is made up of mainly stellate (granular) cells.
5. The ganglionic layer is made up of mainly pyramidal cells. The size of pyramidal cells increase as we go deeper in the cortex and the largest cells are seen in the ganglionic layer. These are called the Giant Pyramidal cells of Betz. These are characteristics of motor cortex.
6. The multiform or polymorphous layer is made up of cells of various shapes and sizes.

Blood Supply of Cerebrum (Figs. 12.16A to C)

Superolateral Surface (Fig. 12.16A)

- Middle cerebral artery—majority of superolateral surface.

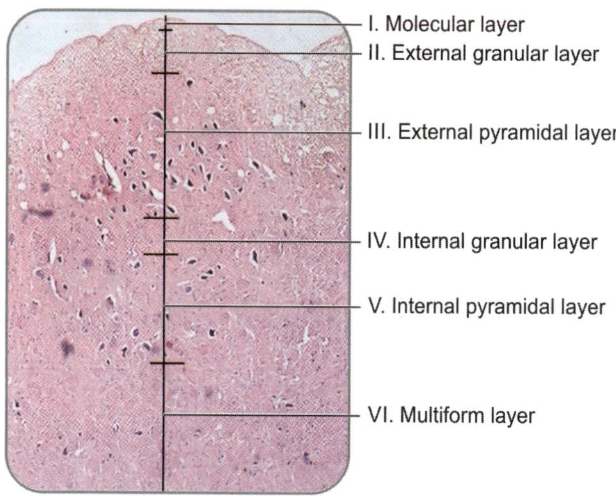

Fig. 12.15A: Photomicrograph of histology of cerebrum.

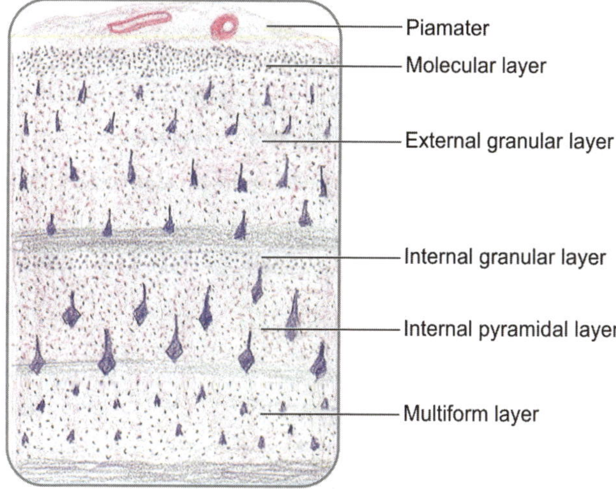

Fig. 12.15B: Diagrammatic representation of histology of cerebrum.

- Anterior cerebral artery—one inch wide, along the superomedial surface.
- Posterior cerebral artery—areas belonging to the occipital lobe, inferior temporal gyrus.

Medial Surface (Fig. 12.16B)

- Anterior cerebral artery—supplies majority of medial surface.
- Posterior cerebral artery—supplies the occipital surface.
- Middle cerebral artery—a small area of the temporal surface.

Inferior Surface (Fig. 12.16C)

- Posterior cerebral artery—majority of inferior surface (tentorial surface).
- Middle cerebral artery—lateral part of orbital surface.
- Anterior cerebral artery—medial part of orbital surface.

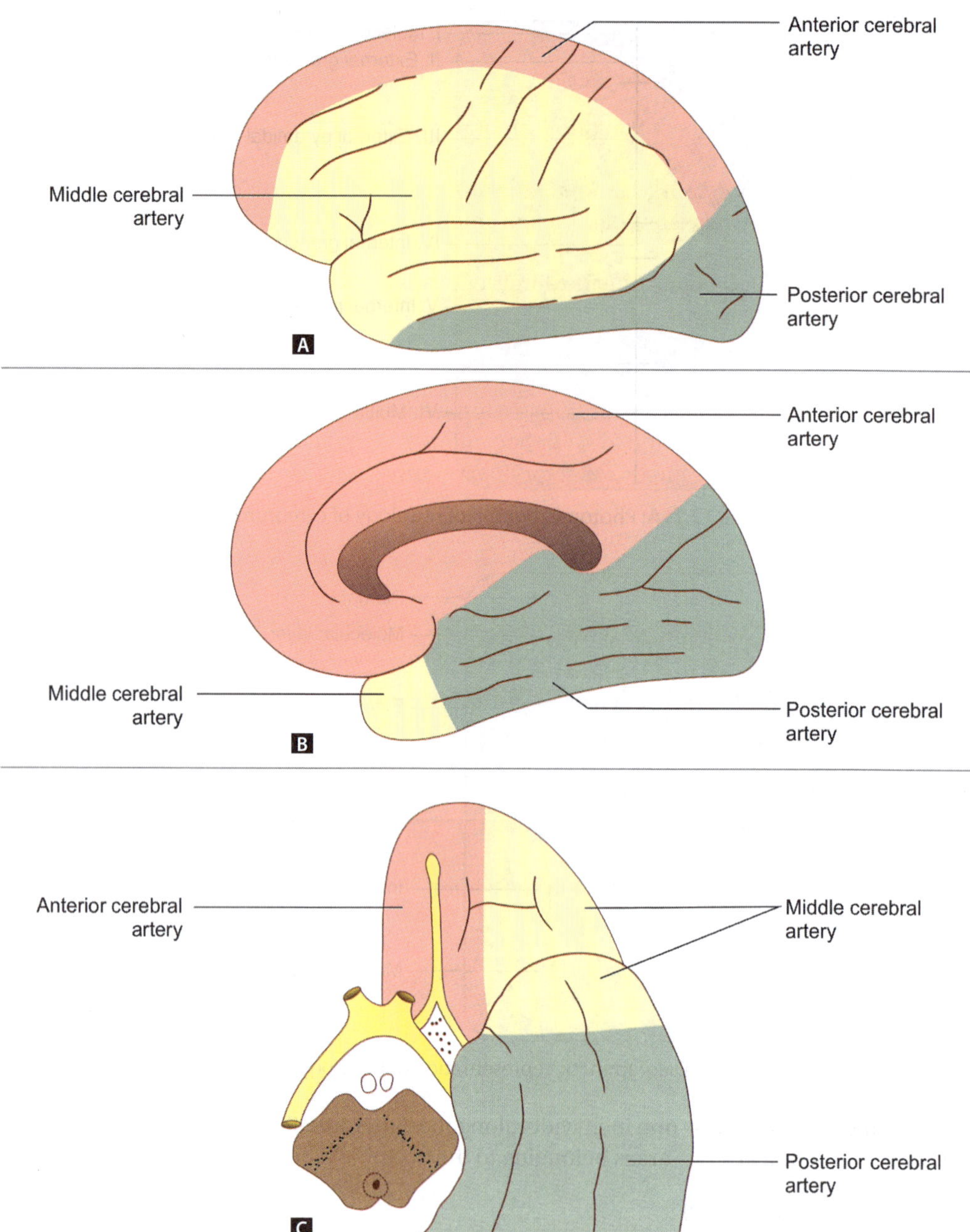

Figs. 12.16A to C: Blood supply of the cerebral hemispheres: (A) Superolateral surface; (B) Medial surface; (C) Inferior surface.

Venous Drainage

Veins of the Cerebrum

- Superficial veins—superior and inferior cerebral veins, superficial and deep middle cerebral vein.
- Deep veins—internal cerebral (union of thalamostriate and choroidal vein), great cerebral (union of 2 great cerebral veins), basal veins (union of anterior cerebral, deep middle cerebral and striate veins).
- Veins draining the brain open into the dural venous sinuses which finally drain into internal jugular vein.

The Limbic System

Includes—cingulate gyrus, piriform area, parahippocampal gyrus, medial and lateral olfactory gyri, gyrus ambiens, gyrus semilunaris, hippocampus with dentate gyrus, indusium griseum, amygdaloid nucleus, septal nuclei, olfactory nerve, tract, roots, fornix, stria terminalis, and anterior commissure.

Function: Concerned with basic emotions—fear, anger, etc.

VENTRICLES (FIG. 12.17)

- Interior of the brain is made up of cavities called the ventricles.
- Each hemisphere has a lateral ventricle.
- Cerebrum contains a median cavity called third ventricle.
- Each lateral ventricle opens into the third ventricle through an interventricular foramen.
- Third ventricle is continuous caudally with the cavity of the midbrain called the cerebral aqueduct.
- The cavity of the pons and medulla is called the fourth ventricle. Cerebral aqueduct opens into fourth ventricle.
- The fourth ventricle is continuous with the central canal of the spinal cord.

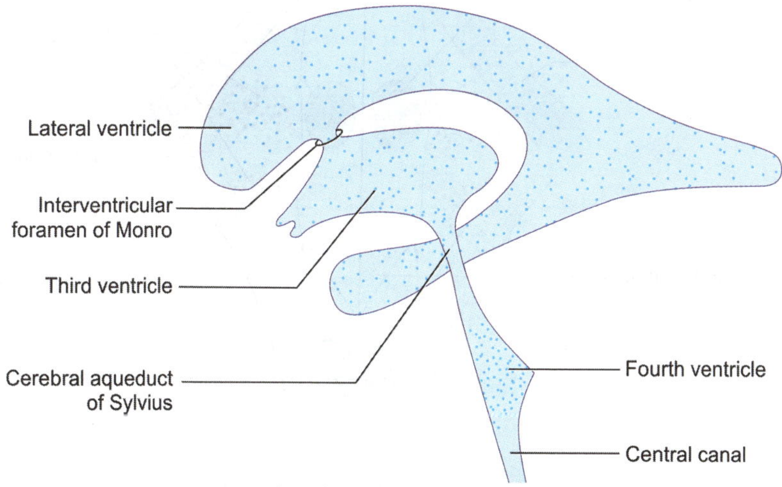

Fig. 12.17: Ventricles of brain.

- The whole of the ventricular system is lined by an epithelial layer of ciliated cuboidal epithelium called the ependyma.
- The ventricles are bathed by the cerebrospinal fluid (CSF).

Lateral Ventricles

- One lateral ventricle is situated in each cerebral hemisphere.
- It has a central part which gives three extensions, anterior, posterior and the inferior horns.
- The anterior horn lies in the frontal lobe, posterior in the occipital lobe and the inferior in the temporal lobe of cerebral hemisphere.

Third Ventricle

- It is the cavity of the diencephalon.
- It has a roof, a floor, anterior, posterior and lateral walls.

Fourth Ventricle (Fig. 12.18)

- It has a roof and a floor.
- The floor is rhomboid shaped and has two parts.
- The upper triangular part is formed by the posterior surface of pons. It has a swelling called the facial colliculus. This is formed by the abducent nucleus and the fibers of facial nerve curving around it.
- The lower triangular part is formed by the upper part of medulla. It has the vagal and the hypoglossal triangles that have the nuclei of the vagus and hypoglossal nerves.
- Both the upper and the lower parts show impression of the vestibular nuclei.

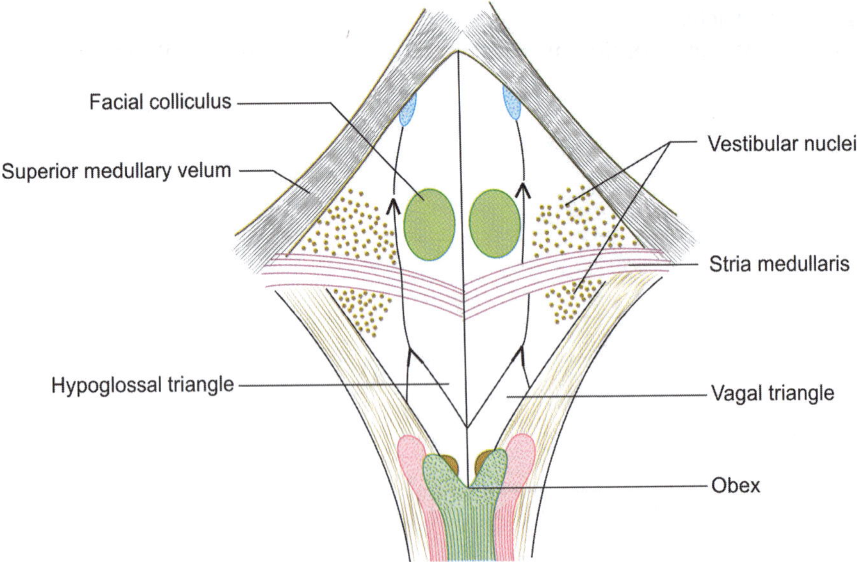

Fig. 12.18: Floor of the fourth ventricle.

Applied Anatomy

The ventricles of the brain can be studied by taking radiographs after injecting a radio-opaque dye into the ventricular system. This procedure is called ventriculography.

CEREBROSPINAL FLUID

- CSF fills the subarachnoid space.
- It also extends into ventricles of brain and central canal of spinal cord.
- It is formed by choroid plexuses of the ventricles.
- It provides a fluid cushion which protects brain from injury. It also helps to carry nutrition to brain and remove waste products.
- Total volume of CSF is 140 mL, out of which 25 mL is in the ventricles.
- Consists of 99% water and contains sodium, chloride, potassium, bicarbonate, glucose and proteins.
- Epithelium of choroid plexus forms an effective barrier between blood and CSF. This blood-CSF barrier allows only selective passage of substances from blood to CSF and vice versa.

Applied Anatomy

An abnormal increase in quantity of CSF can lead to enlargement of head in children—hydrocephalus.

Blood-Brain Barrier

- Some substances can pass from blood to brain while others cannot. This is called the blood-brain barrier.
- Anatomically the structures that form the barrier are capillary endothelium, basement membrane of endothelium and processes of astrocytes.
- Some areas of the brain are devoid of this barrier. These are the pineal body, hypophysis cerebri, choroid plexus and some specialized areas of walls of third and fourth ventricles.

CRANIAL NERVES (FIG. 12.19)

Olfactory Nerve

- **Location:** Arises in olfactory mucosa, passes through olfactory foramina in the cribriform plate of ethmoid bone, and ends in olfactory bulb. The olfactory tract extends via two pathways to olfactory areas in the temporal lobe of cerebral cortex.
- **Function:** Smell
- **Clinical application:** Loss of sense of smell, called anosmia, may result from head injuries in which cribriform plate of ethmoid bone is fractured and forms lesions along olfactory pathway.

Optic Nerve

- **Location:** Arises in retina of eye, passes through optic foramen, forms optic chiasma, passes through optic tracts, and terminates in lateral geniculate nuclei of thalamus. From thalamus, projections extend to visual areas in the occipital lobe of cerebral cortex.
- **Function:** Vision

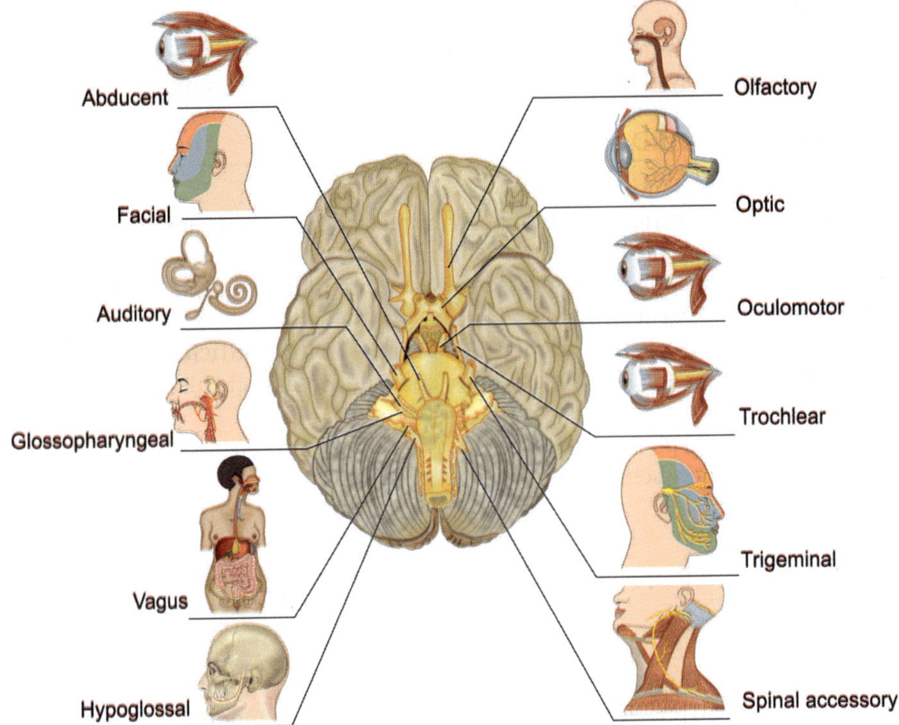

Fig. 12.19: Cranial nerves.

- **Clinical application:** Fractures in orbit, lesions along visual pathway and diseases of nervous system may result in visual field defects and loss of visual acuity. Loss of vision is called anopsia.

Oculomotor Nerve

- **Location**
  - *Motor portion:* Originates in midbrain, passes through superior orbital fissure, and is distributed to levator palpebrae superioris of upper eyelid and four extrinsic eyeball muscles (superior, medial and inferior rectus, inferior oblique); parasympathetic innervation to ciliary muscle of eyeball and sphincter muscle of iris.
  - *Sensory portion:* Consists of fibers from proprioceptors in eyeball muscles that pass through superior orbital fissure and terminate in midbrain.
- **Function**
  - *Motor function:* Movement of eyelid and eyeball, accommodation of lens for near vision, and constriction of pupil.
  - *Sensory function:* Muscle sense (proprioception).
- **Clinical application:** A lesion in the nerve causes strabismus (a deviation of the eye in which both eyes do not fix on the same object), ptosis (drooping) of upper eyelid, pupil dilation, the movement of the eyeball downward and outward on the damaged side, a loss of accommodation for near vision, and diplopia (double vision).

Trochlear Nerve

- **Location**
  - *Motor portion:* Originates in midbrain, passes through superior orbital fissure, and is distributed to superior oblique muscle, an extrinsic eyeball muscle.
  - *Sensory portion:* Consists of fibers from proprioceptors in superior oblique muscles that pass through superior orbital fissure and terminate in midbrain.
- **Function**
  - *Motor function:* Movement of eyeball.
  - *Sensory function:* Muscle sense (proprioception).
- **Clinical application:** In trochlear nerve paralysis, diplopia and strabismus occur.

Trigeminal Nerve

- **Location**
  - It has both motor and sensory function.
  - The sensory part supplies the face and consists of three branches: Ophthalmic, which supplies the upper eyelid. It reaches the face by passing through the superior orbital fissure. It also supplies the scalp up to the vertex, forehead, conjunctiva and the root, tip and the dorsum of the nose. This is done by its branches namely the supraorbital, supratrochlear, lacrimal and infranasal nerves. Maxillary supplies the upper lip, side and ala of nose, the lower eyelid, upper part of cheek and anterior part of temple and reaches the face by passing through the foramen rotundum. Its branches are the infraorbital, zygomaticofacial and zygomaticotemporal. Mandibular supplies the lower lip, chin, lower part of the face, lower jaw except near the angle of mandible and the upper 2/3rds of the lateral part of the auricle. The three branches emerge from the trigeminal ganglion that lies in the trigeminal cave on the apex of the petrous temporal bone.
  - Apart from the face, trigeminal nerve also supplies the nasal cavity, the paranasal air sinuses, eyeball, mouth cavity and the dura mater over the anterior and middle cranial fossae. Sensory portion also consists of fibers from proprioceptors in muscles of mastication.
  - *Motor portion:* Is part of mandibular branch; originates in pons, passes through foramen ovale, and ends in muscles of mastication, anterior belly of digastric and mylohyoid muscles.
- **Function**
  - *Motor function*: Chewing.
  - *Sensory function:* Conveys sensations for touch, pain and temperature from structures supplied; muscle sense (proprioception).
- **Clinical application:** Injury results in paralysis of muscles of mastication and a loss of sensation of touch and temperature. Neuralgia (pain) of one or more branches of trigeminal nerve is called trigeminal neuralgia (tic douloureux).

Abducent Nerve

- **Location**
  - *Motor portion:* Originates from pons, passes through superior orbital fissure, and is distributed to lateral rectus muscle, an extrinsic eyeball muscle.

   - *Sensory portion:* Consists of fibers from proprioceptors in lateral rectus muscle that pass through superior orbital fissure and end in pons.
- **Function**
   - *Motor function:* Movement of eyeball.
   - *Sensory function:* Muscle sense (proprioception).
- **Clinical application:** With damage to this nerve, the affected eyeball cannot move laterally beyond the midpoint and the eye is usually directed medially.

Facial Nerve

This has both sensory and motor function. The nerve is attached to the hindbrain by a motor and a sensory root. The sensory root is also called the nervus intermedius.

- **Location**
   - The two roots emerge from the pons and enter the internal acoustic meatus. They then fuse to form a single trunk and lie in a facial canal in the petrous temporal bone. It leaves the skull by passing out through the stylomastoid foramen. The nerve then enters the posterior aspect of the parotid gland and divides into its five terminal branches at the anterior border of the gland.
   - In the facial canal, the nerve gives the greater petrosal nerve that supplies the lacrimal gland, the nerve to stapedius that supplies the stapedius muscle of the ear and the chorda tympani that carries taste fibers from the anterior 2/3rds of the tongue.
   - As it comes out through the stylomastoid foramen, it gives the posterior auricular nerve that supplies the muscles of the pinna, digastric nerve that supplies the posterior belly of digastric and the stylohyoid that supplies the stylohyoid muscle.
   - The five terminal branches are the temporal, zygomatic, buccal, marginal mandibular and the cervical branch. They supply the muscles of facial expression.
   - *Motor portion:* Originates in pons, passes through stylomastoid foramen, and is distributed to facial, scalp, and neck muscles; parasympathetic fibers are distributed to lacrimal, sublingual, submandibular, nasal and palatine glands.
   - *Sensory portion:* Arises from taste buds on anterior 2/3rds of tongue, passes through stylomastoid foramen, and ends in geniculate ganglion, a nucleus in pons that sends fibers to thalamus for relay to gustatory areas in parietal lobe of cerebral cortex. Also contains fibers from proprioceptors in muscles of face and scalp.
- **Function**
   - *Motor function:* Facial expression and secretion of saliva and tears.
   - *Sensory function:* Muscle sense (proprioception) and taste. Ganglia associated with the facial nerve are:
      - Geniculate ganglion: That carries sensations of taste from the anterior 2/3rds of the tongue.
      - Submandibular ganglion: That carries secretomotor fibers from the submandibular and sublingual glands.
      - Pterygopalatine ganglion: That carries secretomotor fibers from the lacrimal gland.
- **Clinical application:** Injury produces paralysis of facial muscles, called Bell's palsy, loss of taste, and loss of ability to close the eyes, even during sleep.

Vestibulocochlear Nerve

- **Location**
  - *Cochlear branch:* Arises in spiral organ (organ of Corti), forms spiral ganglion, passes through internal auditory meatus, nuclei in the medulla, and ends in thalamus. Fibers synapse with neurons that relay impulses to auditory areas in temporal lobe of cerebral cortex.
  - *Vestibular branch:* Arises in semicircular canals, saccule, and utricle and forms vestibular ganglion; fibers end in pons and cerebellum.
- **Function**
  - *Cochlear branch function*: Conveys impulses associated with hearing.
  - *Vestibular branch function*: Conveys impulses associated with equilibrium.
- **Clinical application:** Injury to cochlear branch may cause tinnitus (ringing) or deafness. Injury to vestibular branch may cause vertigo (a subjective feeling of rotation), ataxia, and nystagmus (involuntary rapid movement of eyeballs).

Glossopharyngeal Nerve

- **Location**
  - The nerve has both sensory and motor functions. It arises as 3–4 rootlets in the medulla that unite to form a single trunk. This then passes through the jugular foramen and passing deep to the styloid process enters the submandibular region where it ends.
  - *Motor portion:* This is the muscular branch that originates in medulla, passes through jugular foramen, and is distributed to stylopharyngeus muscle.
  - *Sensory portion:* Tympanic nerve that forms the tympanic plexus and supplies the middle ear, auditory tube and mastoid air cells. A carotid branch supplies the carotid sinus and carotid body. Lingual branches carry taste and general sensations from posterior 1/3rd of tongue. Pharyngeal branches supply the pharynx and tonsillar branches to the tonsil.
- **Function**
  - *Motor function*: Secretion of saliva.
  - *Sensory function:* Taste, regulation of blood pressure, and muscle sense (proprioception).
- **Clinical application:** Injury results in difficulty during swallowing, reduced secretion of saliva, loss of sensation in the throat, and loss of taste.

Vagus Nerve

This is a mixed nerve. It arises from the medulla and reaches the jugular foramen. Then it leaves the skull and lies on the posterior aspect of carotid sheath. It then enters the thorax and after supplying structures there it passes through the vena caval opening of the diaphragm to end in the abdomen.

- **Location**
  - *Motor portion:* Originates in medulla, passes through jugular foramen, and terminates in muscles of airways, lungs, esophagus, heart, stomach, small intestine, most of large intestine, and gallbladder; parasympathetic fibers innervate involuntary muscles and glands of GIT. The superior and the recurrent laryngeal nerves supply the muscles of the larynx and pharynx.
  - *Sensory portion:* In the jugular foramen it gives the meningeal branch that supplies the posterior cranial fossa and the auricular branch that supplies the skin over the auricle, the external acoustic meatus and the tympanic membrane. The carotid branches supply

the carotid body and the cardiac branches take part in the formation of superficial and deep cardiac plexuses. It gives the parasympathetic supply to all the organs of the abdomen and pelvis.

- **Function**
  - *Motor function:* Smooth muscle contraction and relaxation; secretion of digestive fluids.
  - *Sensory function:* Sensations form visceral organs supplied; muscle sense (proprioception).
- **Clinical application:** Severing of both nerves in the upper body interferes with swallowing, paralyzes vocal cords, and interrupts sensations from many organs.

Accessory Nerve

- **Location**
  - *Motor portion:* Consists of a cranial portion and a spinal portion. Cranial portion originates from medulla, passes through jugular foramen, and supplies voluntary muscles of pharynx, larynx, and soft palate. Spinal portion originates from anterior gray horn of first five cervical segments of spinal cord, passes through jugular foramen, and supplies sternocleidomastoid and trapezius muscles.
  - *Sensory portion:* Consists of fibers from proprioceptors in muscles supplied by motor portion and passes through jugular foramen.
- **Function**
  - *Motor function:* Cranial portion mediates swallowing movements; spinal portion mediates movement of head.
  - *Sensory function:* Muscle sense (proprioception).
- **Clinical application:** If nerves are damaged, the sternocleidomastoid and trapezius muscles become paralyzed, resulting in inability to raise the shoulders and difficulty in turning the head.

Hypoglossal Nerve

- **Location**
  - *Motor portion:* Originates in medulla, passes through hypoglossal canal, and supplies muscles of tongue.
  - *Sensory portion:* Consists of fibers from proprioceptors in tongue muscles that pass through hypoglossal canal and end in medulla.
- **Function**
  - *Motor function*: Movement of tongue during speech and swallowing.
  - *Sensory function*: Muscle sense (proprioception).
- **Clinical application:** Injury results in difficulty in chewing, speaking, and swallowing. The tongue, when protruded, curls towards the affected side and the affected side becomes atrophied, shrunken, and deeply furrowed.

CRANIAL NERVE NUCLEI (FIG. 12.20)

Somatic Efferent Column

This column is situated close to the midline and comprises the following nuclear masses:

- Oculomotor nucleus in the midbrain in the gray matter ventral to the aqueduct of Sylvius at the level of the superior colliculus. The axons from the cells of the nucleus emerge out through the third cranial nerve to supply the striped muscles (superior rectus, medial rectus, inferior

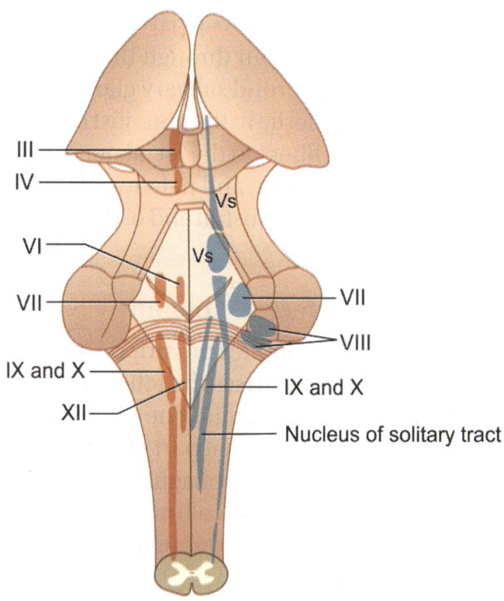

Fig. 12.20: Cranial nerve nuclei.

rectus, inferior oblique muscles of the eyeball and levator palpebrae superioris) which are developed from the first head somite.

- Nucleus of the trochlear nerve situated in the midbrain, in the gray matter ventral to the aqueduct of Sylvius at the level of the inferior colliculus. The axons from the cells of the nucleus emerge out through the trochlear nerve to supply the striped muscle (superior oblique muscle of the eyeball) which is developed from the second head somite.
- Nucleus of the abducent nerve situated in the dorsal part of the lower pons under the facial colliculus. The axons from the cells of this nucleus emerge out through the abducent nerve to supply the lateral rectus muscle of the eyeball, which is developed from the third head somite.
- Nucleus of the hypoglossal nerve situated in the dorsal part of the medulla under the hypoglossal triangle in the floor of the fourth ventricle. The nucleus extends caudally into the closed part of the medulla. The axons from the cells of the nucleus emerge out through the hypoglossal nerve to supply the muscles of the tongue which are developed from the last four head somites.

General Visceral Efferent Column

This column is situated just lateral to the somatic efferent column in the brainstem. The general visceral efferent component consists of two neuron chains. The preganglionic fibers are long and the postganglionic fibers are short. The intermediate ganglia are situated near the organs of supply. These fibers are parasympathetic and supply motor fibers to the smooth muscles or secretomotor fibers to glands. The general visceral efferent column comprises of the following nuclear masses:

- Dorsal nucleus of vagus is situated in the dorsal part of the upper medulla under the vagal triangle of the floor of the fourth ventricle just lateral to the nucleus of the hypoglossal nerve. The fibers are distributed through the vagus and the cranial accessory.

- Inferior salivatory nucleus is situated in the dorsal part of the upper medulla cephalic to the dorsal nucleus of vagus. Its fibers emerge out through the glossopharyngeal nerve and are concerned with the innervation of the parotid salivary gland.
- Superior salivatory and lacrimatory nuclei lie in the pons just cephalic to the inferior salivatory nucleus and contribute secretomotor fibers to the facial nerve to supply the sublingual and submaxillary salivary glands, lacrimal, nasal and palatine glands.
- Edinger-Westphal nucleus lies dorsal to the rostral end of the oculomotor nucleus. It supplies sphincter pupillae and ciliaris muscle.

Special Visceral Efferent (Branchial Efferent) Column

This consists of a single neuron chain and supplies the striped muscles which develop from the branchial arch mesoderm. This column comprises the following nuclear masses:

- **Nucleus ambiguus:** It is situated in the medulla. The fibers emerge out of the cells of this nucleus to pass into the 9th, 10th and the cranial part of the 11th nerves to be distributed to the muscles of the pharynx, larynx and the esophagus.
- Motor nucleus of the facial nerve occupies this column at the level of the lower border of the pons. The fibers emerging out of this nucleus through the facial nerve supply the muscles developed from the second arch mesoderm.
- Motor nucleus of the trigeminal nerve lies in the middle pons cephalic to the motor nucleus of the facial nerve. The emerging fibers of the nucleus are distributed to the muscles developed from the first arch mesoderm, namely, muscles of mastication, anterior belly of digastric, mylohyoid, tensor tympani and tensor palatini through the mandibular division of the trigeminal nerve.

General Visceral Afferent Column

This consists of a long column of nucleus solitarius lying in the tractus solitarius and extending throughout the length of the medulla and lower pons. The fibers enter the brainstem through the 7th, 9th and 10th cranial nerves and their cell bodies are situated in the sensory ganglia of those cranial nerves. The fibers on reaching the tractus solitarius run downwards for a short distance in the tract before ending in relation to nucleus of the tract. Fresh fibers arise from the nucleus, cross over to the opposite side and ascend as the ventral secondary ascending visceral tract (solitario-hypothalamic tract). This tract joins the medial lemniscus and conveys general visceral sensations.

Special Visceral Afferent Column

This column consists of three separate collections of cells (dorsal, visceral, gray) situated in close relation to tractus solitarius at three different levels. The taste fibers enter the brainstem through the 7th, 9th and 10th cranial nerves and their cell bodies are situated in the sensory ganglia of those nerves. The fibers on reaching the tractus solitarius directly end in relation to the cells of the dorsal visceral gray. Fresh fibers arise from these nuclei, cross over to the opposite side and form ventral secondary ascending gustatory tract (solitariothalamic tract). The tract soon joins the medial lemniscus.

General Somatic Afferent Column

This column of nuclei receives fibers concerned with the pain, temperature and general touch from the head and neck region. These fibers reach the brainstem through 5th, 7th, 9th and 10th nerves, and their cell bodies are situated in the ganglia of those nerves. This column comprises the following nuclear masses:

- Chief sensory nucleus of trigeminal nerve in pons. It receives fibers of general touch from the trigeminal area.
- Nucleus of spinal tract of trigeminal nerve which is caudal to the chief sensory nucleus descending through lateral part of pons and medulla oblongata. It is continuous caudally with substantia gelatinosa of the cervical portion of the cord. It receives pain and temperature fibers. The pain fibers lie lateral to temperature fibers in the tract. Fibers from the ophthalmic nerve occupy a ventral position, mandibular nerve fibers lie dorsally and dorsomedially while maxillary fibers lie in the middle of the tract. The fibers originating from the skin near the mouth end in the upper part of the nucleus. Fibers arising from the outer skin areas end in the lower part of the nucleus in an order. Secondary fibers arising from these sensory nuclei cross to the opposite side and collect as a bundle called trigeminal lemniscus which proceeds up, to end in the thalamus and thence into the cortex by further relays.
- Cranial to the chief sensory nucleus of trigeminal nerve in the pons and extending into midbrain are the mesencephalic root of trigeminal nerve and its nucleus. This is made of unipolar cells similar to those of the posterior root ganglion of the spinal nerves. They are said to develop from the neural crest cells but get incorporated within the substance of the neural tube. The mesencephalic tract is the axonal processes of the cells of the nucleus. It is proprioceptive in function and receives impulses from stretch receptors in the muscles of mastication and pressure receptors related to teeth and hard palate. Characteristics of somatic and parasomatic divisions are as following **(Table 12.3)**.

Table 12.3: Characteristics of somatic and parasomatic divisions.

Somatic division	*Parasomatic division*
Forms thoracolumbar outflow.	Forms craniosacral outflow.
Contains sympathetic trunk and prevertebral ganglia.	Contains terminal ganglia.
Ganglia are close to CNS and distant from visceral effectors.	Ganglia are near or within the wall of visceral effectors.
Each preganglionic fiber is short and synapses with many postganglionic neurons that pass to many visceral effectors.	Each preganglionic fiber is long and usually synapses with four or five postganglionic neurons that pass to a single visceral effector.
Distributed throughout the body, including skin, sweat glands, arrector pili muscles attached to hair follicles, adipose tissue, and smooth muscle of blood vessels.	Distribution limited primarily to head and viscera of thorax, abdomen and pelvis. No innervation of sweat glands, arrector pili muscles, adipose tissue, kidneys, and most blood vessels.

Special Somatic Afferent Column

This column comprises cochlear nuclei in the pons receiving the exteroceptive impulses and vestibular nuclei in the pons and medulla receiving proprioceptive impulses.

AUTONOMIC NERVOUS SYSTEM (FIG. 12.21)

Two divisions: Sympathetic and parasympathetic.

The first of the autonomic motor neurons is called preganglionic neuron. Its cell body is in the brain or spinal cord. Its myelinated axon, called preganglionic fiber, passes out of CNS as part of

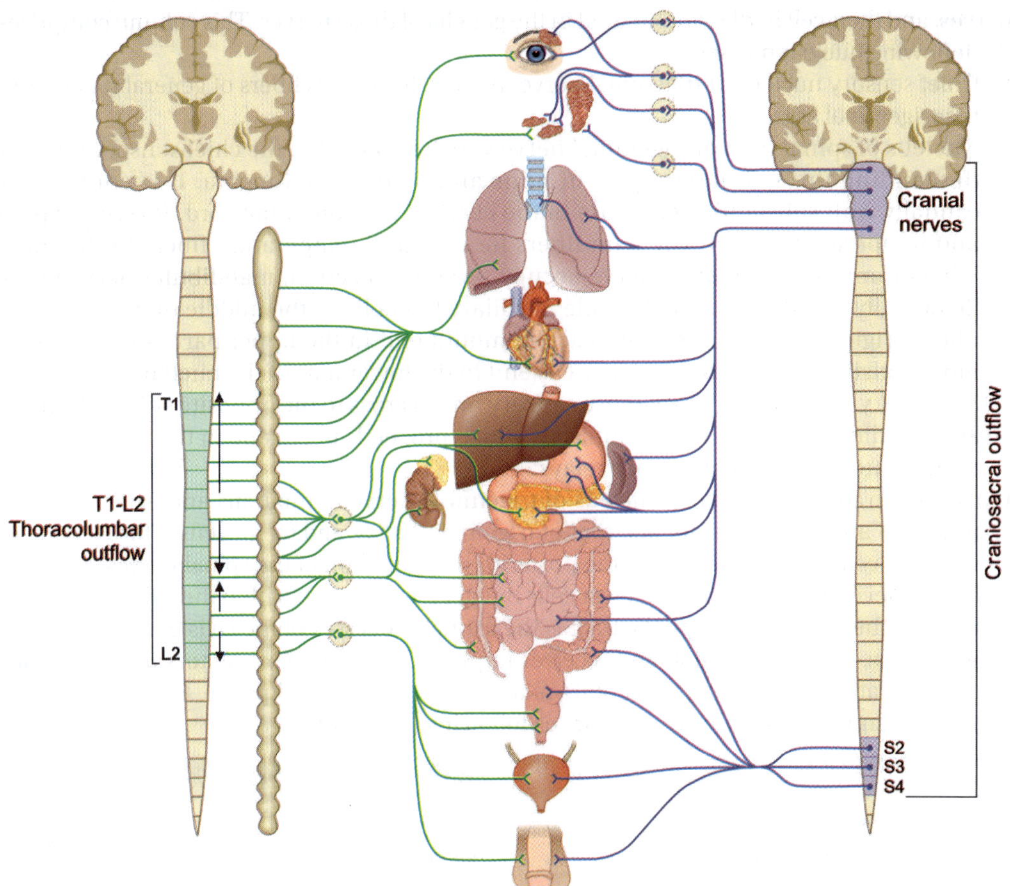

Fig. 12.21: Autonomic nervous system.

a cranial or spinal nerve. The fiber separates from the nerve and extends to an autonomic motor pathway. The postganglionic neuron lies entirely outside the CNS. Its cell body and dendrites are located in an autonomic ganglion, where it makes synapses with one or more preganglionic fibers. The axon of a postganglionic neuron, called a postganglionic fiber, is unmyelinated and terminates in a visceral effector.

PERIPHERAL NERVOUS SYSTEM

Cervical Plexus

It is formed by the ventral primary ramus of upper four cervical nerves, C1, C2, C3 and C4. The four roots are connected to each other to form three loops.

Branches

- The cutaneous branches are lesser occipital (C2), great auricular (C2, 3), anterior cutaneous nerve of neck (C2, 3) and supraclavicular (C3, 4). They supply the skin of face, ear and neck.

- There is a communicating branch from C1 that joins the hypoglossal nerve to supply the thyrohyoid, geniohyoid and superior belly of omohyoid.
- A branch from C2 supplies the sternohyoid and C3-4 supplies the trapezius and communicates with accessory nerve.
- Muscular branches to rectus capitis anterior (C1), rectus capitis lateralis (C1, C2) and longus capitis (C1-3).
- Through the ansa cervicalis it supplies sternothyroid, sternohyoid and inferior belly of omohyoid.

Ansa Cervicalis (Fig. 12.22)

This is a thin nerve loop that lies embedded in the anterior wall of the carotid sheath and supplies the infrahyoid muscles.

Formation

It is formed by a superior and an inferior root. The superior root is the continuation of descending branch of hypoglossal nerve and C1. The inferior root is derived from spinal nerves C2 and C3.

Distribution

The superior root supplies the superior belly of omohyoid. The inferior root supplies sternothyroid, sternohyoid and inferior belly of omohyoid.

Brachial Plexus (Fig. 12.23)

This supplies the upper limb. The plexus is made up of roots, trunks, divisions and cords.

Roots

These are the primary anterior rami of spinal nerves C5, 6, 7, 8 and T1.

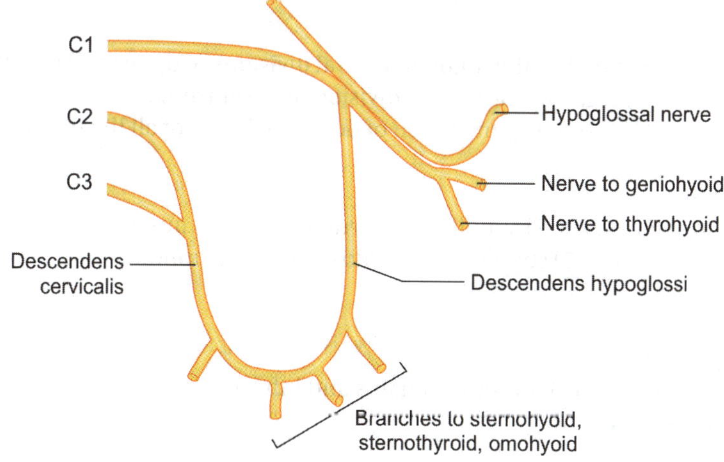

Fig. 12.22: Ansa cervicalis.

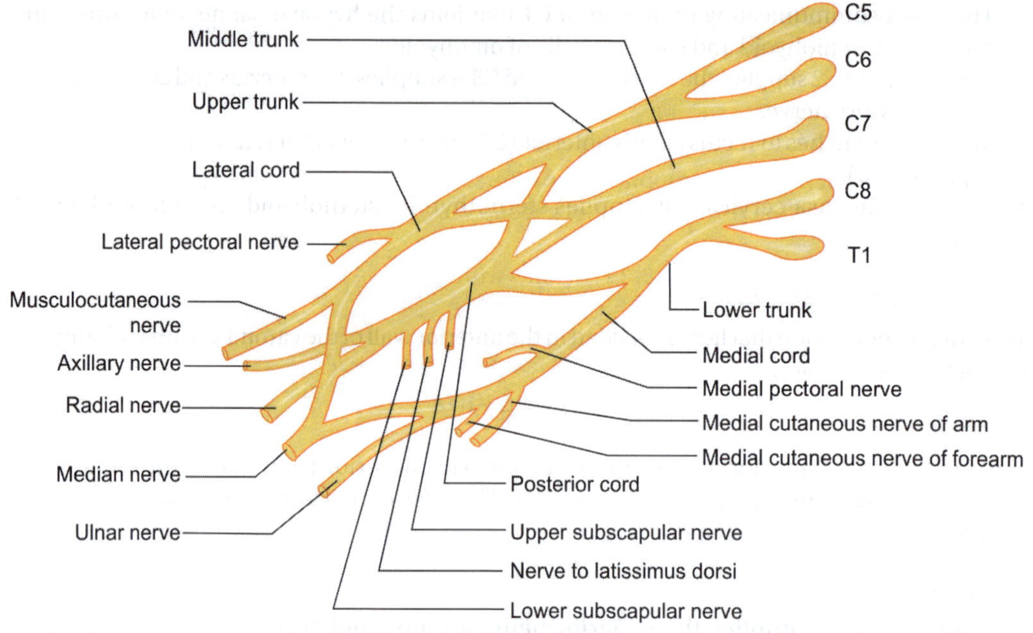

Fig. 12.23: Brachial plexus.

Trunks

- The roots C5 and C6 join to form the upper trunk.
- C7 forms the middle trunk.
- C8 and T1 form the lower trunk.

Divisions

Each trunk divides into a dorsal and a ventral division.

Cords

- The lateral cord is formed by the union of ventral divisions of upper and middle trunks.
- The medial cord is formed by the ventral division of lower trunk.
- The posterior cord is formed by the union of dorsal divisions of all the trunks.

Branches of Roots

- Long thoracic nerve (C5, 6, 7) supplies the serratus anterior muscle.
- Dorsal scapular nerve (C5) supplies rhomboids major and minor.

Branches of Trunks

They arise only from upper trunk.

- Suprascapular nerve (C5, 6) to supraspinatus and infraspinatus muscle.
- Nerve to subclavius (C5, 6).

Branches of Lateral Cord

- **Lateral pectoral nerve (C5, 6, 7):** It supplies the pectoralis major and minor.

- **Musculocutaneous (C5, 6, 7):** It is the main nerve of the front of arm.
- **Lateral root of median (C5, 6, 7):** It joins with medial root of median to form the median nerve.

Branches of Medial Cord

- Medial pectoral (C8, T1). It supplies the pectoralis major and minor.
- Medial cutaneous nerve of arm (C8, T1). It supplies the skin of the medial half of the front of arm.
- Medial root of median nerve (C8, T1). It joins with lateral root of median to form the median nerve.
- Medial cutaneous nerve of forearm (C8, T1). It supplies the skin of the medial half of the front of forearm.
- Ulnar nerve (C8, T1). It is the main nerve of the hand.

Branches of Posterior Cord

- **Upper subscapular (C5, C6):** It supplies the subscapularis muscle.
- **Thoracodorsal (C6, 7, 8):** It is the nerve to latissimus dorsi.
- **Lower subscapular (C5, C6):** It supplies the subscapularis muscle.
- **Radial nerve (C5, 6, 7, 8, T1, T2):** It is the main nerve of the back of arm and forearm.
- **Axillary nerve (C5, C6):** It supplies the shoulder region.

Applied Anatomy

- Injury to the upper trunk of brachial plexus is called Erb's paralysis. It occurs due to undue separation of head from shoulder that is commonly seen in birth injuries and fall on the shoulder. The arm hangs by the side. It is adducted and medially rotated. The forearm is extended and pronated. This is called the policeman's tip hand or the porter's tip hand.
- Injury to lower trunk of brachial plexus leads to Klumpke's paralysis. This causes claw hand and Horner's syndrome (ptosis, miosis, anhydrosis, enophthalmos and loss of ciliospinal reflex).
- Injury to long thoracic nerve paralyzes the serratus anterior muscle. In these cases the medial border of scapula becomes prominent during pushing and punching movements and the deformity is called winging of scapula.

Axillary Nerve

It is a branch of the posterior cord of brachial plexus (C5, 6).

Branches

- **Muscular branches:** It supplies the deltoid and teres minor.
- **Cutaneous branches:** It gives the upper lateral cutaneous nerve of arm that supplies the skin over the lower half of deltoid and upper half of triceps.
- **Articular branches:** To the shoulder joint.
- **Vascular branches:** To the posterior circumflex humeral artery.

Applied Anatomy

- Damage to the nerve causes paralysis of deltoid with loss of abduction of shoulder.
- There is loss of rounded contour of shoulder due to wasting of deltoid muscle.

Musculocutaneous Nerve

It is a branch of the lateral cord of brachial plexus (C5, 6, 7). It is the main nerve of the arm.

Branches

- **Muscular branches:** It supplies the biceps brachii, brachialis and coracobrachialis.
- **Cutaneous branches:** It gives the lateral cutaneous nerve of forearm that supplies the skin over the lateral side of forearm from the elbow to wrist.
- **Articular branches:** To the elbow joint.

Ulnar Nerve

It is a branch of the medial cord of brachial plexus (C8, T1). It gives no branches in the arm and enters the forearm by passing between the two heads of pronator teres. It is also called the musician's nerve as it supplies the muscles of hand that are required for skilled movements.

Branches

- **Muscular branches:** In the forearm, it supplies the flexor carpi ulnaris and medial half of flexor digitorum profundus. In the hand it supplies the hypothenar muscles, palmaris brevis, medial two lumbricals, palmar and dorsal interossei.
- **Cutaneous branches:** It gives palmar branches that supply the skin of medial 1½ fingers on their palmar surfaces, adjoining area of palm and medial 2½ fingers on dorsal surface.
- **Articular branches:** To the elbow and wrist joints.

Applied Anatomy

Injury to ulnar nerve leads to claw hand affecting the little and ring fingers. There is hyperextension at the metacarpophalangeal joint and flexion of interphalangeal joint.

Median Nerve

It is formed by the union of medial root of median (C8, T1) and lateral root of median nerve (C5, 6, 7) of the brachial plexus. It is also called the laborer's nerve as it controls the coarse movements of the hand and wrist.

Branches

- **Muscular branches:** In the forearm, it supplies pronator teres, flexor carpi radialis, palmaris longus and flexor digitorum superficialis. In the hand it supplies the thenar muscles and the lateral two lumbricals.
- Anterior interosseous nerve is given off in the arm and it supplies pronator quadratus, lateral half of flexor digitorum profundus and flexor pollicis longus.
- **Cutaneous branches:** It gives palmar branches that supply the lateral part of palm and lateral 3½ fingers on the palmar aspect.
- **Articular branches:** To the elbow, proximal and distal radioulnar joints.
- **Vascular branches:** To the radial and ulnar arteries.

Applied Anatomy

- Injury to median nerve leads to claw hand affecting the lateral three fingers. There is hyperextension at the metacarpophalangeal joint and flexion of interphalangeal joint.
- Wasting of thenar muscles leads to ape thumb deformity.

Radial Nerve

It is the largest branch of the posterior cord of brachial plexus (C5, 6, 7, 8, T1, T2).

Branches

- **Muscular branches:** It supplies the three heads of triceps, brachialis, and muscles of the back of forearm (brachioradialis, extensor carpi radialis longus and anconeus).
- Posterior interosseous nerve is given at the back of forearm and it supplies the extensor carpi radialis brevis, extensor digitorum, extensor digiti minimi, extensor indicis, abductor pollicis longus, extensor pollicis brevis, extensor pollicis longus, extensor carpi ulnaris and supinator.
- **Cutaneous branches:** In the arm it gives the lower lateral cutaneous nerve of arm that supplies the skin over the lower lateral part of arm, posterior cutaneous nerve of arm that supplies the skin of posterior aspect of arm and posterior cutaneous nerve of forearm that supplies the skin of posterior aspect of forearm. It also supplies the skin of lateral 2½ fingers on their dorsal surfaces.
- **Articular branches:** To the elbow, wrist and distal radioulnar joint.

Applied Anatomy

- Damage to the nerve causes paralysis of extensor muscles of forearm and hand leading to wrist drop.
- This commonly occurs due to compression of the nerve in the radial groove and hence, called crutch palsy or Saturday night palsy.

Intercostal Nerves (Fig. 12.24)

The intercostal nerves are the anterior primary rami of spinal nerves T1 to T11. The anterior primary ramus of T12 forms the subcostal nerve. The upper three nerves also supply the upper limb and the lower five also supply the anterior abdominal wall.

Each nerve passes in the costal groove and lies along with the posterior intercostal vessels. As it reaches the sternum, it pierces the intercostal muscles and membranes to end as the anterior cutaneous nerve of thorax.

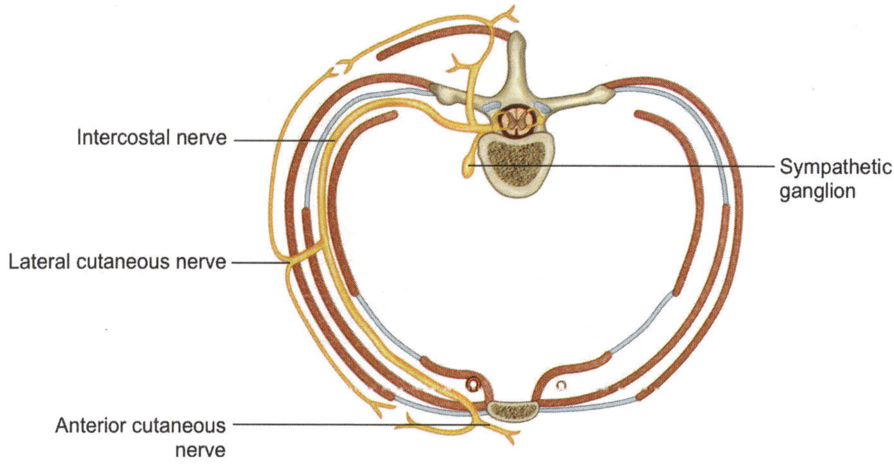

Fig. 12.24: Intercostal nerve.

Branches

- It gives numerous muscular branches to the intercostal muscles, transverses thoracis and serratus posterior superior.
- The collateral branch runs in the intercostal space and supplies the muscles of the space, parietal pleura and periosteum of the rib.
- Lateral cutaneous nerve supplies the lateral half of anterior thoracic wall.
- Anterior cutaneous nerve supplies the skin near the sternum.
- Each nerve is connected to a thoracic sympathetic ganglion by a white (distal) and a gray ramus communicantes (proximal).

Applied Anatomy

Irritation of the intercostal nerves causes severe pain which is referred to the front of the chest or abdomen near the peripheral termination of the nerve. This is called root pain or girdle pain.

Lumbar Plexus (Fig. 12.25)

The lumbar plexus lies in the posterior part of substance of psoas major muscle. It is formed by the ventral ramus of L1, L2, L3 and L4. The L1 receives contribution from subcostal nerve and L4 from lumboscaral trunk.

Branches

- Iliohypogastric nerve (L1) supplies the gluteal region.
- Ilioinguinal nerve (L1) supplies the skin over the root of penis, anterior 1/3rd of scrotum and superomedial part of thigh.
- Genitofemoral nerve (L1-2, ventral division) divides into genital and femoral branches. The genital branch supplies the cremasteric muscle in males and the round ligament and skin

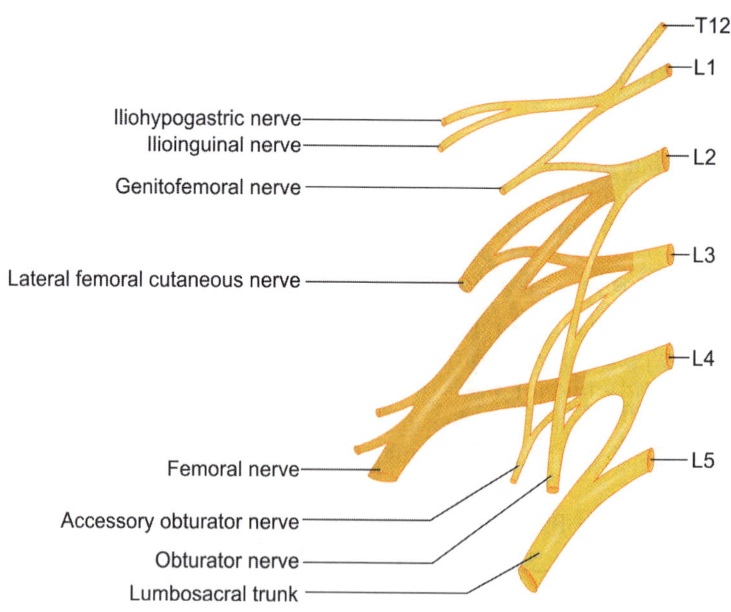

Fig. 12.25: Lumbar plexus.

of labium majus in females. The femoral branch supplies the skin over the femoral triangle of upper part of thigh.

- Lateral cutaneous nerve of thigh (L2, 3 dorsal divisions) supplies the anterolateral side of thigh.
- Femoral nerve (L2, 3, 4 dorsal divisions) supplies the muscles of the anterior compartment of thigh, hip and knee joints.
- Obturator nerve (L2, 3, 4 ventral divisions) supplies the medial compartment of thigh and the knee joint.
- Lumbosacral trunk (L4, 5 ventral rami) takes part in the formation of sacral plexus.

Femoral Nerve

It is a branch of lumbar plexus (L2, 3, 4 dorsal divisions). It is the main nerve of the anterior compartment of thigh. It emerges from below the inguinal ligament in the thigh and is not covered by the femoral sheath. It divides into an anterior and a posterior division by the lateral circumflex femoral artery.

Branches

- **Muscular branches:** The anterior division supplies sartorius. The posterior division supplies quadriceps femoris (consisting of vastus medialis, vastus intermedius, vastus lateralis, rectus femoris) and the articularis genu.
- **Cutaneous branches:** The anterior division gives the medial and intermediate cutaneous nerves of the thigh. The intermediate cutaneous nerve supplies the skin over the intermediate area of front of thigh. The medial cutaneous nerve supplies the skin on the medial side of lower 2/3rds of thigh and upper 1/3rd of leg. The posterior division gives saphenous nerve that supplies the skin of the medial side of leg and foot up to the ball of big toe.
- **Articular branches:** To the hip joint (through nerve to rectus femoris) and knee joint (through nerve to vastus medialis).
- **Vascular branches:** To the femoral artery and its branches.

Obturator Nerve

It is a branch of lumbar plexus (L2, 3, 4 ventral divisions) and mainly supplies the medial compartment of thigh. It enters the thigh by passing through the obturator canal. Within the canal it divides into an anterior and a posterior division.

Branches

- **Muscular branches:** The anterior division supplies pectineus, gracilis and adductor brevis (if not supplied by posterior division). The posterior division supplies obturator externus, adductor magnus and adductor brevis (if not supplied by anterior division).
- **Cutaneous branches:** The anterior division gives a twig to the subsartorial plexus.
- **Articular branches:** To the hip joint through the anterior and posterior divisions (branch is genicular branch).
- **Vascular branches:** To the popliteal artery and its branches.

Sacral Plexus

It is formed by the lumbosacral trunk and ventral rami of S1, S2 and S3 and a part of S4.

Branches

- Sciatic nerve (L4, 5, S1, 2, 3). It is the largest division of the sacral plexus. It divides into a ventral division which is tibial and a dorsal division which is common peroneal nerve.
- Posterior cutaneous nerve of thigh (S1, 2, 3). It supplies the skin up to the middle of back of leg.
- Superior gluteal nerve (L5, S1). It supplies the gluteus medius and minimus and tensor fascia lata.
- Inferior gluteal nerve (L5, S1, S2). It supplies the gluteus maximus.
- Nerve to pyriformis (S1, S2). Supplies the pyriformis.
- Perforating cutaneous nerve (S2, 3). Supplies the skin over the posteroinferior quadrant of gluteal region.
- Nerve to quadratus femoris (L5, S1). Supplies quadratus femoris and superior gemellus.
- Nerve to obturator internus (L5, S1). Supplies obturator internus and inferior gemellus.
- Pudendal nerve (S2, 3, 4). Supplies the perineum and external genitalia.
- Pelvic splanchnic nerves (S2, 3, 4). They supply the pelvic organs.
- Muscular branches to levator ani, coccygeus and external anal sphincter.

Sciatic Nerve (L4, 5, S1, 2, 3)

It is the thickest nerve in the body and largest division of the sacral plexus. It divides into a ventral division which is tibial and a dorsal division which is common peroneal nerve.

Branches

- **Muscular branches:** The tibial component supplies semitendinosus, semimembranosus, long head of biceps femoris and ischial head of adductor magnus. The common peroneal supplies only the short head of biceps femoris.
- **Articular branches:** To the hip joint.

Applied Anatomy

- Compression of sciatic nerve against femur or unusual stretching after sitting for a long time can cause sleeping foot.
- Compression and irritation of one or more nerve roots that form the sciatic nerve causes shooting pains in the region of gluteal region that radiates along the back of thigh, lateral side of leg and dorsum of foot.

Tibial Nerve

It is the ventral branch of sciatic nerve (L4, 5, S1, 2, 3). It is the main nerve of the posterior compartment of leg given at the level of superior angle of popliteal fossa.

Branches

- **Muscular branches:** In the popliteal fossa it supplies the plantaris, popliteus, soleus and gastrocnemius (medial and lateral heads). In the leg it supplies flexor hallucis longus, flexor digitorum longus and tibialis posterior.
- **Cutaneous branches:** Sural nerve that supplies the skin over the lower half of back of leg and the whole of the lateral border of foot up to the tip of little toe. It also gives the medial calcaneal branches to the skin of back and lower surface of heel.
- **Articular branches:** In the popliteal fossa it gives the superior and inferior medial and middle genicular to supply the knee joint. It also gives branches to the ankle joint.

- **Medial plantar nerve:** It is one of the terminal divisions of tibial nerve. It supplies the muscles of the sole and the medial side of the skin of sole.
- **Lateral plantar nerve:** It is the other terminal division of tibial nerve. It supplies the muscles of the sole and the lateral side of the skin of sole.

Common Peroneal Nerve

It is the dorsal branch of sciatic nerve (L4, 5, S1, 2, 3). It is given at the apex of popliteal fossa. It moves laterally and at the neck of fibula divides into a deep peroneal and a superficial peroneal nerve.

Branches

- **Muscular branches:** To the short head of biceps femoris.
- **Cutaneous branches:** It gives the peroneal communicating nerve that joins with the sural nerve and the lateral cutaneous nerve of calf that supplies the lateral side of back of leg.
- **Articular branches:** In the popliteal fossa it gives the superior and inferior lateral and recurrent genicular branches that supply the knee joint.

Deep Peroneal Nerve

It is the nerve of the anterior compartment of leg and dorsum of foot.

Branches

- **Muscular branches:** Tibialis anterior, extensor hallucis longus, extensor digitorum longus, peroneus tertius and extensor digitorum brevis.
- **Cutaneous branches:** To adjacent sides of the first and second toes.
- **Articular branches:** To the ankle joint, tarsal joints and the tarsometatarsal and metatarsophalangeal joints of big toe.

Applied Anatomy

Injury to the nerve causes loss of dorsiflexion of foot. This is called foot drop.

Superficial Peroneal Nerve

It is the nerve of the lateral compartment of leg.

Branches

- **Muscular branches:** Peroneus longus and brevis.
- **Cutaneous branches:** To the lower 1/3rd of leg and greater part of the dorsum of foot.

Applied Anatomy

Injury to the nerve causes loss of eversion of foot.

APPLIED ANATOMY

Spinal Cord

- **Lumbar puncture:** Drawing cerebrospinal fluid for diagnostic purposes below second lumbar vertebra.
- Lesion of ascending tracts in spinal cord leads to loss of different sensations (touch, pressure, pain, temperature, proprioception) depending upon the level and type of tract.

- Lesion of descending tracts of spinal cord may lead to loss of motor function depending on the level and type of tract.
- **Upper motor neuron lesion:** Spastic paralysis, exaggerated tendon reflexes, rigidity, positive Babinski's sign.
- **Lower motor neuron lesion:** Flaccid paralysis, absent tendon reflexes, muscle atrophy.

Medulla Oblongata

- **Wallenberg's syndrome:** Ipsilateral/same side—paralysis of pharynx, larynx, loss of taste on posterior 1/3rd of tongue, Horner's syndrome (miosis, ptosis, enophthalmos, anhydrosis, sympathetic inactivity), loss of pain and temperature on face, analgesia, ataxia; contralateral/opposite side—dissociated hemianesthesia (loss of pain, temperature).
- **Anterior medullary syndrome:** Contralateral hemiplegia, ipsilateral paralysis of tongue.

Pons

- **Pontine hemorrhage:** Common in uncontrolled hypertension, pupils become pinpointed, bilateral paralysis of face and limbs.
- **Pontocerebellar angle tumor:** Tinnitus, progressive deafness and vertigo.

Midbrain

- **Hydrocephalus:** Blockage of cerebral aqueduct leads to increase in fluid.
- **Weber's syndrome:** Contralateral hemiplegia.

Cerebellum

- Lesion in cerebellum leads to inability to maintain the equilibrium of body.
- **Dysdiadochokinesia:** Difficulty in performing rapid movements involving opposite group of muscles.
- **Dysarthria:** Speech defects.
- **Nystagmus:** Repeated jerky movements of eyeballs.

Cerebrum

- **Ventriculography:** X-ray of ventricles.
- **Hydrocephalus:** Increase in cerebrospinal fluid leading to enlargement of head.

Injuries to Cranial Nerves

- **Olfactory:** Anosmia (loss of smell).
- **Optic:** Anopsia (loss of vision), visual field defects, loss of visual acuity.
- **Oculomotor:** Strabismus (both eyes do not fix on same object), ptosis (drooping of upper eyelid), pupil dilatation, diplopia (double vision).
- **Trochlear:** Diplopia, strabismus.
- **Trigeminal:** Paralysis of muscles of mastication, loss of touch and temperature on face, trigeminal neuralgia (pain of one or more branches of trigeminal nerve).
- **Abducent:** Eyeball cannot move laterally beyond midpoint and usually directed medially.
- **Facial:** Bell's palsy (paralysis of facial muscles), loss of taste and ability to close the eyes.
- **Vestibulocochlear:** Tinnitus (ringing), deafness, vertigo (rotation), ataxia, nystagmus.
- **Glossopharyngeal:** Difficulty during swallowing, reduced saliva, loss of sensation in throat, loss of taste.

- **Vagus:** Difficulty swallowing, paralysis of vocal cords, interrupts sensations from many organs.
- **Accessory:** Paralysis of sternocleidomastoid and trapezius.
- **Hypoglossal:** Difficulty in chewing, speaking, swallowing, affected side of tongue becomes atrophied, shrunken, deeply furrowed.

Injuries to Peripheral Nerves

- **Erb's paralysis:** Policeman's tip hand (arm adducted and medially rotated, forearm extended and pronated).
- **Klumpke's paralysis:** Claw hand, Horner's syndrome.
- **Winging of scapula:** Medial border of scapula becomes prominent during pushing and punching.
- **Axillary nerve injury:** Paralysis of deltoid leading to loss of abduction of shoulder, wasting of deltoid.
- **Ulnar nerve injury:** Claw hand (hyperextension at metacarpophalangeal joint, flexion of interphalangeal joints in medial two fingers).
- **Median nerve injury:** Claw hand (hyperextension at metacarpophalangeal joint, flexion of interphalangeal joints in lateral three fingers), ape thumb deformity (wasting of thenar muscles).
- **Radial nerve injury:** Wrist drop (paralysis of extensor muscles of forearm and hand).
- **Saturday night palsy/crutch palsy:** Compression of radial nerve in radial groove leading to temporary wrist drop.
- **Sciatica:** Compression of sciatic nerve or branches leading to sleeping foot, shooting pain in the region of gluteal region, back of thigh, lateral side of leg, dorsum of foot.
- **Deep peroneal nerve injury:** Foot drop (loss of dorsiflexion).
- **Superficial peroneal nerve injury:** Loss of eversion of foot.

SUMMARY

Central Nervous System

Spinal Cord

- **Extent:** Foramen magnum to lower border of L1 vertebra.
- **Coverings:** Dura mater, arachnoid mater, pia mater.
- **Tracts:** Descending tracts (corticospinal/pyramidal, rubrospinal, tectospinal, vestibulospinal, reticulospinal, olivospinal); ascending tracts (lateral spinothalamic, ventral spinothalamic, spinocerebellar, spinoreticular, spinovestibular, spinotectal).

Brainstem

- **Parts:** Medulla oblongata, pons, midbrain, and all three are connected to cerebellum by inferior, middle and superior cerebellar peduncles.
- Medulla oblongata forms lower part of brainstem and is very important for the functions like heart rate, blood pressure, reflexes, and involuntary controls such as vomiting, coughing and sneezing. When blood supply to this region is interrupted it leads to stroke which can result in death.
- Pons forms the middle part of brainstem with the following function, regulates the breathing and deep sleep, involved in transmission of signals to and from cerebrum or cerebellum, sensations like hearing, taste, and balance.
- Midbrain forms upper part of brainstem; serves as relay center for visual, auditory and motor system information; regulates autonomic functions like digestion, heart rate and breathing rate.

Cerebellum

- Present in the posterior cranial fossa.
- Maintains the equilibrium, muscle tone and coordination.
- **Fissures:** Primary, posterolateral, horizontal.
- **Lobes:** Anterior, posterior, flocculonodular.
- Central core of white matter surrounded by thin layer of gray matter arranged in the form of branching tree called arbor vitae cerebella. Embedded in the white matter are dentate, emboliform, globose and fastigial nuclei.
- **Cerebellar peduncles:** Superior, middle and inferior.

Cerebrum

- Present in anterior, middle and posterior cranial fossae.
- **Parts:** 2 cerebral hemispheres, each hemisphere with 4 lobes—frontal, parietal, temporal, occipital; 3 poles—frontal, temporal, occipital; 3 borders—superomedial, inferomedial, inferolateral; 3 surfaces—superolateral, inferior, medial.
- Surfaces present irregular elevations called gyri and linear depressions called sulci.
- **Functional areas:** Motor/area 4 (precentral gyrus, paracentral lobule); Broca's motor speech area/area 44, 45 (inferior frontal gyrus); sensory area/area 1, 2, 3 (postcentral gyrus, paracentral lobule); visual area/area 17 (occipital lobe); auditory area/area 41 (superior temporal gyrus); Wernicke's sensory speech area/area 22 (superior temporal gyrus); olfactory area/area 28 (parahippocampal gyrus).
- White matter—association fibers (connects same cerebral cortex), projection fibers (connects cerebral cortex with lower centers), commissural fibers (connects two cerebral hemispheres).
- **Blood supply:** Arteries—anterior, middle, posterior cerebral arteries; veins—superficial (superior and inferior cerebral veins, superficial and deep middle cerebral veins), deep (internal cerebral, great cerebral, basal veins).

Ventricles

- Cavities inside the cerebral hemispheres and between brainstem and cerebellum filled with cerebrospinal fluid (CSF) and choroid plexus which produce CSF.
- **Parts:** Lateral ventricle, third ventricle, and fourth ventricle. Lateral ventricle → interventricular foramina, third ventricle → cerebral aqueduct → fourth ventricle → central canal of spinal cord.

Cranial Nerves

Cranial nerve	*Motor/ sensory*	*Distribution*	*Function*
Olfactory	Sensory	Olfactory mucosa	Smell
Optic	Sensory	Retina	Vision
Oculomotor	Motor	Levator palpebrae superioris, superior rectus, middle rectus, inferior rectus, inferior oblique	Movement of eyelid and eyeball, accommodation of lens for near vision, constriction of pupil
	Sensory	Eyeball	Proprioception of eyeball
Trochlear	Motor	Superior oblique	Movement of eyeball
	Sensory	Superior oblique	Proprioception
Trigeminal	Motor	Muscles of mastication, anterior belly of digastric muscles, mylohyoid	Chewing
	Sensory	Muscles of mastication	Proprioception
Abducent	Motor	Lateral rectus	Movement of eyeball
	Sensory	Lateral rectus	Proprioception

Cranial nerve	*Motor/ sensory*	*Distribution*	*Function*
Facial	Motor	Muscles (Facial, platysma, scalp); Glands (Lacrimal, sublingual, submandibular, nasal, palatine)	Facial expression, secretion of saliva and tears
	Sensory	Taste buds in anterior 2/3rds of tongue, muscles of face and scalp	Taste, proprioception
Vestibulocochlear	Vestibular	Semicircular canals, saccule, utricle	Equilibrium
	Cochlear	Spiral organ of corti	Hearing
Glossopharyngeal	Motor	Stylopharyngeus, lingual glands	Acts on pharynx, secretion of saliva
	Sensory	Middle ear, auditory tube, mastoid air cells, carotid sinus, posterior 1/3rd of tongue	Equilibrium, taste, regulation of blood pressure, proprioception
Vagus	Motor	Muscles of respiration, lungs, esophagus, heart, GIT, larynx, pharynx	Smooth muscle contraction and relaxation; secretion of digestive fluids
	Sensory	Posterior cranial fossa; skin over auricle, external acoustic meatus, tympanic membrane; carotid body; organs of abdomen and pelvis	Sensations from visceral organs, proprioception
Accessory	Motor	Muscles of pharynx, larynx, soft palate, sternocleidomastoid, trapezius	Swallowing, movement of head
	Sensory	Muscles of pharynx, larynx, soft palate, sternocleidomastoid, trapezius	Proprioception
Hypoglossal	Motor	Muscles of tongue	Movement of tongue
	Sensory	Muscles of tongue	Proprioception

QUESTIONS

Long Essays

- Describe the cerebrum giving its gross anatomy, sulci and gyri, functional areas, connections, blood supply and applied aspects.
- Describe cerebellum giving its gross anatomy, connections, blood supply, histology and applied aspects.
- Describe pons giving its external and internal features.
- Describe midbrain giving its external and internal features.
- Describe medulla oblongata giving its external and internal features.
- Describe circle of Willis and its applied aspects.
- Describe the venous drainage of brain.
- Describe course, distribution and applied aspects of cranial nerves.
- Describe basal ganglia.
- Describe cranial nerve nuclei.
- Describe external and internal features of spinal cord.

CHAPTER

Sensory Organs

LEARNING OBJECTIVES

The student should be able to:

- Describe skin under gross features, nerve endings and functions, histology of thin and thick skin.
- Describe the appendages of skin.
- Name the parts of ear.
- Name the parts of middle ear, tympanic cavity, middle ear ossicles and muscles.
- Name the parts of inner ear, auditory pathway.
- Name the parts of eye and lacrimal apparatus.
- Names of extraocular muscles and nerve supply.
- Describe histology of cornea and retina.
- Describe visual pathway.

SKIN

Skin is the covering of the entire external surface of the body, including external auditory meatus and outer surface of tympanic membrane.

It is continuous with mucous membrane at the orifices of the body.

The color of skin is determined by five pigments:

1. Melanin, brown in color, present in germinative zone of epidermis.
2. Melanoid, diffuse.
3. Carotene, yellow to orange in color, in stratum corneum and fat cells of dermis and superficial fascia.
4. Hemoglobin, purple.
5. Oxyhemoglobin, red, in cutaneous vessels.

Skin is marked by three types of surface irregularities: (1) Tension lines, (2) flexure lines and (3) papillary ridges.

Receptors

- **Free nerve endings:** Terminals of sensory nerves do not show any particular specialization of structure, e.g., connective tissue, epithelium of skin, cornea.
- **Tactile corpuscles (of Meissner):** Responsible for touch, e.g., dermal papillae.

- **Lamellated corpuscles (of Pacini):** Responsible for vibration and pressure, e.g., subcutaneous tissue of palm and sole.
- Bulbous corpuscle (of Krause)
- **Tactile menisci (Merkel cell receptor):** Responsible for pressure, e.g., sheaths of hair follicles.
- Ruffini endings.

Appendages of Skin

Nail, hair, sweat glands and sebaceous glands.

Nail

Nails are hardened keratin plates (cornified zone) on the dorsal surface of the tips of fingers and toes, acting as a rigid support for the digital pads of terminal phalanges.

Parts

- Root is the proximal hidden part which is buried into the nail groove and is overlapped by the nail fold of the skin.
- Free border is the distal part free from the skin.
- Body is the exposed part of the nail which is adherent to the underlying skin. The proximal part of the body presents a white opaque crescent called lunule. Each lateral border is overlapped by a fold of skin, called nail wall. The skin beneath root and body is called nail bed. The germinative zone of the nail bed beneath the root and lunule is thick and proliferative (germinal matrix) and is responsible for the growth of the nail. The rest of the nail bed is thin (sterile matrix) over which the growing nail glides.

Hair

Hairs are keratinous filaments derived from invaginations of the germinative layer of epidermis into dermis.

Hair is absent in palms, soles, dorsal surface of distal phalanges, umbilicus, glans penis, inner surface of prepuce, labia minora, inner surface of labia majora.

Parts

- Implanted *root* and a projecting *shaft*.
- Root is surrounded by a *hair follicle* (a sheath of epidermis and dermis) and is expanded at its proximal end to form *hair bulb*.
- Each hair bulb is invaginated at its end by *hair papilla* (vascular connective tissue) which forms the neurovascular hilum of the hair and its sheath. Hair grows at the hair bulb, by proliferation of its cells capping the papilla.
- Arrectores pilorum muscles (smooth muscles supplied by sympathetic nerves) connect the undersurface of the follicles to the superficial part of the dermis. Contraction of these muscles leads to erection of hair, squeezes out the sebum, and produces 'goose skin'.
- Hair follicle is made up of an outer dermal coat and an inner epidermal coat.
- Shaft is made up, from within outwards, of medulla, cortex (main part) and cuticle.

Sweat Glands

Sweat glands are distributed all over the skin, except lips, glans penis and nail bed. They are of two types:

1. **Eccrine glands:** Distributed in almost every part of the skin.

2. **Apocrine glands:** Confined to axilla, eyelids, nipple and areola of breast, perianal region, external genitalia.

Sebaceous Glands

They produce oily secretion (sebum), are widely distributed all over the dermis, except palms and soles. They are abundant in scalp and face, and numerous around the apertures of ear, nose, mouth and anus. Their ducts open into hair follicles, with exception of lips, glans penis, inner surface of prepuce, labia minora, nipple and areola of breast, tarsal glands of eyelids, where the ducts open on the surface of skin.

Histology of Skin (Figs. 13.1A and B and 13.2A and B)

- Consists of epidermis and dermis.
- Epidermis, the avascular layer, is lined by stratified squamous keratinized epithelium consisting of stratum basale with columnar cells; stratum spinosum with polyhedral cells; stratum granulosum with cells having keratohyalin granules; stratum lucidum with cells having pyknotic or no nucleus; stratum corneum or the keratin layer. Stratum corneum is thin in thin skin and thick in thick skin.
- Dermis, the vascular layer, consisting of connective tissue with blood vessels, lymphatics and nerves. It has a superficial papillary layer which forms conical, blunt projections (dermal papillae) which fit into reciprocal depressions on the undersurface of epidermis and a deep reticular layer, with white fibrous tissue.
- In dermis of thin skin, many sweat glands and sensory nerve endings, pilosebaceous apparatus consisting of hair follicle, arrectores pilorum with sebaceous gland are seen.
- In dermis of thick skin, many sweat glands and sensory nerve endings are present, sebaceous glands and hair follicles are absent.

Applied Anatomy of Skin

- Skin is pale in anemia, yellow in jaundice, blue in cyanosis.
- Boil (furuncle) is an infection and suppuration of hair follicle and sebaceous gland.

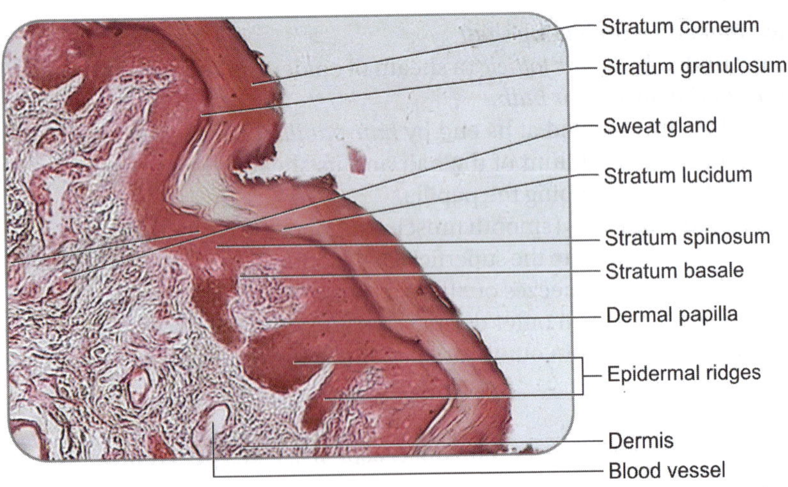

Fig. 13.1A: Photomicrograph of histology of thick skin.

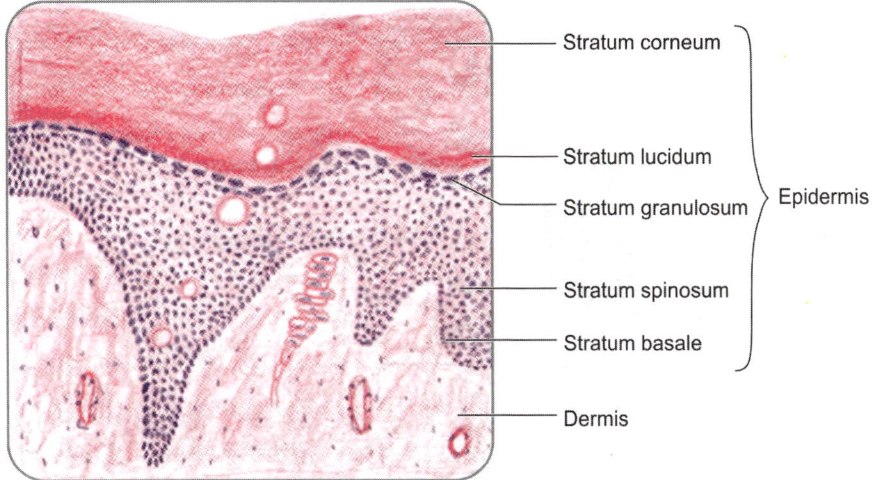

Fig. 13.1B: Diagrammatic representation of histology of thick skin.

- Skin incisions should be made parallel to lines of cleavage. This will result in smaller scars.
- Sebaceous cyst is common in scalp. It is due to the obstruction of mouth of a sebaceous duct, caused either by trauma or infection.
- Common skin diseases are fungal (like ringworm), allergic (like urticaria, eczema, dermatitis) and parasitic (like scabies).
- Loss of touch sensibility is anesthesia, loss of pain sensibility is analgesia, loss of temperature sensibility is thermanesthesia. Exaggerated sensibility is hyperesthesia, and perverted sensibility, paresthesia. Trophic changes result from loss of its sensibility.
- **Skin grafting:** *Split-thickness*, where greater part of epidermis with tips of dermal papillae is used and full thickness, where both epidermis and dermis are used.

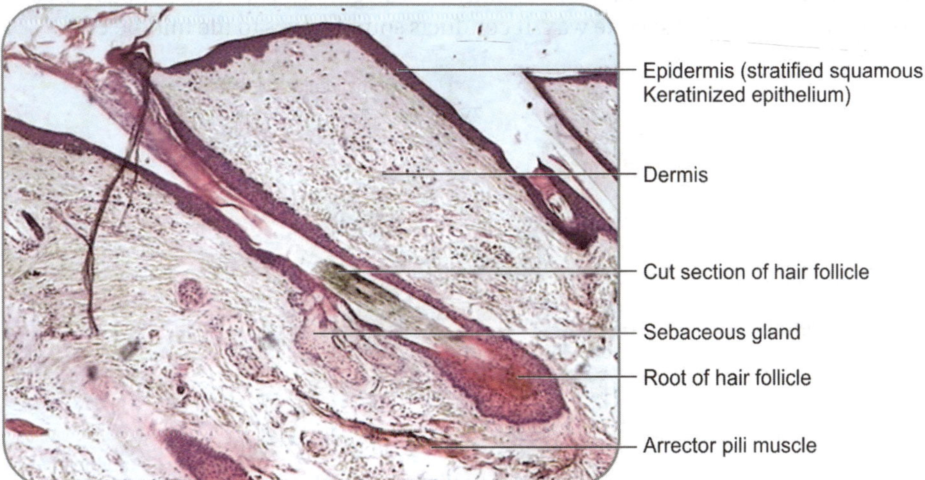

Fig. 13.2A: Photomicrograph of histology of thin skin.

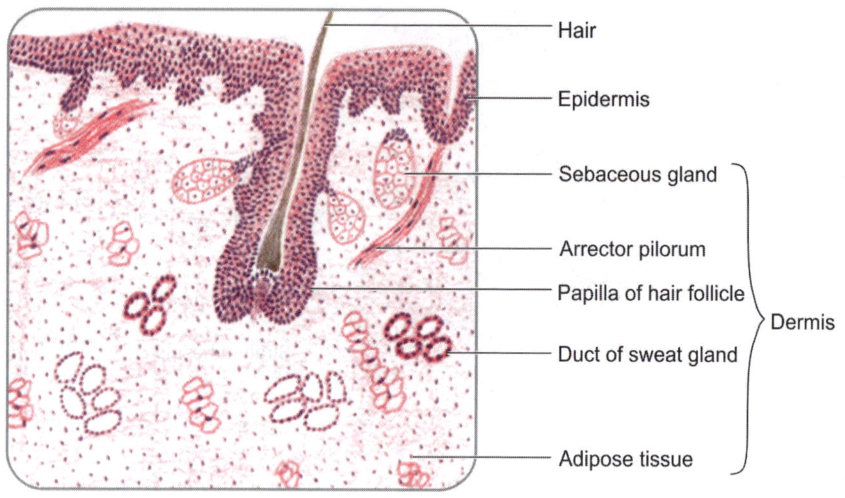

Fig. 13.2B: Diagrammatic representation of histology of thin skin.

EAR (FIG. 13.3)

The ear is the organ of hearing and maintenance of balance.

Parts

It is made up of three parts: External, middle and inner ear.

External Ear

- It is made up of the auricle or pinna and the external acoustic meatus.
- Auricle is the part seen on the surface. It is made up of elastic cartilage and covered by skin.
- External acoustic meatus is an S-shaped canal. It is about 24 mm long, the medial 2/3rd (16 mm) is bony and the lateral 1/3rd (8 mm) is cartilaginous. The cartilaginous part contains ceruminous glands that secrete wax. It conducts sound waves to the middle ear.

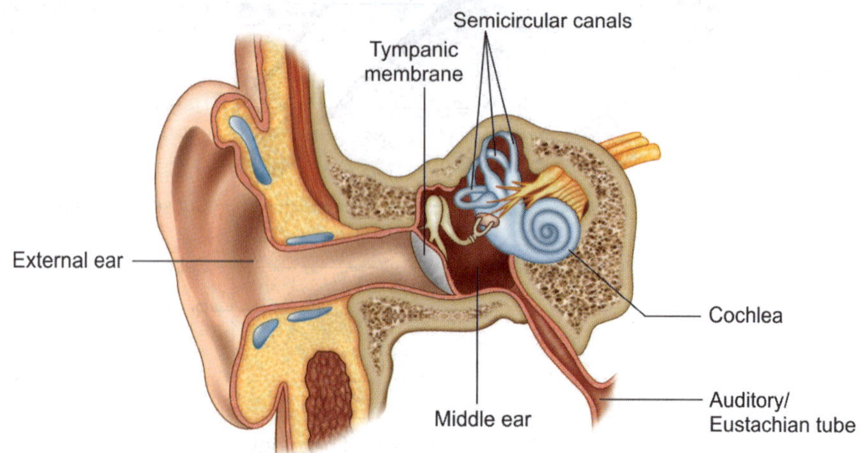

Fig. 13.3: Ear.

Middle Ear

- It is a cube shaped cavity.
- It is separated from the external ear from a thin membrane called the tympanic membrane.
- The tympanic membrane **(Fig. 13.4)** has an outer and an inner surface. The outer surface is covered by skin and is concave. The inner surface has the attachment of the handle of malleus and is convex.
- The site of maximum convexity lies at the tip of the handle of malleus and is called the umbo. This throws a cone of light on the inferior aspect of the membrane.
- The greater part of the membrane is tense and called pars tensa. A small part of it on the superior aspect is flaccid and called pars flaccida.

The *walls* of the middle ear are:

- Roof which is made up of thin plate of bone called the tegmen tympani.
- Floor is related to the bulb of the internal jugular vein.
- Anterior wall has three openings, uppermost is for tensor tympani muscle, middle for opening of auditory tube and lowermost is separated from internal carotid artery by a thin plate of bone.
- The posterior wall is related to the mastoid process and facial nerve.
- The lateral wall is the tympanic membrane.
- The medial wall is related to the inner ear.

Contents:

- The middle ear has three small bones called the ear ossicles **(Fig. 13.5)**. These are the malleus, the incus and the stapes. The malleus articulates with the tympanic membrane. The stapes has a footplate that rests on the inner ear on a window called the oval window.
- The middle ear has two small muscles called the tegmen tympani and the stapedius. They both act to dampen the intensity of high-pitched sound waves.

Sound waves are conducted to the middle ear by vibrations of the tympanic membrane. Sound is then carried by the ear ossicles to the inner ear.

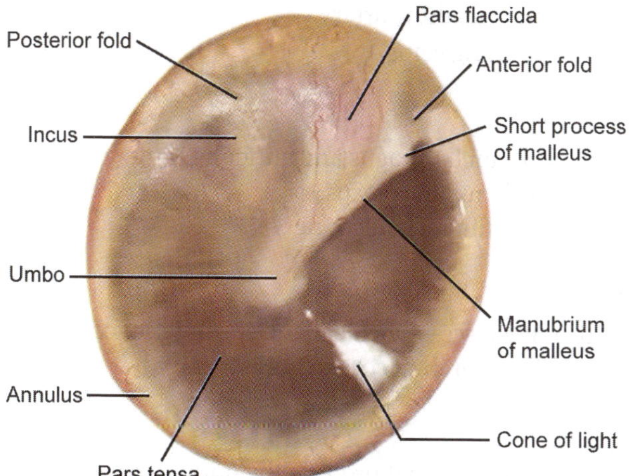

Fig. 13.4: Tympanic membrane.

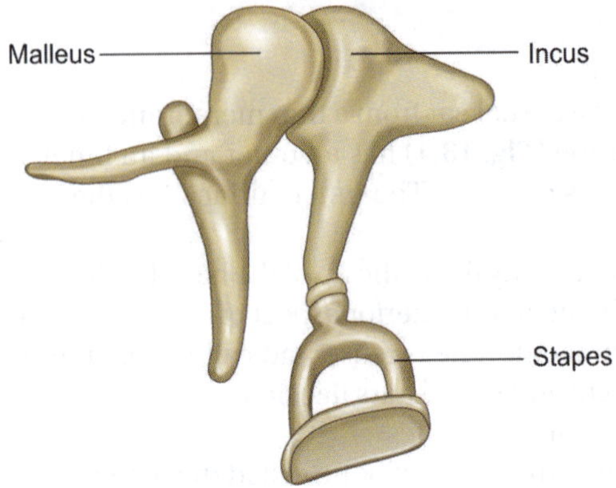

Fig. 13.5: Ear ossicles.

Inner Ear

- The inner ear lies in the petrous part of the temporal bone.
- It consists of a bony labyrinth within which is the membranous labyrinth. The bony labyrinth is filled with a fluid called the perilymph. The bony labyrinth consists of cochlea, vestibule and the semicircular canals.
- Within bony labyrinth, the membranous labyrinth floats in its own fluid called the endolymph. The membranous labyrinth is made up of the duct of cochlea, utricle and saccule and the semicircular ducts.
- Duct of cochlea contains organ of hearing called organ of Corti.
- Utricle and saccule are organs of balance and help in the maintenance of equilibrium.

Blood Supply

- Outer ear is supplied by posterior auricular and superficial temporal arteries.
- Middle ear is supplied by maxillary and posterior auricular arteries.
- Inner ear is supplied by labyrinthine artery.
- Veins drain into corresponding veins.

Nerve Supply

- Outer ear is supplied by branch of vagus and auriculotemporal nerves.
- Middle ear is supplied by tympanic plexus.
- Inner ear is supplied by vestibulocochlear nerve.

Auditory Pathway

Sound → organ of Corti → 8th nerve → cochlear nuclei → inferior colliculus → medial geniculate body → auditory radiations → cerebral cortex (auditory area).

Applied Anatomy

- Ceruminous glands secrete wax that protects the outer ear. Excessive wax production may lead to blockage of the ear. The method of removal of wax is called syringing.

- Infection of middle ear is called otitis media. In this condition, pus is removed from the ear by making a cut in the tympanic membrane. This procedure is called myringotomy.
- Auditory tube opens into middle ear. Hence, infections of the throat can infect the middle ear and vice versa.

EYE (FIG. 13.6)

- Eyeball is the organ of vision.
- It is like a spherical ball about 2.5 cm in size. It is made up of three layers:
  1. The outermost layer is called *fibrous coat*. It gives strength to the eyeball and maintains its shape. It is made up of the transparent cornea (anterior 1/6th) and the thick white fibrous sclera (posterior 5/6th).
  2. The middle layer is called the *vascular layer*. It is made up of choroid, ciliary body and iris. It is also called the uveal tract. The ciliary body suspends the lens. The iris has an aperture in the middle called the pupil. It is through the pupil that the light enters the eyeball. Lens is a transparent biconvex structure with a refractive power of 15D.
  3. The innermost layer is called the nervous layer. It is made up of retina which has a layer of rods and cones that is the site for perception of light. Light rays travel from the retina to the visual cortex of the brain.

Aqueous Humor

- Aqueous humor is a clear fluid that fills both anterior and posterior chambers. Anterior chamber is the space present between cornea and iris, posterior chamber is the space between iris and lens.
- **Vitreous body:** This is a colorless jelly-like substance that fills the posterior 4/5th of the eyeball.

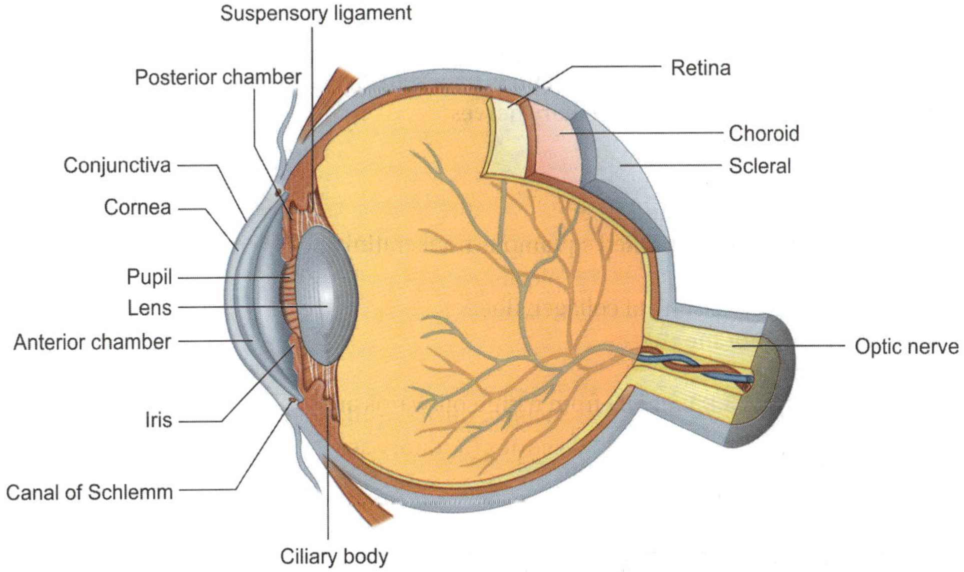

Fig. 13.6: Layers of eyeball.

Extraocular Muscles

They are medial, lateral, superior and inferior rectus, superior and inferior oblique. Superior oblique is supplied by trochlear nerve, lateral rectus by abducent nerve, and the rest by oculomotor nerve.

Eyelids and Lacrimal Apparatus

- Free margins of upper and lower eyelids enclose the palpebral fissure, the ends of which are called angles of the eye or canthi.
- Lateral 5/6th of the free margin of eyelids are flat and carry eyelashes or cilia.
- Medial 1/6th are rounded, devoid of hairs and called lacrimal part, because the lacrimal canaliculi pass through this part.
- On the lacrimal part is a small conical projection called lacrimal papilla with an opening, lacrimal punctum at its apex.
- Layers of eyelid are skin, superficial fascia, muscle layer (orbicularis oculi), tarsal plate, tarsal glands, palpebral conjunctiva.
- Lacrimal apparatus consists of lacrimal gland, lacus lacrimalis, lacrimal canaliculi, lacrimal sac, and nasolacrimal duct.

Visual Pathway

Light → retina → optic nerve → optic chiasma → optic tract → lateral geniculate body → optic radiations → visual cortex.

Blood Supply

- Cornea and sclera are avascular and nourished by aqueous humor.
- Retina is supplied by the central artery of retina, a branch of ophthalmic artery.
- Choroid, ciliary body and iris is supplied by branches of ophthalmic artery.
- Venous drainage is into ophthalmic veins.

Nerve Supply

The cornea is richly supplied by nerves and is pain sensitive. It is supplied by the branches of the ophthalmic nerve and the short ciliary nerves.

Histology

Layers of cornea (**Figs. 13.7A and B**) are:

i. Anterior epithelium—stratified squamous nonkeratinized
ii. Bowman's membrane
iii. Corneal stroma consisting of collagen fibers
iv. Descemet's membrane
v. Endothelium

Layers of retina (**Figs. 13.8A and B**) from within outwards are:

i. Pigment cell layer
ii. Layer of processes of rods and cones
iii. Outer limiting membrane
iv. Outer nuclear layer made of nuclei of rods and cones.
v. Outer plexiform layer made up of synapses of rods and cones and dendrites of bipolar cells.
vi. Inner nuclear layer made of nuclei of bipolar cells.

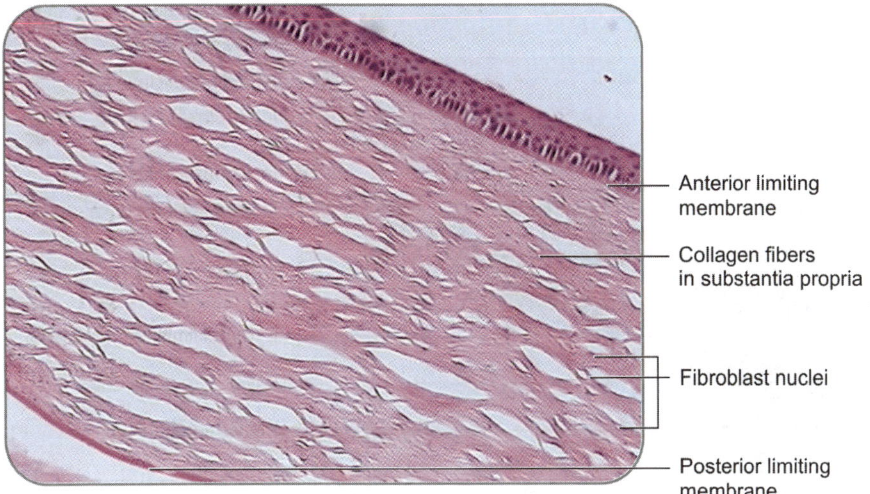

Fig. 13.7A: Photograph of histology of cornea.

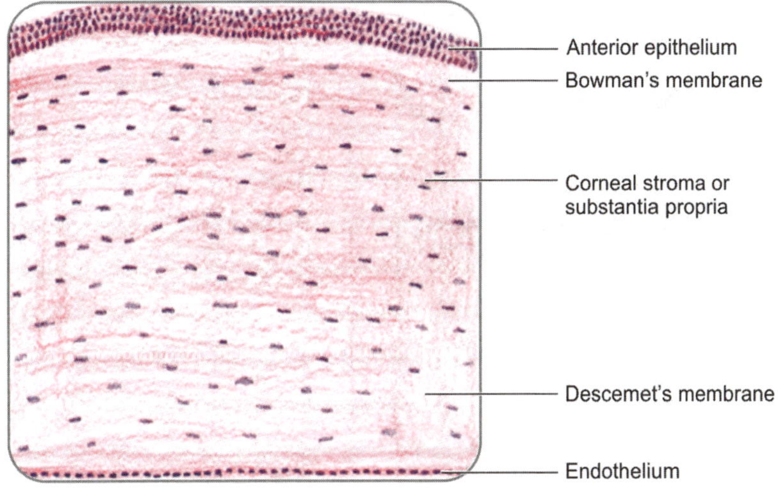

Fig. 13.7B: Diagrammatic representation of histology of cornea.

vii. Inner plexiform layer made of synapses of bipolar cells and dendrites of ganglion cells.
viii. Ganglion cell layer
ix. Layer of optic nerve fibers.
x. Inner limiting membrane.

Applied Anatomy

- Disruption of optic pathway may lead to loss of sight.
- Cornea may get abraded to form corneal ulcers which are very painful due to a rich nerve supply.

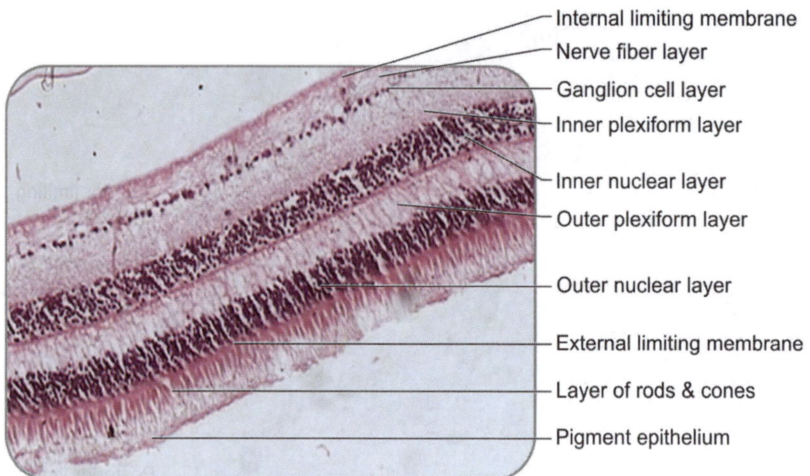

Fig. 13.8A: Photograph of histology of retina.

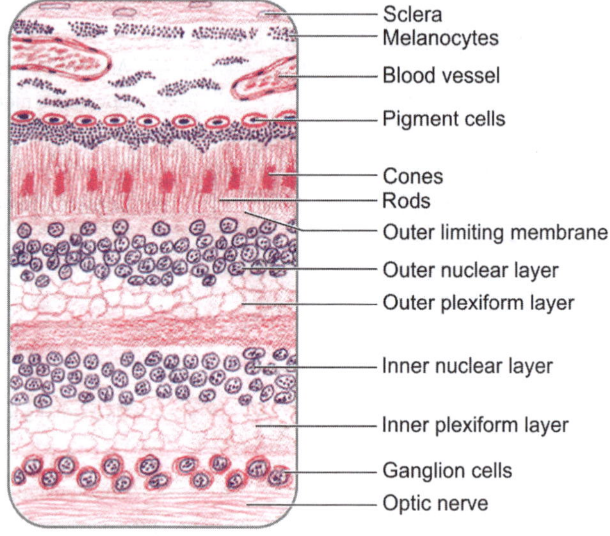

Fig. 13.8B: Diagrammatic representation of histology of retina.

- Opacity of lens is called cataract.
- Increase in intraocular pressure is called glaucoma.

APPLIED ANATOMY

- **Skin color:** Pale in anemia, yellow in jaundice, blue in cyanosis.
- **Boil:** Infection and suppuration of hair follicle and sebaceous gland.
- **Sebaceous cyst:** Obstruction of sebaceous duct leading to an increase in sebum.
- **Anesthesia:** Loss of touch sensation.

- **Analgesia:** Loss of pain sensation.
- **Thermanesthesia:** Loss of temperature sensation.
- **Hyperesthesia:** Exaggerated sensation.
- **Paresthesia:** Perverted sensation.
- **Syringing of ear (removal of wax):** Excessive wax production may lead to blockage of ear.
- **Otitis media:** Infection of middle ear.
- **Myringotomy:** Removal of pus from middle ear by making a cut in tympanic membrane.
- Infections may spread between throat and middle ear due to the communication between them.
- **Cataract:** Opacity of lens.
- **Glaucoma:** Increase in intraocular pressure.
- Disruption of optic pathway leads to loss of sight.

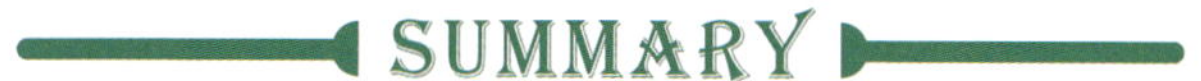

Skin

- Skin is the largest organ of the body.
- **Receptors of skin:** Free nerve endings, tactile corpuscles, corpuscles of Pacini, bulbous corpuscle of Krause, Merkel cell receptor, Ruffini endings.
- **Appendages of skin:** Hair, nail, sweat glands, sebaceous glands.

Ear

- Ear is the organ of hearing and helps in maintenance of balance.
- **Parts:** External (conducts sound waves to middle ear), middle (sound waves carried to inner ear through ear ossicles), inner (sound waves are processed in organ of Corti and transmitted to brain for interpretation through vestibulocochlear nerve).
- **Blood supply:** Arteries-posterior auricular and superficial temporal (outer ear), maxillary and posterior auricular (middle ear), labyrinthine (inner ear); veins-corresponding veins.
- **Nerve supply:** Vagus and auriculotemporal (outer ear), tympanic plexus (middle ear), vestibulocochlear (inner ear).

Eye

- **Eyeball coverings:** Outer fibrous coat (cornea, sclera), middle vascular coat (choroid, ciliary body, iris), inner nervous coat (retina with rods and cones).
- **Lens:** Transparent biconvex structure.
- **Aqueous humor:** Clear fluid in anterior chamber (between cornea and iris) and posterior chamber (between iris and lens).
- **Vitreous humor:** Jelly-like substance between lens and retina.
- **Extraocular muscles:** Four recti (medial, lateral, superior, inferior), two oblique (superior, inferior), levator palpebrae superioris.
- **Blood supply:** Arteries-cornea (avascular), ophthalmic artery; veins: Ophthalmic veins.
- **Nerve supply:** All muscles supplied by oculomotor except superior oblique (trochlear) and lateral rectus (abducent).

QUESTIONS

Short Essays

- Microscopy of thick skin
- Microscopy of thin skin
- Nerve endings of skin
- Labeled diagram of eyeball
- Layers of retina.

Short Answers

- Name appendages of skin
- Parts of eye
- Parts of lacrimal apparatus
- Name of extraocular muscles and nerve supply
- Visual pathway
- Histology of cornea.

CHAPTER 14

General Embryology

LEARNING OBJECTIVES

The student should be able to:

- Describe mitosis and meiosis, spermatogenesis and oogenesis.
- Describe ovulation and tests for ovulation.
- Describe fertilization, implantation and germ layer formation.

INTRODUCTION

Embryology is the study of formation and development of embryo from the moment it is formed to the time when it is born.

CELL DIVISION

Multiplication of cells takes place by division of pre-existing cells. This is an essential feature of formation of embryo.

There are two types of cell divisions: Mitosis and meiosis.

Mitosis (Fig. 14.1)

Mitosis is also called the equational division. At the end of the division, the number of chromosomes in the cell remains the same.

Stages

- **Interphase:** Time between two cell cycles. Amount of DNA in the cell doubles.
- **Prophase:** Chromatin of cell becomes coiled to form chromosomes. Centrioles separate and move to opposite poles of cell. They produce a number of microtubules that pass from one centriole to the other and form a spindle. The nuclear membrane and nucleoli disappear.
- **Metaphase:** With formation of spindle, chromosomes now arrange themselves in the center of the cell. They get attached to spindles at the centromere. Chromosomes are the thickest and the shortest during metaphase.

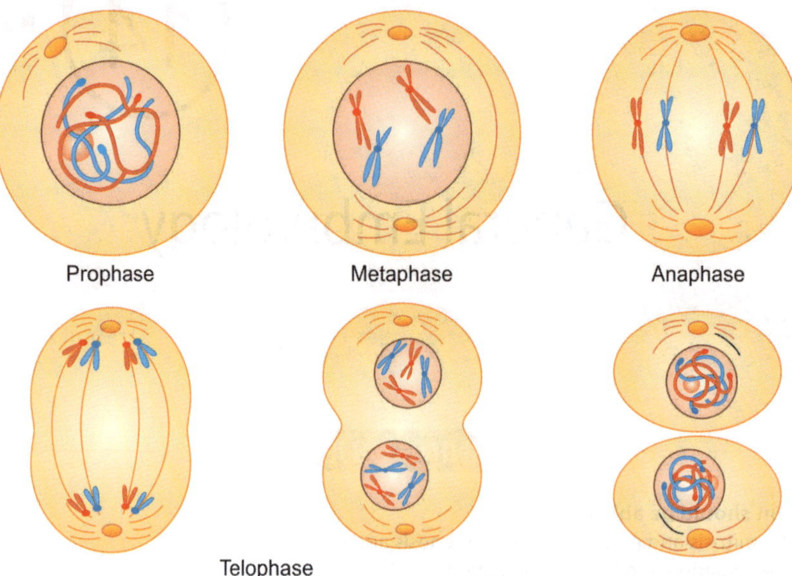

Fig. 14.1: Mitosis.

- **Anaphase:** Centromere of each chromosome splits longitudinally into two so that chromatids become independent chromosomes. The cell has 46 pairs of chromosomes, which now move to opposite directions of the cell.
- **Telophase:** Two daughter cells containing 46 chromosomes each are formed by formation of nuclear membrane in the cell. Centrioles and nucleoli form in each cell. Chromosomes uncoil.

Meiosis (Fig. 14.2)

Meiosis is also called the reductional division. At the end of the division, the number of chromosomes in the cell becomes half.

Stages

Meiosis I and II.

Interphase

Time between two cell cycles.

Meiosis I

Prophase I

It is divided into the following phases:
- **Leptotene:** The chromatin of the cell becomes coiled to form chromosomes.
- **Zygotene:** There are 46 pairs of chromosomes in each cell. Two chromosomes of each pair come to lie parallel to each other and form a bivalent.
- **Pachytene:** The chromosomes become distinct and the bivalent has four chromatids in it forming a tetrad. There is crossing over of the chromosomes with exchange of genetic material.

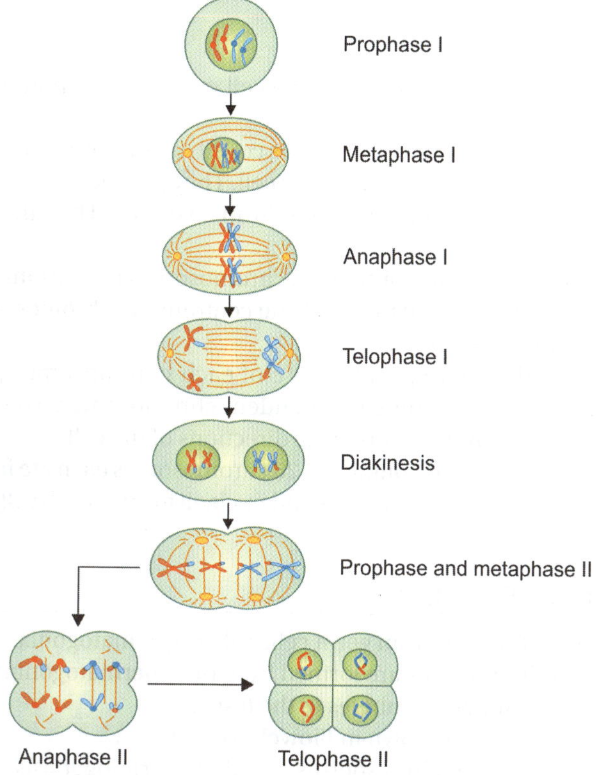

Fig. 14.2: Meiosis.

- **Diplotene:** The two chromosomes now break and separate, each carrying some part of the other. These points of crossing over are called chiasmata. The centrioles separate and move to the opposite poles of the cell. They produce a number of microtubules that pass from one centriole to the other and form a spindle. The nuclear membrane and the nucleoli disappear.

Metaphase I

With formation of spindle, chromosomes now arrange themselves in the center of the cell. They get attached to the spindles at centromere. Chromosomes are the thickest and the shortest during metaphase.

Anaphase I

During this phase, the centromere of each chromosome does not split. The cell has 46 chromosomes, which now move to opposite directions of the cell. Hence, at the end each, cell has 23 chromosomes.

Telophase I

Two daughter cells containing 23 chromosomes each are formed by the formation of nuclear membrane in the cell. Centrioles and nucleoli form in each cell. The chromosomes uncoil.

Meiosis II

It is a replication of mitosis.

- **Interphase:** This is the time between the two cell cycles. The amount of DNA in the cell doubles in this phase.
- **Prophase II:** The chromatin of the cell becomes coiled to form chromosomes. The centrioles separate and move to the opposite poles of the cell. They produce a number of microtubules that pass from one centriole to the other and form a spindle. The nuclear membrane and the nucleoli disappear.
- **Metaphase II:** With the formation of spindle, chromosomes now arrange themselves in the center of the cell. They get attached to spindles at centromere. Chromosomes are the thickest and the shortest during metaphase.
- **Anaphase II:** During this phase, centromere of each chromosome splits longitudinally into two so that chromatids become independent chromosomes. The cell has 23 pairs of chromosomes, which now move to opposite directions of the cell.
- **Telophase II:** Two daughter cells containing 23 chromosomes each are formed by formation of nuclear membrane in the cell. Centrioles and nucleoli form in each cell. The chromosomes uncoil.

SPERMATOGENESIS (FIG. 14.3)

- This is the formation of sperms from germ cells called spermatogonia.
- At the end of each cycle, 4 sperms are formed from one spermatogonium.
- It takes place in the seminiferous tubules of the testis.
- Stages in spermatogenesis are shown in **Flowchart 14.1.**
- The maturation of spermatids into sperms is called spermiogenesis. This takes place by changes in the structure of the spermatid.

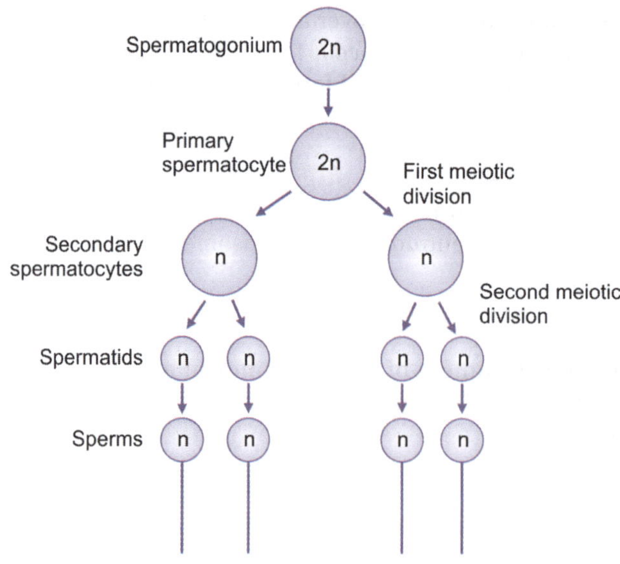

Fig. 14.3: Spermatogenesis.

Flowchart 14.1: Stages in spermatogenesis.

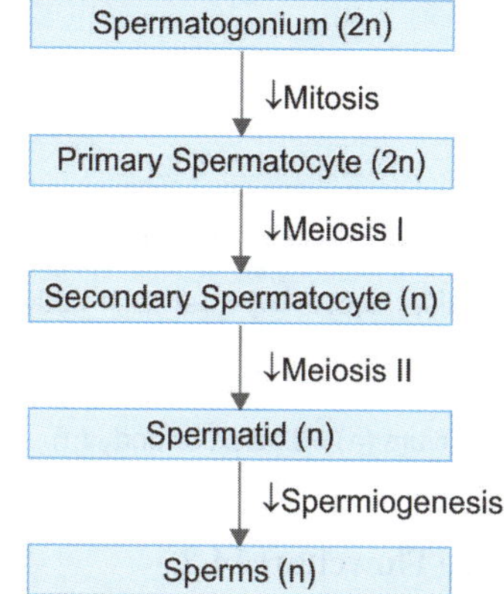

- Each mature sperm has a head, a tail, a neck and a middle piece.
  - Nucleus of the spermatid elongates to form the head of the sperm.
  - Golgi apparatus forms the acrosomal cap.
  - Mitochondria form the middle piece.
  - One of the centrioles comes to lie in the neck.
  - The other centriole forms the axial filament that emerges as the tail.

OOGENESIS (FIG. 14.4)

- Oogenesis is the production of ovum from the oogonium.
- It takes place in the ovaries.
- At the end of each cycle only one ovum is formed from each oogonium.

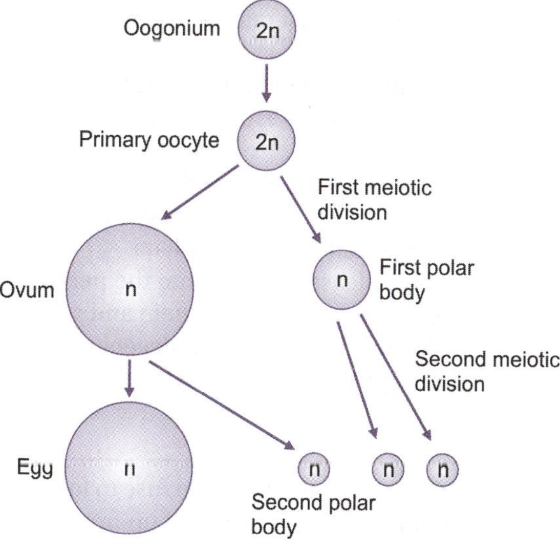

Fig. 14.4: Oogenesis.

Flowchart 14.2: Stages in oogenesis.

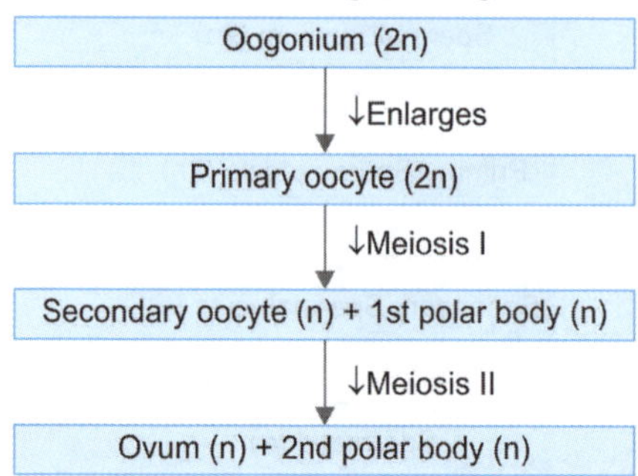

- Stages in oogenesis are shown in **Flowchart 14.2.**
- During the process there is unequal distribution of cytoplasm, i.e. the ovum contains all the cytoplasm and the polar bodies contain none.
- Oogenesis is arrested at the prophase I stage. During ovulation meiosis I is completed and secondary oocyte is formed.
- Ovulation is the process whereby the secondary oocyte is released from the ovary.
- During fertilization, meiosis II is completed and the mature ovum is formed.

Changes that take place in the ovum for ovulation to take place are:

- **Primordial follicles:** They consist of ovum lined by simple squamous epithelium.
- **Primary follicles:** The lining epithelium that surrounds the ovum changes from squamous to columnar.
- **Secondary follicles:** The stromal cells around the ovum now collect around the ovum to form layers of cells called follicular cells and now the ovum becomes a secondary follicle. Small intercellular spaces start appearing and is filled with follicular fluid.
- **Graafian follicle:** Between the follicular cells that surround the ovum, small spaces merge and form a single large cavity. This is called the antrum and is filled by fluid. The ovum now lies in a fluid-filled cavity and it is the most mature and ready for ovulation. This structure is called the Graafian follicle.
- The stromal cells surrounding the Graafian follicle differentiate into two layers, the theca interna just around the follicle that secretes estrogen and theca externa that is like a capsule surrounding the follicle.
- The ovum is now released from the ovary. Before this takes place, it is covered by a thick membrane called the zona pellucida. This has protective function. Some follicular cells are also shed along with the ovum and called corona radiata.
- **Corpus luteum:** After ovulation (release of ovum into the peritoneal cavity), the follicular cells enlarge; accumulate a yellow pigment called lutein and start secreting progesterone.
- **Corpus albicans:** The corpus luteum after some time degenerates to leave fibrous scar tissue forming a structure called the corpus albicans.

FERTILIZATION

- This is the process whereby the sperm and the ovum fuse to form a zygote.
- After the release of ovum from the ovary, it is picked up from the peritoneal cavity by the fimbriae of the fallopian tube.

- If sexual intercourse takes place at this time, the sperms swim to the uterine tube and one of them fuses with the ovum.
- The fertilization takes place in the ampulla of the uterine tube and the fusion of two haploid gametes restores the diploid number.
- The acrosomal cap of the sperm undergoes a chemical reaction called the acrosomal reaction to be able to fuse with the ovum.
- Similarly after one sperm fertilizes the ovary, the zona pellucida undergoes a chemical change such that no more sperms can fertilize the ovum. This is called the zona reaction.
- The cell formed immediately divides to form two daughter cells that again divide to form more daughter cells. This process is called cleavage.
- There is continuous division such that a ball of 16 cells called the morula is formed.
- The morula contains an inner cell mass that is surrounded by another layer of cells called the trophoblast.
- This then accumulates fluid in it to form the blastocyst.
- It is the blastocyst stage at which the zygote is implanted in the uterine cavity.

Functions of Zona Pellucida

- It prevents the fertilization of ovum by more than one sperm.
- The trophoblast has the ability to stick to the uterine tissue. This is prevented by the zona pellucida. Hence, the zygote is not implanted at abnormal sites.
- It provides nutrition to the ovum.

Formation of Three Germ Layers

The inner cell mass differentiates to form the three layers called the endoderm, mesoderm and the ectoderm.

Derivatives of Ectoderm

- Skin and its appendages
- Mucous membrane of mouth, palate, nasal cavities and paranasal sinuses
- Lower part of anal canal
- Terminal part of male urethra
- Epithelium of cornea, conjunctiva, ciliary body and iris
- Sweat, sebaceous, salivary, mammary and lacrimal glands
- Hypophysis cerebri and adrenal medulla

Derivatives of Mesoderm

- Connective tissue, adipose tissue, cartilage and bone
- Muscles
- Heart and blood vessels
- Urinary system, trigone of bladder
- Reproductive system of males and females
- Mesothelium lining the pleural, pericardial and peritoneal cavities
- Dura mater.

Derivatives of Endoderm

- Lining epithelium of gastrointestinal tract, respiratory tract, gallbladder and extrahepatic biliary apparatus.

- Epithelium of urinary bladder except trigone, female and male urethra.
- Thyroid, parathyroid and thymus glands.
- Liver, pancreas and glands of gastrointestinal tract.

SUMMARY

Difference between mitosis and meiosis:

Features	*Mitosis*	*Meiosis*
Occurrence	Somatic cells, early cell division of germ cells	Final cell divisions of germ cells
Chromosome number	46 (2n)/diploid	23 (n)/haploid
Number of cell cycles	One	Two, meiosis 1, meiosis 2
Cell division	Equational (chromosome number same in parent and daughter)	Meiosis 1 is reductional division (chromosome number reduced to half in daughter), meiosis 2 equational division
Phases of cell cycle	Prophase, metaphase, anaphase, telophase	Prophase 1 has 5 stages (leptotene, zygotene, pachytene, diplotene, diakinesis), rest same as in mitosis
Duration	24 hours	Few days to years

Difference between oogenesis and spermatogenesis:

Features	*Oogenesis*	*Spermatogenesis*
Commencement	Intrauterine life	Puberty
Duration	10 to 50 years	60 to 65 days
Number of mitoses in gamete formation	20 to 30	30 to 500
Daughter cells per meiosis	1 ovum, 3 polar bodies	4 spermatids
Gamete production in adult life	1 ovum per month	100 to 200 million per ejaculation

Derivatives of germ layers

Ectoderm	*Mesoderm*	*Endoderm*
Skin and appendages; mucous membrane of mouth, palate, nasal cavities, paranasal sinuses; lower part of anal canal; terminal part of male urethra; epithelium of cornea, conjunctiva, ciliary body, iris; sweat, sebaceous, salivary, mammary, lacrimal glands; hypophysis cerebri; adrenal medulla.	Connective tissue, adipose tissue, cartilage, bone; muscles; heart and blood vessels; urinary system, trigone of bladder; male and female reproductive system; mesothelium lining the pleural, pericardial and peritoneal cavities; dura mater.	Lining epithelium of GIT, respiratory tract, gallbladder, extrahepatic biliary apparatus; epithelium of urinary bladder except trigone, female and male urethra; thyroid, parathyroid, thymus glands; liver, pancreas.

QUESTIONS

Short Essays

- Mitosis
- Meiosis
- Fertilization
- Spermatogenesis
- Oogenesis
- Ovulation
- Derivatives of ectoderm
- Derivatives of mesoderm
- Derivatives of endoderm

Short Answers

- Name the germ layers.
- Give the functions of zona pellucida.

CHAPTER 15

Nursing Care Related to Anatomy

LEARNING OBJECTIVES

The student should be able to:

- The importance of learning anatomy is explained for budding nurses.
- Practical examples are included in order to gain knowledge on how anatomy can help nurses in the nursing care profession.

Nurses may be wondering why we have to learn Anatomy. What is the relation between nursing care and anatomy? There is a cause behind it. When the patient comes to clinic or nursing home or hospital, once the consultation with the doctor is over, it is the nurse who is going to deal a lot of time with them. In so many procedures nurse will be assisting the doctor. The nurse needs to explain the patients about their condition and what treatment they have to undergo. Some treatments are focused on the functions of organs and body. In order to understand what is wrong, first the normal structure and function of a particular organ should be understood. Without knowing the normal structure, relations and functions of the body parts, the diseases and their effects on the organs cannot be mastered.

To develop good relationship between nurses and patients, the patient should place trust in nursing staff. The nursing staff to have the trust from patient, should utilize all their knowledge and skills to ensure patient's well-being and assist the patient to come back to normal health. In the process, there are different roles the nurse has to play. Sometimes she has to explain and make the patient understand about the abnormal condition with normal anatomy, sometimes she has to assist the doctor in the surgical procedure, sometimes she needs to do a few of the procedures on her own.

What one cannot understand cannot be explained to others. It will only lead to confusion and mistrust on the patient's part if the nurse appears to doubt herself. By having enough knowledge on the human parts and normal functions, the nurse may be able to explain that to the patients in simple ways which they can understand.

In view of this, to make nurses know why Anatomy is important, one or two examples in each system are highlighted. Most of the systems are interconnected. Example, when a fracture is being treated, it should be looked for related nerve injury, the bone and location fractured, related joint, related blood vessels, muscles related to it, etc. So the systems involved in treating fracture are skeletal, circulatory, muscular and nervous systems.

Some of the procedures mentioned in this chapter may not be practiced by the nurses in India, but are practiced in abroad and may be helpful for those who go abroad.

CONNECTIVE TISSUE, SKELETAL AND MUSCULAR SYSTEM

Fracture

To provide management to a fracture, the nurse has to assess many aspects:

- Five Ps (**P**ain, **P**ulse, **P**allor, **P**aresthesia, **P**aralysis)
- Mechanism of injury
- Move injured parts
- Circulatory impairment (cyanosis, coldness, decreased peripheral pulses, edema not relieved by elevation, pain or cramping)
- Neurologic impairment (lack of sensation or movement, pain or tenderness, or numbness and tingling).

To assess all these, the nurse should know:

- Which bone is fractured, part of the bone fractured, to repair by realignment or reduction
- The blood vessel related to the bone, to assess pulse, color and temperature
- The nerve related to the bone, to prevent compression syndromes by testing sensation and motor function
- Muscles related to the bone, to assess the muscle weakness and pain which can prevent tissue damage.

Example: If the injury has occurred in the arm, the nurse should know:

- Arm bone fractured is humerus, by seeing the swelling in the upper part of arm, it is known that upper part of humerus is fractured.
- The nerves related to upper part of humerus are axillary, radial, musculocutaneous, median. The muscles supplied by these nerves should be known.
- Any one of these nerves may be injured. If axillary nerve is injured, the muscles affected will be deltoid.
- How to know if the nerve is injured and the muscle is paralyzed. Ask the patient to move the arm away from the body (abduction) up to the level of the shoulder slowly; if the patient cannot raise the arm then it is known the deltoid is paralyzed.
- The joint involved here will be shoulder joint and the movements occurring at shoulder joint should be known to mobilize the part. The movements occurring at shoulder joint will be flexion, extension, adduction, abduction, medial and lateral rotation, and circumduction.

Joints

Why should nurses know about joints and movements? When talking about joint dislocations, it is important to know the muscles involved in movements and the nerves supplying the joints and muscles.

Dislocation of Shoulder Joint

To explain the condition to the patient, the nurse should know:

- **The bones forming the joint:** Head of humerus and glenoid cavity of scapula. The bone dislocated will be head of humerus, fracture may be associated with dislocation.

- **The muscles responsible for movements:** Supraspinatus, infraspinatus, teres minor, subscapularis, deltoid, pectoralis major, minor, latissimus dorsi, long head of biceps brachii.
- **The nerves supplying the joint and muscles:** Axillary, musculocutaneous, suprascapular nerve, nerve to pectoralis major, minor, nerve to latissimus dorsi. Commonly injured nerve is axillary, followed by suprascapular and radial nerves.
- The nerve which is very closely related to humerus is axillary nerve. So during the dislocation, an axillary nerve may be injured which may lead to paralysis of deltoid in turn leading to loss of abduction above the shoulder level.

SIMS Position

- This position is used mainly for postpartum perineal examination, perrectal examination and enemas.
- In this position the patient lies on her left side, left hip and left knee are straight, the right hip and right knee are flexed.
- Here the nurse should know about the joints and movements, to make the patient lie down in recumbent position, even if this position is used for other procedures and treatments by the gynecologists.

LYMPHATIC SYSTEM

Nurses who have good understanding of the lymphatic system can understand different reactions and illnesses.

Infection and the Lymphatic System

- Lymph vessels and lymph nodes often become inflamed as the result of infection.
- An infection in the hand may cause inflammation of the lymph vessels as high as axilla (armpit).
- The nurse should know the drainage of lymph in the upper limb in order to explain how the infection from hand spreads to axilla. The lymph from the upper limb drains into axillary group of lymph nodes, so when there is infection in the hand of forearm or arm, it spreads to axilla.
- A sore throat may cause inflammation and swelling of lymph nodes in the neck, since the lymph from in and around the throat drains into submandibular nodes below the jaw and cervical nodes posteriorly.

Carcinoma or Tumor

- The nurse should provide adequate information about carcinoma or tumor to the patient.
- Usually the carcinoma or tumors will spread from one part to another part of the body through lymph vessels and lymph nodes.
- So the nurse should know the lymph nodes draining the specific region of the body.

Example: Lymphatics from breast drain into internal mammary nodes, axillary nodes, supraclavicular nodes and subdiaphragmatic nodes. The internal mammary nodes also drain into opposite subdiaphragmatic nodes. The subdiaphragmatic nodes are connected to the lymph nodes which drain ovary in females. So the carcinoma of breast on one side may spread to opposite side breast and also to ovary forming secondary carcinoma.

CARDIOVASCULAR SYSTEM

Heart Abnormalities

- Abnormal configuration, tumors and calcifications in the heart, aorta and pericardial effusions are detected through fluoroscopy.
- During the procedure barium is given by mouth so the outline of esophagus is seen.
- To identify these structures the nurse should know the normal position of the heart, relations of aorta and esophagus, and the covering of the heart, i.e. pericardium.
- The nurse needs to explain the patient about coronary artery disease, the effect of it to the heart, so that the patient can take steps to improve his condition. Now if she has to explain, she has to know what coronary artery disease is. If she has to know about the disease she should know the normal anatomy of the coronary arteries and the parts of the heart supplied by it.

Arteries

- Arteriosclerotic disease is characterized by thickening and loss of elasticity of the arterial walls.
- If this is to be identified by the nurse, she has to know the normal 3 layers (tunica intima, tunica media, tunica adventitia) and composition of the arterial wall.

Blood Pressure Reading

When doing the procedure of blood pressure reading, the cuff connected to sphygmomanometer has to be placed around the upper arm and the stethoscope over the brachial artery to listen to the pulse. For this, the nurse should know the extent of the brachial artery to place the stethoscope. The stethoscope has to be placed in the bend of the elbow where the brachial artery can be palpated in the cubital fossa.

Pulse Reading

- The nurse usually feels the pulse of the patient. To take the pulse, the nurse should know which artery is present at which location.
- Pulse can be taken in different parts of the body like temporal artery in front of the ear, carotid artery in the neck, brachial artery in the cubital fossa, radial artery in the wrist at the base of thumb, apex of the heart (apical pulse), femoral artery in the groin, popliteal artery at the back of the knee and the dorsalis pedis artery at the foot.
- Nurse may be requested by the doctor to take radial and apical pulse simultaneously. A significant difference in the pulse is indicative of vascular disease.

RESPIRATORY SYSTEM

Abnormalities of Lungs, Pulmonary Vessels

Fluoroscopy is used to look for abnormal configuration, tumors and calcifications in pulmonary vessels, to find congestion of the lungs, and to detect pleural effusions.

Paranasal Air Sinuses—Sinusitis

- Sinusitis is characterized by pain in the paranasal air sinuses and nasal congestion.
- Diagnosing the location of the pain is very important, because all the sinuses may not be infected at a time. Frontal pain or headache indicates frontal sinus involvement. Pain in and around the eyes is associated with the ethmoid sinuses. Maxillary sinusitis is characterized by pain lateral to the nose, sometimes accompanied by aching in the upper teeth. In sphenoid sinusitis, an occipital headache may occur.
- To examine the sinuses for tenderness, avoiding the eyes, fingertips are used to direct manual pressure upward over the frontal sinuses. With the thumbs, direct pressure upward over the lower edge of the maxillary bones to examine the maxillary sinuses.
- To do this procedure the nurse should know how many paranasal air sinuses are present and where in the body it is present. Paranasal air sinuses are the air spaces present in the bones. Pair of frontal air sinuses present in the frontal bone, ethmoidal air sinuses in the ethmoid bone, maxillary air sinuses in the maxilla and sphenoidal air sinuses are present in the body of sphenoid bone. All these 4 pairs of air sinuses surround and open into the nasal cavity.

DIGESTIVE SYSTEM

When obtaining the history of a gastrointestinal patient, a detailed interview should be conducted about the dietary habits, bowel habits, and GI complaints (signs and symptoms).

Examination of the digestive system in detail from mouth to intestine:

- Lips, tongue, and mucous membranes, should be examined for cuts, sores, or discoloration.
- Teeth for any discolored, cracked, chipped, loose, or missing teeth.
- Gums for its healthiness and breathe for unusual odors (fruity, foul, alcohol, and so forth).
- While examining the abdomen, to know the location of the viscera, abdomen is viewed as four quadrants or nine regions.
- Organs can be palpated for size, contour.
- Palpate for masses and irregularities in and around the abdominal organs.
- To do this examination the nurse should know the parts and location of the digestive system (mouth, pharynx, esophagus, stomach, intestines, rectum and anal canal) and its accessory organs (liver, gallbladder and pancreas which open into the duodenum).

Gastric and Intestinal Intubation

- It is the process of passing a tube through the nose or mouth, then through the esophagus, and into the stomach or intestine.
- Instruct the patient to tilt the head back and insert the tube into one of the nares.
- When the tube begins to curve down into the pharynx, the patient should be instructed to tilt the head forward slightly. This position facilitates passage of the tube by closing the trachea and opening the esophagus for ease of swallowing.
- Tube can be advanced up to the desired distance.
- If the nurse has to assist the doctor in this procedure or do it on her own, she has to know which part of the digestive system continues with what. The distance of the part from the nares or from the teeth should be known while inserting the tube. Constrictions of the esophagus to be studied, so that there will be no damage to the organs while inserting the tube.

URINARY SYSTEM

Urinalysis

- It is the examination and analysis of urine.
- It is routinely performed to detect abnormalities. The results of urinalysis are used by the physician in diagnosis of urinary conditions.

During Collection of Clean Catch Urine, Nurse has to Instruct the Patient

- Ask the patient to separate her labia to expose the urethral orifice. Keeping the labia separated prevents labial or vaginal contamination of the urine specimen.
- Cleanse the area around the urethral orifice with antiseptic towelettes.
- To give these instructions, the nurse should know the parts of external genitalia (labia majora, labia minora, clitoris, vaginal orifice, urethral orifice) and know the location of urethral orifice.

Urinary Tract Infections

- **Urethritis:** Infection of the urethra
- **Cystitis:** Infection of the urinary bladder
- **Prostatitis:** Infection of the prostate gland
- **Pyelonephritis:** Infection of the kidney.

REPRODUCTIVE SYSTEM

Nurses need to know the anatomy of the male and female reproductive systems to assess the health of these systems, to care for conditions that might affect the reproductive organs.

Female Reproductive System

Endometriosis

- It is the abnormal growth of cells (endometrial cells) similar to those that form the inside of the uterus, but in a location outside of the uterus.
- This ectopic tissue can appear anywhere in the body, but it usually remains in the pelvic area, around the ovaries, fallopian tubes, uterosacral ligaments, and uterovesical peritoneum.
- The nurse to explain the condition of endometriosis to the patient, has to know what is endometrium and the location of it. Endometrium is the innermost layer of the wall of uterus.

Pelvic Inflammatory Disease (PID)

- PID refers to any acute, subacute, recurrent, or chronic infection of the oviducts and ovaries, with adjacent tissue involvement. It includes inflammation of the cervix (cervicitis), uterus (endometritis), fallopian tubes (salpingitis), and ovaries (oophoritis), which can extend to the connective tissue lying between the broad ligaments (parametritis).
- The nurse to explain PID to the patient needs to know what are the organs which will be affected or which can be affected in PID, since there are so many organs present in the pelvis which are closely related to each other.

Male Reproductive System

Hydrocele

- A fluid-filled sac partially surrounding the testis. Manifests itself as a swelling on the side of the scrotum.
- The nurse to explain about hydrocele to the patient, should know about testis, scrotum, and relation of testis to scrotum. Testis male reproductive organ is located in the blind sac called scrotum.

Benign Prostatic Hypertrophy (BPH)

- Swelling of the prostate gland which surrounds the base of the male bladder and urethra causing difficulty urinating, dribbling and nocturia. Possible transurethral resection of the prostate (partial internal removal of prostatic tissue) may be done.
- The nurse may have to assist doctor in the prostatic surgery. The location of prostatic gland, relation of prostate to urinary bladder and urethra to be considered during surgery. Prostatic gland surrounds the neck of the urinary bladder in the male and urethra from the bladder passes through the prostate.

ENDOCRINE SYSTEM

Syndrome of Inappropriate ADH Hypersecretion (SIADH)

- If the nurse needs to explain the patient about the syndrome of inappropriate ADH hypersecretion (SIADH), where the pituitary secretes too much of antidiuretic hormone secretion (ADH) , the nurse should know what are the hormones produced by pituitary gland, and which part of the brain controls the pituitary. The pituitary is controlled by hypothalamus of the brain. The hypothalamus produces releasing or inhibitory hormones which act on pituitary to either release the hormone or inhibit the hormone.
- In SIADH, aldosterone is suppressed, increasing renal excretion of sodium and leads to the retention of fluid within the cells.
- The nurse should advise patient on the need to maintain the fluid balance in the body.

Hypothyroidism or Hyperthyroidism

- The thyrotropin-releasing hormone from hypothalamus acts on pituitary to secrete thyroid-stimulating hormone which in turn acts on thyroid gland to secrete thyroid hormones. Hypo- or hyperthyroidism can be associated to goiter which is enlargement of thyroid gland.

NERVOUS SYSTEM

Sciatic Nerve Injury

- If sciatic nerve or any of its branches is injured, and the patient should be assessed for motor function, the nurse should know which part of the body is supplied by sciatic nerve.
- The nurse should know that sciatic nerve and its branches supply the lower limb. So to test the nerve injury, the movements have to be assessed in lower limb.
- For this, the nurse should know different types of movements and in which joint it occurs, since the movements have to be performed or instructed for the patient.

- When the patient performs all the movements normally, then there is no injury to the nerve or the muscle. But when the patient cannot perform the actions at any one of the joints, then there is some problem with the nerve and muscles.
  Example: The patient is asked to perform the movements at each joint of lower limb to know at what level the nerve is injured. To assess at what level the injury is whether to the trunk or the branches, the nurse should know the movements occurring at each joint to instruct the patient what movements he has to perform at what joint. The patient is asked to abduct and adduct at the hip joint, flex and extend at the knee joint, plantar and dorsi flex at the ankle joint. If the patient cannot plantar flex the ankle joint, then injury is in tibial nerve, if the patient cannot dorsi flex the ankle joint, the injury is in the deep peroneal nerve. To assess the abnormalities, the first thing a nurse should know is the normal anatomy of the joints, movements, muscles causing movements and the nerves supplying the joint and muscles.

SENSORY ORGANS

The nurse should be very careful while dealing with the sensory organs.

Eye

Instilling Eye Drops or Ointments

- With the free hand, gently pull down the lower lid of the affected eye, exposing the conjunctival sac. Instill the prescribed amount of drops or a thin ribbon of ointment into the conjunctival sac. Medication should not be instilled directly onto the eyeball.
- When instilling the ointment the nurse should know what is conjunctiva (protective coat over the eyeball and the palpebrae), conjunctival sac (the region where the palpebral conjunctiva is continuous with bulbar conjunctiva) since the drops should be instilled in that region and not directly onto the eyeball.

Ear

Instilling Ear Drops

- With the nondominant hand, straighten the external ear canal by gently pulling up and back on the ear for an adult, or down and back for a child.
- The nurse should know why the external ear has to be pulled up and back in adult and down and back in children. In both cases, the external ear is not straight canal, it is a curved S-shaped canal in adults and in children it is curved upward.

Irrigating the Ear

- Straighten the ear canal. Point the tip of the irrigating syringe upward and toward the back of the ear canal. Direct a steady stream of solution into the ear, aiming toward the roof of the ear canal.
- The nurse should know why the syringe should be aimed at the roof and not medially. The medial wall of external ear is made of tympanic membrane (eardrum) which might be ruptured if the fluid is directed towards it.

SUMMARY

Understanding anatomy is essential for nurses as it forms the foundation of effective and safe patient care. Knowledge of the human body's structure helps nurses accurately assess health conditions, administer medications correctly, interpret symptoms, and assist in clinical procedures. It allows them to communicate effectively with doctors and other healthcare professionals using precise medical terminology. Moreover, a clear grasp of anatomy enhances a nurse's ability to educate patients about their conditions, surgeries, and treatments. In emergency situations, anatomical knowledge is critical for quick decision-making and life-saving interventions. Overall, studying anatomy equips nurses with the confidence and competence needed to deliver high-quality, holistic care.

CHAPTER 16

The Crucial Role of Anatomy in Physiotherapy Education

LEARNING OBJECTIVES

The student should be able to:

- The importance of learning anatomy is explained with Practical examples for budding physiotherapists.

INTRODUCTION

Anatomy is the cornerstone of medical education, and for Bachelor of Physiotherapy (BPT) students, it holds a place of paramount importance. Understanding the human body's structure is essential for physiotherapists, who rely on this knowledge to diagnose, treat, and rehabilitate patients effectively. This chapter will explore why BPT students need to learn anatomy, supported by practical examples that illustrate its application in the field of physiotherapy.

Foundation for Clinical Practice

Anatomy provides the fundamental knowledge required for clinical practice in physiotherapy. It is impossible to assess or treat a patient without a clear understanding of the body's structures. For instance, when a patient presents with shoulder pain, a physiotherapist must be able to identify the bones, muscles, tendons, and ligaments involved. This knowledge enables them to pinpoint the source of pain, whether it be a rotator cuff tear, impingement syndrome, or tendinitis.

Example: A patient with shoulder pain could have issues with the rotator cuff muscles, specifically the supraspinatus, infraspinatus, teres minor, or subscapularis. Understanding the anatomy of these muscles allows the physiotherapist to conduct targeted assessments and create a specific rehabilitation plan.

Understanding Biomechanics

Biomechanics is the study of movement and the forces that act on the body. To fully grasp biomechanics, BPT students must first understand the anatomical structures involved in movement. Anatomy helps physiotherapists comprehend how muscles, bones, and joints interact to produce movement, which is crucial for developing effective treatment plans.

Example: When analyzing gait abnormalities, a physiotherapist needs to understand the role of muscles like the gluteus medius and minimus in stabilizing the pelvis during walking.

A weakness in these muscles can lead to a gait deviation known as Trendelenburg gait, which the physiotherapist can then address through targeted exercises.

Essential for Accurate Diagnosis

Accurate diagnosis is the first step toward effective treatment. Without a thorough understanding of anatomy, BPT students would struggle to identify the underlying causes of a patient's symptoms. Anatomy enables them to distinguish between different types of injuries and conditions, such as differentiating between a herniated disc and muscular strain in a patient with lower back pain.

Example: Consider a patient with sciatica. A solid grasp of the anatomy of the lumbar spine, intervertebral discs, and the sciatic nerve is necessary to determine whether the pain is due to a disc herniation, spinal stenosis, or piriformis syndrome. Each of these conditions requires a different treatment approach.

Enhancing Manual Therapy Skills

Manual therapy is a key component of physiotherapy, involving hands-on techniques to manipulate muscles, joints, and soft tissues. To perform these techniques effectively, BPT students must have a deep understanding of anatomy. Knowing the precise location and function of muscles, bones, and nerves allows physiotherapists to apply the correct pressure and technique.

Example: In treating a patient with carpal tunnel syndrome, a physiotherapist needs to know the anatomy of the wrist, particularly the transverse carpal ligament and the median nerve. This knowledge allows them to apply techniques like myofascial release or nerve gliding exercises to alleviate the patient's symptoms.

Facilitating Communication with Other Healthcare Professionals

Physiotherapists often work as part of a multidisciplinary team, collaborating with doctors, nurses, and other healthcare professionals. A strong understanding of anatomy enables BPT graduates to communicate effectively with their colleagues, ensuring that patient care is coordinated and comprehensive.

Example: When discussing a patient's rehabilitation plan with an orthopedic surgeon, a physiotherapist must be able to understand and discuss the surgical procedure performed, such as an anterior cruciate ligament (ACL) reconstruction. Knowing the anatomy of the knee joint, including the ACL, menisci, and surrounding muscles, allows for a more informed discussion and better patient outcomes.

Developing Patient Education Skills

Educating patients about their condition and the treatment process is a crucial aspect of physiotherapy. Patients are more likely to adhere to their treatment plan if they understand their condition and how the therapy will help. Anatomy knowledge allows BPT students to explain complex concepts in a way that patients can understand, fostering trust and cooperation.

Example: A physiotherapist explaining a herniated disc to a patient can use their anatomy knowledge to describe how the disc's nucleus pulposus has protruded through the annulus fibrosus, compressing a nearby nerve root. This explanation can help the patient understand the source of their pain and the importance of exercises designed to relieve pressure on the nerve.

SUMMARY

Anatomy is not just a subject that BPT students need to pass; it is the bedrock of their future practice as physiotherapists. From diagnosing injuries to developing treatment plans, anatomy informs every aspect of their work. By mastering anatomy, BPT students equip themselves with the knowledge and skills necessary to provide high-quality care, improve patient outcomes, and excel in their profession.

SUMMARY

INDEX

Page numbers followed by *f* refer to figure, *fc* refer to flowchart and *t* refer to table

G

H

I

J

Q

R

S